SURGERY OF THE ARTHRITIC HAND AND WRIST

SURGERY OF THE ARTHRITIC HAND AND WRIST

Editors

Arnold-Peter C. Weiss, MD

Professor, Department of Orthopaedics
Brown University School of Medicine
Rhode Island Hospital
Providence, Rhode Island

Hill Hastings, II, MD

Clinical Associate Professor, Department of Orthopaedics
Indiana University Medical Center
Indiana Hand Center
Indianapolis, Indiana

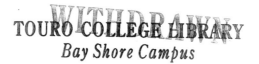
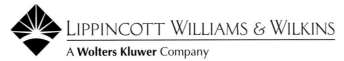
LIPPINCOTT WILLIAMS & WILKINS
A **Wolters Kluwer** Company
Philadelphia • Baltimore • New York • London
Buenos Aires • Hong Kong • Sydney • Tokyo

BS

Acquisitions Editor: Robert Hurley
Developmental Editor: Michael Standen
Supervising Editor: Mary Ann McLaughlin
Production Editor: Diane Ratto
Manufacturing Manager: Ben Rivera
Cover Designer: Christine Jenny
Compositor: Michael Bass & Associates
Printer: Maple Press

© 2002 by LIPPINCOTT WILLIAMS & WILKINS
530 Walnut Street
Philadelphia, PA 19106 USA
LWW.com

Printed in the USA

Library of Congress Cataloging-in-Publication Data
Weiss, Arnold-Peter C.
   Surgery of the arthritic hand and wrist / Hastings, Hill II
      p.; cm.
   Includes bibliographical references and index.
   ISBN 0-7817-1821-X
     1. Hand—Surgery. 2. Arthritis—Surgery. 3. Arthritis—Treatment. 4. Hand—Diseases—Treatment. I. Weiss, Arnold-Peter C. II. Hastings, H. (Hill)
   [DNLM: 1. Hand—surgery. 2. Arthritis—surgery. 3. Wrist Joint—surgery.
  WE 830 S961 2001]
  RD778.S87 2001
  617.5'75059—dc21
                                       2001038687

10 9 8 7 6 5 4 3 2 1

10/01/03

CONTENTS

Contributing Authors vii

Preface viii

Section 1: THE FOUNDATION 1

1 Pathophysiology of Osteoarthritis: A review of current findings 3
K. Shaw Lamberson

2 Pathophysiology of Rheumatoid Arthritis 10
Edward V. Lally

3 General Clinical Considerations in Rheumatoid Surgery 27
John A. McAuliffe

Section 2: THE HAND 39

4 Distal Interphalangeal Joint 41
Scott H. Kozin

5 Proximal Interphalangeal Joint 65
Michael Sauerbier and Ronald L. Linscheid

6 Metacarpophalangeal Joint 75
Stephen D. Trigg

7 Thumb Interphalangeal and Metacarpophalangeal Joints 92
Edward Diao

8 Thumb Carpometacarpal Joint 106
Robert J. Strauch and Melvin P. Rosenwasser

9 Carpometacarpal Joints (excluding the thumb) 111
Martin I. Boyer and Drew Engles

Section 3: THE WRIST 119

10 Limited Wrist Arthrodesis 121
Michael Sauerbier and Richard A. Berger

11 Limited Wrist Arthroplasty 140
Thomas B. Hughes, Jr. and Mark E. Baratz

12 Total Wrist Arthrodesis 155
Kavi Sachar and Hill Hastings, II

13 Total Wrist Arthroplasty 166
Brian D. Adams and Joseph G. Khoury

14 Distal Radioulnar Joint 177
Keith A. Glowacki and William H. Bowers

Index 197

Contributing Authors

Brian D. Adams, MD   Professor, Department of Orthopaedic Surgery, University of Iowa, Iowa City, Iowa

Mark E. Baratz, MD   Professor, Medical College of Pennsylvania/Hahnemann University; Vice Chairman, Department of Orthopaedics, Allegheny General Hospital, Pittsburgh, Pennsylvania

Richard A. Berger, MD, PhD   Professor, Departments of Orthopedic Surgery and Anatomy, Mayo Medical School; Consultant, Departments of Orthopedic Surgery and Anatomy, Mayo Clinic, Rochester, Minnesota

William H. Bowers, MD   Assistant Clinical Professor, Department of Orthopaedics, Medical College of Virginia; Chief, Medical Staff, Health South Medical Center, Richmond, Virginia

Martin I. Boyer, MD, MSc, FRCS(S)   Assistant Professor, Department of Orthopaedic Surgery, Washington University School of Medicine, St. Louis, Missouri

Edward Diao, MD   Associate Professor, Department of Orthopaedic Surgery, University of California San Francisco; Chief, Division of Hand, Upper Extremity and Microvascular Surgery, UCSF Medical Center, San Francisco, California

Drew Engles, MD   Attending Physician, Department of Orthopaedic Surgery, Central Dupage Hospital, Winfield, Illinois

Keith A. Glowacki, MD   Assistant Professor, Department of Orthopaedic Surgery, Virginia Commonwealth University/Medical College of Virginia; Chief, Department of Orthopaedics, Health South Hospital, Richmond, Virginia

Thomas B. Hughes, Jr, MD   Department of Orthopaedic Surgery, Brown University; Rhode Island Hospital, Providence, Rhode Island

Joseph G. Khoury, MD   Resident Physician, Orthopaedic Surgery, University of Iowa, Iowa City, Iowa

Scott H. Kozin, MD   Assistant Professor, Department of Orthopaedic Surgery, Temple University; Hand Surgeon, Shriners Hospital for Children, Philadelphia, Pennsylvania

Edward V. Lally, MD   Associate Professor, Department of Medicine, Boston University School of Medicine, Boston, Massachusetts; Director, Division of Rheumatology, Department of Medicine, Roger Williams Medical Center, Providence, Rhode Island

K. Shaw Lamberson, MD   Clinical Research Physician, US Womens Health and Reproductive Medicine, Eli Lilly, Indianapolis, Indiana

Ronald L. Linscheid, MD   Professor of Orthopedic Surgery-Emeritus, Mayo Medical School; Emeritus Staff, Department of Orthopedic Surgery, Mayo Clinic, Rochester, Minnesota

John A. McAuliffe, MD   Acting Chairman, Chief, Section of Hand Surgery, Department of Orthopaedics, Cleveland Clinic Florida, Weston, Florida

Melvin P. Rosenwasser, MD   Professor of Hand Surgery, Department of Orthopaedic Surgery, Columbia University; Attending Orthopaedic Surgeon, New York Presbyterian Hospital, Columbia Campus, New York, New York

Kavi Sachar, MD   Hand Surgery Associates, Denver, Colorado

Michael Sauerbier, MD, PhD   Lecturer & Consultant, Department of Hand, Plastic and Reconstructive Surgery, Burn Center, BG Trauma Center, Center Ludwigshafen, University of Heidelberg, Ludwigshafen, Germany

Robert J. Strauch, MD   Assistant Professor of Clinical Orthopaedic Surgery, Columbia University, Columbia University College of Physicians and Surgeons; Assistant Attending in the Orthopaedic Surgery, Columbia University, Department of Orthopaedic Surgery, Columbia University College of Physicians and Surgeons, New York, New York

Stephen D. Trigg, MD   Assistant Professor, Department of Orthopedic Surgery, Mayo Medical School; Consultant, Hand and Orthopedic Surgery, Mayo Clinic, Jacksonville, Florida

Preface

Surgery for arthritic conditions of the hand and wrist has been blessed by the presence of both time-proven techniques and newer innovations in complex reconstructions. A large percentage of the adult population will suffer from some condition involving joint degeneration causing pain and loss of function. As the population ages over the next few decades, coupled with the advancing age of baby boomers and improved overall health care, surgery for all arthritic conditions is likely to dramatically increase. This text summarizes treatment options available for these conditions in an anatomic location approach, allowing a rapid, in-depth understanding of the thought process required for successful outcomes.

The editors wish to thank the selected authors, all recognized experts in their topics, for providing a constructive framework to understand and assimilate the basic and advanced principles of arthritic surgery of the hand and wrist. We are also deeply indebted to our parents, for providing each of us with the support and encouragement required to stimulate a healthy learning desire, our wives, for being an invaluable source of emotional and practical support during our careers, and our children, who understand that our love for them eclipses that for hand surgery, even though we hold our surgical specialty dear.

With improving technology in implant design, increasingly clever procedures to reconstruct arthritic destruction, and advances in the biological treatment of these conditions, this book will only enjoy a finite usefulness, as have those that have come before. This book brings the most up-to-date review of this area available and will provide the basis for a lifetime understanding of the basic principles for care of these conditions.

Arnold-Peter C. Weiss, MD
Providence, Rhode Island

Hill Hastings, II, MD
Indianapolis, Indiana

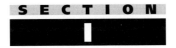

SECTION

I

THE FOUNDATION

PATHOPHYSIOLOGY OF OSTEOARTHRITIS: A REVIEW OF CURRENT FINDINGS

K. SHAW LAMBERSON

INTRODUCTION

Osteoarthritis (OA) is the most common rheumatologic disease in humans. It afflicts more than 40 million Americans, with X-rays showing the disease evident in more than 80% of those 55 years of age and older. In those over age 75, more than 80% have symptoms of OA, making it one of the most expensive and debilitating diseases in terms of cost of diagnosis and therapy, complications of therapy, and lost productivity (1,2). The disease process involves the entire joint, including subchondral bone, ligaments, capsule, synovial membrane, articular cartilage, and periarticular muscles. Eventually, the articular cartilage degenerates with fissures, fibrillations, ulcerations, and the loss of full thickness of the joint surface.

Initially, it may seem difficult to distinguish OA from simple wear and tear of the joints, but there are notable differences that distinguish OA.

1. OA is not necessarily age-related and can be triggered by trauma, congenital deformity, etc.
2. OA is asymmetrically distributed and often involves only one part of the joint.
3. OA relates more clearly to impact loading than to frictional wear and tear.
4. OA pain and joint dysfunction progresses in a steady, albeit asymmetrical fashion.

Once established, OA may result in low-grade inflammation but show few systemic effects. In general, it may be said that the osteoarthritic process results from normal cartilage that has been subjected to abnormal loads, or abnormal weight-bearing tissues.

Although often called "degenerative," osteoarthritis reflects a dynamic process that manifests itself in an imbalance between destruction and repair. This process involves cartilage softening and fibrillation, exposure of the subarticular bone plate, and fragmentation of the subchondral trabec-

ulae accompanied by hyperactive new bone formation, osteophytosis, and bone remodeling (3).

Normally, the osteoarthritic phenomena is characterized by destruction and/or degradation followed by the body activating a repair process. However, in some people—especially the elderly—the body makes little or no attempt to effect these primary repairs. As a result, X-rays show a more rapid deterioration than usual, which resembles damage found in erosive arthritis (4). In addition, certain "modifiers" influence the rate of pathologic and clinical progression, including:

1. Recurrent synovitis, due to shedding of articular debris or the appearance of calcium-containing crystals in the joint.
2. Avascular necrosis of the subchondral bone.
3. Joint instability.
4. Prolonged use of powerful anti-inflammatory preparations that may depress bone healing (5–7).

These factors may help explain the apparent differences in osteoarthritis in a particular joint, but, complicating the clinical diagnosis can be differences in the pattern of joint involvement. For example, differences may arise depending upon whether a joint has suffered a specific insult—monarthritis—or through a pauciarticular arthritis involving only large, weight-bearing joints, or a polyarthritis involving numerous sites (8).

Classification

The classifications for osteoarthritis include several categories, among them:

1. Primary or idiopathic, as when it appears without prior history of insult to the joint.
2. Secondary, when it follows an abnormality or injury (Table 1.1).

In most cases, both primary and secondary factors are important. Thus, patients following a meniscectomy of the

TABLE 1.1. CLASSIFICATION OF OSTEOARTHRITIS

Primary (Idiopathic)

1. Generalized
   a. Spinal apophyseal, hands and knees
   b. Hands (Heberden's nodes, Bouchard's nodes)
2. Localized
   a. Spinal apophyseal
   b. Hand (base of thumb, interphalangeal)
   c. Knee
   d. Hip
   e. Foot (first metatarsophalangeal joint, midfoot, hindfoot)
   f. Other (ankle, wrist, elbow, shoulder)

Secondary

1. Post-traumatic
   a. Postoperative
   b. Acute
   c. Repetitive
2. Post-inflammatory
   a. Inflammatory arthropathies
   b. Infection
3. Connective tissue
   a. Mucopolysaccharidoses
   b. Hypermobility syndromes
4. Dysplastic
   a. Congenital joint displacements
   b. Chondrodysplasias
   c. Developmental disorders
   d. Epiphyseal dysplasias
5. Endocrine and metabolic
   a. Ochronosis
   b. Crystal deposition disorders
   c. Hemochromatosis
   d. Acromegaly
6. Structural failure
   a. Osteochondritis
   b. Osteonecrosis

knee may suffer secondary OA, but also have a higher than usual incidence of primary and generalized osteoarthritis (9). The explanation may be that primary factors—endocrine, metabolic, genetic—alter the physical properties of the articular cartilage. That in turn may determine who develops osteoarthritis. Meanwhile, secondary factors, such as trauma or eccentric stress, help determine when and where it will occur (10).

Epidemiology

As the most common arthritic disease, osteoarthritis affects all races, all sexes, and even all age groups. Still, it remains most prevalent in older people. It can be said if you live long enough, you most likely will develop some form or degree of osteoarthritis (1,11,12).

In the United States, osteoarthritis causes more work disabilities in men over 50 years of age than any other disease except ischemic heart disease. Each year it accounts for more hospitalizations than rheumatoid arthritis (RA). The prevalence of OA varies among different populations (Table 1.2), but represents a universal problem for humans.

Men and women are equally apt to develop osteoarthritis, but more joints are affected in women than in men. As a result, generalized OA shows up more often in women than in men. It is more likely to occur in some joints, including the fingers, hip, knee, and spine, than in others, such as the elbow, wrist, or ankle (8,13). This may simply reflect congenital or childhood abnormalities of some joints, or it may be related to joint biomechanics and local anatomy (14).

Occupations that repeatedly subject particular joints to trauma and stress can also lead to OA in these joints. Such continuous overuse or abuse of a joint can cause the subsequent development of osteoarthritis (15). Also, an isolated severe trauma to a joint can lead to OA at the joint site in later life.

Gender and race play roles in the onset and severity of osteoarthritis (31–35). Studies show that the frequency of OA is about equal in men and women from age 45 to 55. However, after age 55, osteoarthritis is much more common in women (16). Women are more prone to a type of inflammatory form of OA in the hands that produces Heberden's and Bouchards nodes involving the distal interphalangeal (DIP) and proximal interphalangeal (PIP) joints (17). Studies of mice suggest that estrogens may protect against the development of OA (18,19). However, studies of rabbits (20) and of postmenopausal women (21) taking replacement estrogens show estrogen failed to slow down disease progression or offer other significant benefits in fighting OA.

Other notable factors associated with the development of osteoarthritis can include a history of trauma, rare inherited genetic mutations of collagen, other bone and joint disorders, a history of inflammatory arthritis, and other metabolic disorders.

TABLE 1.2. OCCURRENCE OF OSTEOARTHRITIS IN VARIOUS POPULATIONS

	Age (years)	Female (%)	Male (%)
U.S. Whites (31)	40 and over	44	43
English population (32)	35 and over	70	69
Pima Indians (33)	30 and over	74	56
Alaskan Eskimos (31)	40 and over	24	22
South African Blacks (34)	35 and over	53	60
Jamaican rural population (35)	35 to 64	62	54
Blackfeet Indians (33)	30 and over	74	61

MOLECULAR BASIS OF THE DISEASE

Osteoarthritis primarily attacks the cartilage. As summarized by Moskowitz et al. (22), the cartilage consists primarily of collagens, proteoglycans, and water. It is a shiny, slippery, pearl–blue-white tissue that covers the articulating ends of the bone. The thickest articular cartilage, on the surface of the patella, varies between 6 and 8 mm; all other surfaces are only 3 to 4 mm thick. This cartilage is easily compressible, exuding a thin layer of sticky, gelatinous, viscid synovial fluid on pressure. Microscopically, normal articular cartilage is composed of three zones that are based on the shapes of chondrocytes and the distribution of the Type II collagen: (a) the superficial or tangential zone; (b) the intermediate zone; and (c) the basal zone.

The tangential zone has flattened chondrocytes tangentially arranged and condensed collagen fibers and relative sparse proteoglycans. The intermediate layer is the thickest layer, with rounded chondrocytes that tend to be oriented and perpendicular or vertical columns paralleling the collagen fibers. The basal layer is the deepest layer and in it the chondrocytes are round.

Deep in the basal zone in an adult joint is a "blue line" that is called the tidemark. (Fig. 1.1). Embryologically, this line separates the true articular from the deeper cartilage that

is a remnant of the cartilage anlage or precursor. The anlage participated in endochondral ossification during growth in childhood.

The tidemark separates superficial and uncalcified cartilage from deeper cartilage and also is the division between nutritional sources for the chondrocytes. Above the tidemark, chondrocytes are nourished by synovial fluid diffusion. Below the tidemark, calcified cartilage is supplied by epiphyseal vessels.

Furthermore, the tidemark is the zone in which the chondrocyte renewal took place in childhood; above the tidemark, cells migrated upward to replenish the articular cartilage, and below the tidemark cells migrated into the calcified zone. Cell replication took place during childhood but ceased when the epiphyseal plate closed and longitudinal growth stopped. The tidemark is seen only in an adult, nongrowing joint.

Chondrocytes stand alone rather than in clusters. Each chondrocyte in the articular cartilagen has its own lacuna and is surrounded by a prominent proteoglycan bluish ring. A layer of lamellar bone, called the subchondral bone plate, runs deep to the calcified cartilage and supports it. Both cortex and underlying trabeculae of the marrow space are contiguous with the structure. Depending on its location, the bone marrow itself is either hematopoietic or fatty.

The normal synovium is rich with blood vessels but never totally covers or adheres to the articular cartilage. The synovium is composed of two zones: (a) a synovial lining layer one to two cells thick and (b) a deeper layer of supporting tissues, either loose fibrous tissue with significant vascular supply, or fat. The synovial cells have secretory and phagocytic functions. A normal synovium features some scattered mast cells that are the only inflammatory cells present.

Clinical Consequences

Clinically, arthritis results from the breakdown of normal functioning cartilage within a joint that may have been caused by altered anatomy or physiology. The loss of joint stability almost always results in pain and limits the ability of the articulating surfaces to move over one another easily. Freedom of movement may be limited by either loss of cartilage or a change in the joint shape. Most forms of arthritis exhibit a change in shape resulting from cartilage and bone loss.

Osteoarthritis, however, differs markedly inasmuch as it is the addition of new bone and cartilage that becomes a key characteristic of the disease. While the patient may suffer bone and cartilage loss, too, it is the addition of osteophytes, commonly called bone spurs, that marks the disease. These bone-covered cartilage caps, or "spurs," commonly occur at the joint periphery, but also can form beneath the articular surface.

The shapes of the osteophytes are determined by the mechanical tension on the joints. They originate at tendinous and capsular attachments. Where extra cartilage appears on the articular surface of a diseased joint, there can be marked

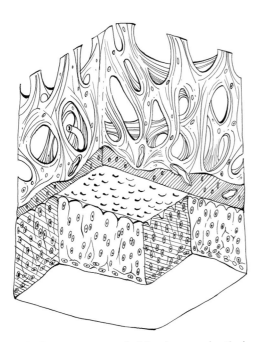

FIGURE 1.1. Demonstrates underlying bone and articular cartilage connected by a thin layer of calcified cartilage. The basophile line with embedded chondrocytes is delineated by the tidemark or calcified front, which subsequently regulates its formation. Through the process of endochondral ossification, blood vessels permeate from the marrow spaces into the calcified cartilage, which is slowly replaced with bone. (Redrawn from Moskowitz RW, et al. *Osteoarthritis: Diagnosis and medical/surgical management,* 2nd ed. Philadelphia: WB Saunders, 1992, with permission.)

reduplication and irregularity of the tidemark. An examination of the surrounding tissue shows evidence of increased bony hardening (endochondral ossification) that expands the subchondral bone periphery but does not result in the formation of an osteophyte.

The microscopic evidence for increased ossification includes increased irregularity of the bone cartilage junction, increased vascular penetration of the calcified cartilage, and the development of immature bone at the bone-cartilage interface. Visual evidence of injury to cartilage is seen mainly in the collagenous component of the extra cellular cartilage matrix. Where the surface would normally have a smooth appearance, instead the articular cartilage becomes rough and eroded. There seem to be three distinct stages or patterns that lead to changes that result in damage to the cartilage surface and underlying tissue. These stages include (a) fibrillation, (b) erosion, and (c) cracking.

Fibrillation, which can be euphemistically described as shredding, occurs while cartilage is still present and is marked by surface disruptions and tears running parallel to the tangential surface of the cartilage. These tears can deepen, eroding the cartilage, until they become cracks that expose the subchondral bone. Sites with the most loss of cartilage are notable for prominence and thickness of the subchondral bone.

In the early stages of OA, it's important to note that the disease process of these lesions tends to affect only one of the apposed articular surfaces. (This contrasts with eburnation, where both surfaces are affected.) In addition, a softening of the cartilage can result from an increase in water content and a decrease in the proteoglycan of the cartilage matrix. Chondromalacia and fibrillation usually occur together, although chondromalacia may occur prior to fibrillation.

BONE STRUCTURES

While OA primarily affects the cartilage, it can also impact joint structures and the underlying bone. As joint cartilage erodes, localized overloading and stress wear away the bone. In turn, as the bone is denuded, the body sends in an army of cells called osteoblasts to generate new bone. In OA, these osteoblasts overdo it and create too much bone density, called sclerosis. X-rays show this bone-on-bone phenomena as due to the absence of cartilage where there was once joint space between the bones.

Also, increased local stress on the bone can result in "focal pressure necrosis." Where overlying cartilage is gone, subarticular cysts can appear. According to Landells, such cysts may arise as a result of the transmission of intra-articular pressure through defects in the articulating bony surface into the marrow spaces of the subchondral bone. The cysts increase in size until the pressure within them is equal to the intra-articular pressure (23). Cysts may also occur because of focal tissue deadening or necrosis (24).

In later stages of OA, cartilage can regenerate and cover the surface of a joint; pressure may again rise but be more evenly distributed, resulting in a regression or even disappearance of the cysts. Fragments of cartilage or bone separated from a damaged joint surface may be digested, incorporated into the synovial membrane, or may simply form loose bodies within the joint cavity. Sometimes cartilage cells grow on these loose bodies and they grow in size. As they do, the centers become calcified and necrotic. Occasionally, they attach to the synovial membrane and are invaded by blood vessels. That results in endochondral ossification and the bodies turn bony. Since in most incidences of OA there exists some degree of loose body formation, it's important to distinguish those loose bodies from primary synovial chondromatosis (25).

Another common finding of microscopic examination of the ligamentous and capsular tissue in an arthritic joint often shows scar tissue from the repair of lacerations. It cannot be determined from microscopic examination whether this scar tissue preceded or resulted from the arthritic process.

Injury and OA

A by-product of injuries that affect the joints can be the breakdown of cartilage and bone and a flood of debris to the joint cavity. Phagocytic cells in the synovial membrane work to remove the debris from synovial fluid. As a result, the membrane can become both hyperplastic and hypertrophic. That's because the breakdown of the bone and cartilage matrix provoke an inflammatory response. Accordingly, even when the injury is purely a mechanical one, some degree of inflammatory response can be expected.

Under normal conditions the synovial membrane helps provide nutrition for the articular cartilage. But a chronically inflamed or scarred synovial membrane of OA may not be able to do this work as well as a healthy membrane. Disturbance of the synovial membrane's ability to supply nutrients as well as increase enzymatic activity may explain why OA tends to become chronic in nature. Further damage can occur as the synovial membrane becomes hypertrophied and hyperplastic, and synovial tissue extends into the joint cavity where it can be further damaged by the joint itself.

SYNOVIAL FLUID

Examination of the synovial fluid itself can help determine both the cause and stage of arthritis. Where the disease is present the fluid becomes altered. If there is an increase in volume and the hyaluronic acid has diminished, there will be a decrease in viscosity—all signs of inflammatory arthritis. However, in degenerative forms like OA, the amount of hyaluronic acid increases, resulting in extremely viscous fluid. The volume may also increase but not to the degree of inflammatory arthritis.

CLINICAL MANIFESTATIONS OF OA

It starts with what many patients describe as a "nagging pain." They may cite a specific location, or it may come from a referred source. While seldom very severe, the pain has a constant quality, often increasing in intensity according to the weather or amount of physical activity of the patient. With less activity and rest, the pain may subside, except in the more advanced stages where even bed rest may be accompanied by pain.

Depending upon the stage of the disease, the cause and amount of pain will vary according to the stage the osteoarthritis has reached. Some patients experience mild joint pain and intermittent episodes of mild to moderate synovitis. However, a more constant feature includes raised intraosseous pressure due to vascular congestion of the subchondral bone (26). Muscular fatigue, joint contracture, and capsular fibrosis may occur in later stages.

Patients often complain of stiffness, which in early stages may be intermittent, particularly after a person has resumed activity after a period of rest. However, as the disease progresses this stiffness—probably due to a combination of joint incongruity and capsular fibrosis—can become permanent. Swelling and deformity may appear in the superficial joints such as the finger or knee joints. Knobby fingers resulting from advancing stages of OA may make it difficult to grip large objects or open jars. This loss of function can also result in problems with walking, grooming, and fatigue. OA in the knees and hips may limit mobility and restrict walking distance; problems in the shoulders and hands can hinder the ability to reach up to the head for simple grooming. This in turn may affect the quality of life the patient experiences.

Examination

While a patient may note pain in only one or two joints, an examination may reveal that others are affected as well. The peripheral joints, especially the fingers, readily exhibit swelling and deformity. Superficial joints may show local signs of inflammation (redness, warmth, and swelling), as well as tenderness, synovial thickening, intra-articular fluid, and marginal osteophytes. At first, joint movement may be restricted in one direction, then later more generally. Creaking joints and palpable crepitus are common and are probably due to irregularities of the articular surface. In advanced cases, muscle wasting may be present as well as joint instability.

Imaging

Radiography

Although not the most detailed form of imaging, X-rays are the most useful in identifying stages of OA. That's because the radiographic appearances of OA are so consistent in character that more refined imaging may not be necessary. The typical features include asymmetric narrowing of the joint space, sclerosis of the subchondral bone under the area of cartilage loss, cysts close to the subchondral bone place, osteophytes at the joint margins, and bone remodeling (Figs. 1.2 and 1.3). Also present may be signs of previous traumas or injury, including old fractures, osteonecrosis, or congenital dysplasia.

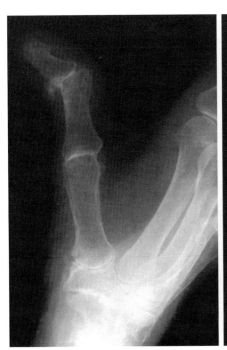
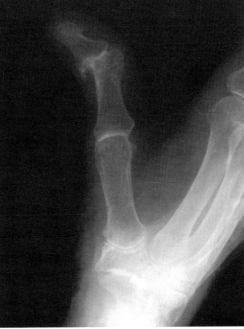

FIGURE 1.2. Osteoarthritis of the thumb. Note claps and radial deviation at interphalangeal joint with marginal osteophytes and subchondral sclerosis. Similar sclerosis is present at the peri-trapezial joints.

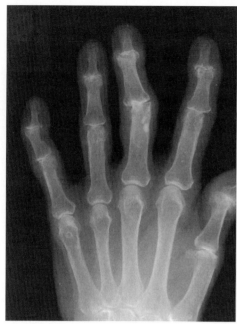 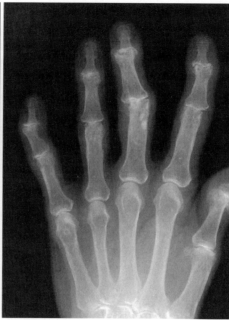

FIGURE 1.3. Osteoarthritis of the index through small digits. Note subchondral cysts at proximal interphalangeal joint of the middle finger and the sclerotic remodeling that has occurred at the ulnar base of the middle phalanx.

Radionuclide

Scanning with technetium-99m (99m-Tc)-HDP shows increased activity during the bone phase in the subarticular region of any affected joint (27). This may show up years before changes that would show up on common X-rays appear. This increased activity reflects the vascular reaction and osteoblastic activity in the early stages of the disease.

Laboratory Investigations

At present there exists no reliable early diagnostic test for OA (28). Our best early means of detection include sampling synovial fluid for nonspecific features of mild inflammation: increased volume, decreased viscosity, mild pleocytosis, and a slight increase in protein (29). Meanwhile, laboratory analysis helps exclude other disorders in the differential diagnosis.

NONOPERATIVE MANAGEMENT OF DISEASE

The goal of therapy for OA patients usually focuses on diminishing their pain and keeping them active. The main therapy includes nonspecific, non-pharmacologic measures such as rehabilitation, education, and support. Intervention with appropriate nutrition and exercise is also critical. Where a patient is overweight, it has been shown that significant weight loss can help decrease the progression of OA of the knee. However, weight loss has not been shown to halt the progression of OA in the hip. Unfortunately, no therapy alters the natural progression of the disease.

Pharmacologic therapy includes simple analgesics followed by nonsteroidal anti-inflammatory drugs (NSAIDs) if the analgesics do not work. While NSAIDs are analgesic and anti-inflammatory, the evidence to date does not show that these drugs modify the natural course of the disease. However, they do provide relief from pain and decrease the amount of inflammation present. For patients with morning stiffness or gel phenomenon, the nonsteroidals can provide relief patients do not get from analgesics alone. In these patients, some form of NSAID therapy will be required.

Hyaluronan, a hyaluronic acid preparation, injected into the osteoarthritic knee joint has been shown to provide relief in some patients for various periods of time. These preparations currently are not approved for use in joints other than the knee.

Many patients have turned to alternative treatments for their OA such as the nutritional supplements glucosamine sulfate and chondroitin sulfate. Numerous trials have suggested that some degree of efficacy appears probable for these preparations. One study from China concluded that glucosamine sulfate was as effective as ibuprofen in treatment of OA of the knee (30). Numerous herbs have also been used throughout the centuries for the treatment of OA.

With exercise, rehabilitation therapy, splinting when appropriate, and either simple analgesics or NSAIDs, OA patients can find significant relief. However, if these measures fail and the patient is increasingly debilitated day and night, surgical intervention may be appropriate.

SUMMARY

Osteoarthritis is a common disease of the articular cartilage. It affects both males and females, almost all ethnic groups, and is multifactorial in its etiology. Many obvious factors such as infection, trauma, and congenital abnormality can cause OA. However, there are many patients for whom the origin of their arthritis is not obvious. These individuals are usually diagnosed as having idiopathic OA.

The arthritic process leads to erosion of articular cartilage, development of bone spurs, and joint deformity. This results in loss of motion, instability, and chronic pain. Diagnosis of the disease involves physical examination, and laboratory analysis of synovial fluid from the affected joint, as well as X-rays that provide a reliable means of discerning the presence and severity of the disease.

While modern pharmacologic therapy as well as other modalities such as physical therapy and assistive devices may provide some comfort, there remains little evidence to suggest that the natural course of the disease can be circumscribed. At its worst, osteoarthritis leads to substantial pain and disability that may persist even with diminished activity. In such cases, surgical intervention may be appropriate.

REFERENCES

1. Peyron JG. The epidemiology of osteoarthritis. In: Moskowitz RW, Howell DS, Goldberg VM, Mankin HJ, eds. *Osteoarthritis: Diagnosis and management.* Philadelphia: WB Saunders, 1984:9–27.
2. Gordon T. Osteoarthrosis in U.S. adults. In: Bennett PH, Wood PHN, eds. *Population studies of the rheumatic diseases.* New York: Excerpta Medica Foundation, 1968:391–397.
3. Sokoloff L. Osteoarthritis as a remodeling process. *J Rheumatol* 1987;14:7–10.
4. Cobby M, Cushnaghan J, Creamer P, et al. Erosive osteoarthritis: is it a separate disease entity? *Clin Radiol* 1990;42:258–263.
5. Gibilisco PA, Schumacher HR, Hollander JL, et al. Synovial fluid crystals in osteoarthritis. *Arthritis Rheum* 1985;28:511–515.
6. Solomon L. Drug-induced arthropathy and necrosis of the femoral head. *J Bone Joint Surg* 1973;55B:246–261.
7. Rashad S, Revell P, Hemingway A, et al. Effect of non-steroidal anti-inflammatory drugs on the course of osteoarthritis. *Lancet* 1989;2(8662):519–522.
8. Cushnaghan J, Dieppe P. Study of 500 patients with limb joint osteoarthritis: I. analysis by age, sex, and distribution of symptomatic joint sites. *Ann Rheum Dis* 1991;50:8–13.
9. Doherty M, Watt I, Dieppe P. Influence of primary generalized osteoarthritis on the development of secondary osteoarthritis. *Lancet* 1983;2(8340):8–11.
10. Dieppe P, Kirwan J. The localization of osteoarthritis. *Br J Rheumatol* 1994;33:201–203.
11. Lawrence JS. *Rheumatism in populations.* London: William Heinemann Medical Books, 1977.
12. Heine J. Uber die Arthritis deformans. *Arkh Patol Anat* 1926; 260:521.
13. Van Saase JL, Van Romunde LKJ, Cats A, et al. Epidemiology of osteoarthritis: Zoetermeer survey. Comparison of radiological osteoarthritis in a Dutch population with that in 10 other populations. *Ann Rheum Dis* 1989;48:271–280.
14. Swann AC, Seedham BB. The stiffness of normal articular cartilage and the predominant acting stress levels: implications for the aetiology of osteoarthrosis. *Br J Rheumatol* 1993;32: 16–25.
15. Fife RS. Osteoarthritis. In: Hazzard WR, Bierman EL, Blass JP, et al., eds. *Principles of geriatric medicine and gerontology*, 3rd ed. New York: McGraw-Hill, 1994:981–986.
16. Acheson RM, Collart AB. New Haven survey of joint diseases. *Ann Rheum Dis* 1975;34:379–387.
17. Stecher RM. Heberden's nodes: a clinical description of osteoarthritis of the finger joints. *Ann Rheum Dis* 1955;14:1–10.
18. Silberberg R, Thomasson R, Silberberg M. Degenerative joint disease in castrate mice. *Arch Pathol* 1958;65:442–444.
19. Silberberg M, Silberberg R. Role of sex hormones in the pathogenesis of osteoarthrosis of mice. *Lab Invest* 1963;12:285–289.
20. Sokoloff L, Varney DA, Scott JF. Sex hormones, bone changes and osteoarthritis in DBA/2JN mice. *Arthritis Rheum* 1965;8: 1027–1038.
21. Hannon MT, Felson DT, Anderson JJ, et al. Estrogen use and radiographic osteoarthritis of the knee in women: the Framingham Osteoarthritis Study. *Arthritis Rheum* 1990;33:525–532.
22. Bullough PG. The pathology of osteoarthritis. In: Moskowitz RW, Howell DS, Goldberg VM, Mankin HJ, eds. *Osteoarthritis: Diagnosis and medical/surgical management*, 2nd ed. Philadelphia: WB Saunders, 1992:39–69.
23. Landells JW. The bone cysts of osteoarthritis. *J Bone Joint Surg* 1953;35B:643.
24. Rhaney K, Lamb DW. The cysts of osteoarthritis of the hip. A radiological and pathological study. *J Bone Joint Surg* 1955;37B:663.
25. Villacin AB, Brigham LN, Bullough PG. Primary and secondary synovial chondrometaplasia. *Hum Pathol* 1979;10:439–451.
26. Arnoldi CC, Linderholm H, Mussbichler H. Venous engorgement and intraosseous hypertension in osteoarthritis of the hip. *J Bone Joint Surg* 1972;54B:409–421.
27. Hutton CW, Higgs ER, Jackson PC, et al. 99mTc HMDP bone scanning in generalised nodal osteoarthritis. II. The four hour bone scan image predicts radiologic change. *Ann Rheum Dis* 1986; 45:622–626.
28. Altman RD. Laboratory findings in osteoarthritis. In: Moskowitz RW, Howell DS, Goldberg VM, Mankin HJ, eds. *Osteoarthritis: Diagnosis and management.* Philadelphia: WB Saunders, 1992: 313–328.
29. Fawthrop F, Hornby J, Swan A, et al. A comparison of normal and pathological synovial fluid. *Br J Rheumatol* 1985;24:61–69.
30. Qiu GX, Gao SN, Giacovelli G, et al. Efficacy and safety of glucosamine sulfate versus ibuprofen in patients with knee osteoarthritis. *Arzneimittelforschung* 1998;48(5):469–474.
31. Blumberg BS, Bloch KJ, Black RL, Dotter C. A study of the prevalence of arthritis in Alaskan Eskimos. *Arthritis Rheum* 1961; 4:325–341.
32. Lawrence JS, Bremner JM, Bier F. Osteoarthrosis: prevalence in the population and relationship between symptoms and x-ray changes. *Ann Rheum Dis* 1966;25:1–24.
33. Bennet PH, Burch TA. Osteoarthrosis in the Blackfeet and Pima Indians. In: Bennet PH, Wood PHN, eds. *Population studies of the rheumatic diseases.* Amsterdam: Excerpta Medica Foundation, 1968:407–412.
34. Solomon L, Beighton P, Lawrence JW. Osteoarthrosis in a rural South African Negro population. *Ann Rheum Dis* 1976;35: 274–278.
35. Bremner JM, Lawrence JS, Miall WE. Degenerative joint disease in a Jamaican rural population. *Ann Rheum Dis* 1968;27: 326–332.

2

PATHOPHYSIOLOGY OF RHEUMATOID ARTHRITIS

EDWARD V. LALLY

INTRODUCTION

Rheumatoid arthritis (RA) is a chronic systemic autoimmune disorder with variable clinical expression, including the potential for destructive arthritis and for significant extra articular manifestations (1–3). It is the prototypical inflammatory joint disorder characterized by immunogenetic susceptibility, by profound abnormalities of humoral and cell-mediated immunity, and by immunologically driven chronic synovitis. The immunologic and inflammatory cascade that leads to chronic rheumatoid synovitis appears to be antigen driven, although currently the putative antigen (or antigens) remains unknown. Within the past decade, insights regarding the etiopathogenesis of RA have emerged from the arena of molecular biology at an accelerated pace. It is evident that RA can be understood on the basis of class II major histocompatability complex (MHC) gene product expression and its selective influence on immunologically active cells and their soluble products. The present chapter will discuss pathologic and immunopathogenetic mechanisms in RA against the backdrop of major developments in the understanding of genetic factors and soluble mediators that affect articular damage.

EPIDEMIOLOGY

RA is the most common type of chronic inflammatory arthritis and the most common systemic inflammatory disease (1–3). The disease has a worldwide distribution with no geographic region or ethnic group spared its effects (4). As a historical perspective, RA is a relatively new disorder, having been reported only within the past 400 years. No evidence of its existence was found in Europe, Asia, or Africa prior to the seventeenth century (5). Depending on the clinical criteria used to classify the disease, the usual quoted prevalence rate is approximately 1% worldwide and an incidence rate of 0.03% (3). Although data are conflicting, the annual incidence appears to be about 2 to 4 new cases per 10,000 adults.

Although RA can develop at any age, the peak age of onset is between the ages of 30 and 60. However, a significant number of cases develop in individuals over the age of 65 (6). Women are two to three times more likely to be affected than men. With older age at onset, the gender discrepancy diminishes.

Based on two studies (7,8), it has been suggested recently that there is a decline in the occurrence of RA. These observations were not confirmed in a more recent study in central Massachusetts (9), and methodological differences may have accounted for different conclusions in the previous reports. Insufficient data currently exist to substantiate or refute the observation that RA is becoming less common.

For many decades, RA was considered to be a nonfatal disorder and even likely to extend life. "It has often been said that the way to live a long life is to acquire rheumatism" (10). However, several studies have now shown conclusively that RA is associated with significantly shortened survival (3). The disease decreases life expectancy by 3 to 10 years in both men and women. Factors associated with increased mortality include persistent synovitis, rheumatoid factor positivity, poor functional status, and lower levels of education. RA also impacts negatively on the quality of life, work capability, and health care costs.

ETIOLOGY

The cause of RA is unknown. To date, no specific agent (or agents) has been identified as being causal for RA, although an array of potential candidates has been scrutinized. It is likely (although not proven) that an infectious agent (or agents) is responsible for at least the initiation of RA. Several animal models of chronic arthritis implicate microbial etiologies (Table 2.1). Synovitis develops secondary to *Erysipelothrix insidiosa* infection in swine, to streptococcal cell-wall products in rats and guinea pigs, and to *Mycoplasma arthritides* in mice and rabbits (11). In humans, there are striking clinical and pathologic similarities between RA and arthritis associated with, or secondary to infection with, streptococcal species, several viruses (vaccinia, hepatitis B, rubella, parvovirus B19), as well as the infectious agent causing Lyme disease (*Borrelia burgdorferi*) (Table 2.1). Furthermore, the

TABLE 2.1. INFECTIOUS AGENTS IMPLICATED IN RA

Animal Models	Human Models
Bacteria	Bacteria
▪ *Erysipelothrix insidiosa*	▪ Acute rheumatic fever
▪ Streptococcal cell walls	▪ Lyme arthritis
Mycoplasma	Viruses
▪ *Mycoplasma arthritides*	
Mycobacteria	
▪ Adjuvant arthritis	
Viruses	

worldwide distribution of RA without specific geographic clustering and the prevalence of 1% to 2% of the population would implicate a relatively ubiquitous infectious agent (11).

Several microbial species including pyogenic bacteria, mycoplasmas, and viruses have been studied extensively. It is also possible that two or more agents act to trigger rheumatoid arthritis. Bacterial and mycoplasma species have been studied, but attempts to isolate specific agents from synovial fluid or the synovial membrane have been unsuccessful, and no specific humoral response to bacteria or mycoplasma has been consistently demonstrated.

It has been shown that T-lymphocytes from patients with RA show increased reactivity to a fraction of mycobacteria cross-reactive with cartilage (12). Also, antigens from four different mycobacterial species injected intradermally in patients with leprosy showed augmented reactions in patients that were HLA-DR4-positive, the allele associated with RA (13). It has been speculated that a mycobacterial 65-kd heat shock protein (hsp65) is involved with rodent models of arthritis and with human RA, but no conclusive evidence in this regard has been forthcoming (14).

More interest has focused on viral species (Table 2.2). Throughout the 1970s and early 1980s, Epstein-Barr virus was studied extensively in relationship to a causal role for RA (15–17). In spite of several provocative theories, no proof currently exists that Epstein-Barr virus causes RA. Other DNA viruses including cytomegalovirus, herpes simplex virus 1 and 2, herpes virus 6, adenovirus and parvovirus B19

TABLE 2.2. VIRUSES IMPLICATED IN RA

DNA Viruses	RNA Viruses
▪ Epstein-Barr virus	▪ Rubella
▪ Cytomegalovirus	▪ Mumps virus
▪ Herpes simplex virus	▪ Measles virus
▪ Adeno virus	
▪ Parvovirus B19	
▪ Human herpes virus 6	

have all been studied but none was definitively implicated in the etiology of RA (18-21). With the recent advent of molecular biology, and specifically, nucleic acid analysis, viral species have been studied in more detail in the joints of patients with RA. Genomic RNA for rubella, mumps virus, and measles virus was analyzed in the peripheral blood mononuclear cells and synovial fluid cells in patients with early RA (22). These studies did not suggest a causal role for these viruses in RA.

Currently there is no conclusive evidence to support at least a single infectious agent in the etiopathogenesis of RA. It is also possible that a variety of infectious agents are capable of triggering RA but are not responsible for the perpetuation of the disease. The best contemporary hypothesis is that a common infectious pathogen, or pathogens, is responsible for acute synovitis in a large number of patients, but that only immunologically susceptible individuals progress to develop chronic rheumatoid synovitis. Current theories, however, do not rule out the possibility that noninfectious agents, either alone or in combination, act as triggers for the onset of RA.

IMMUNOGENETICS

RA has long been suspected as a disease of genetic susceptibility and altered immune regulation. Twin and family studies have suggested that heredity plays a large role in RA. In monozygotic twins, the concordance rate for RA is between 30% and 50% when one twin is affected, compared to 1% concordance for the general population. However, the pattern of inheritance does not fit a simple monogenic model.

The presence of autoantibodies (particularly rheumatoid factors) in the circulation and in the joint tissue as well as the presence of immunologically active cells in the synovial membrane implicate immunologically driven synovitis. Several lines of evidence point to RA as an example of a delayed-type hypersensitivity reaction focused mainly in synovial lined structures. The link between genetics and immunopathology of RA is found in the immune response genes.

In humans, the major histocompatability complex (MHC) is located on the short arm of chromosome #6. This is analogous in mice to the immune response genes located in the histocompatability (H_2)-associated I region. In the human MHC, four human leucocyte antigen (HLA) loci (A, B, C, and D) contain genetic information that codes for cell surface antigens. Alleles at the A, B, and C loci (Class I alleles) encode for cell surface peptides that are expressed on the surface of all nucleated cells and platelets and are also found free in the circulation. The D locus encodes cell surface antigens (Class II) that have a much more restricted distribution, being found on the surface of immunologically active cells, especially B-cells, macrophages, and activated T-cells.

In 1978, Stastny first reported the association of RA with HLA-DR4 (23). Seventy percent of patients with adult RA studied by Stastny were DR4-positive compared to 28% of controls. Individuals that were HLA-DR4 positive had a 4- to 5-fold relative risk for RA. Subsequently, this observation was refined to identify specific alleles at the DR4 locus that were responsible for the associated risk. Major differences in subtypes of DR4 are determined by the DRB1 locus, which encodes for the DR β1 chain. Only certain DRB1 subtypes have been associated with RA, and these include DRB1*0401, *0404/0408, *0410, *0101, *0102, *1001, and *1402 (Table 2.3) (24–29). Other closely related DR-subtypes are not associated with RA (Table 2.3). It is hypothesized that the reason that these subtypes are associated with RA has to do with their role in presenting antigen to T-cells.

The surface expression of Class II molecules on antigen-presenting cells (typically macrophages) has critical importance for the manner in which pathogenic peptides in RA are presented to T-cells in the context of the T-cell receptor. The shared epitope hypothesis of Winchester and Gregersen states that specific amino acid substitutions in the "groove" or cleft of the antigen-presenting site of the Class II molecule causes the same antigen to be presented in different ways to the inducer T-cells (30,31). Specifically, the critical region involves a common sequence of amino acids #70-74 within the third hypervariable region of the Class II molecule. This region forms the base or floor of the antigen-presenting site (Fig. 2.1). The HLA-DRB1 subtypes associated with RA share a common amino acid sequence in this region that is different from other subtypes. According to this hypothesis, because the groove of the antigen-presenting site is stoichiometrically altered due to the amino acid differences, an antigen peptide would be presented in a different configuration to the T-cell receptor. Because of this antigen T-cell receptor interaction, a critical series of immunologic events characteristic of RA is set in motion. Individuals lacking these critical alleles would present the same peptide antigen to the T-cell receptor, but no such immunologic cascade would ensue.

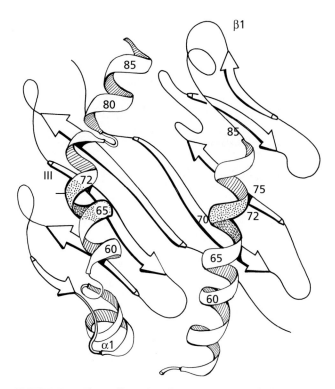

FIGURE 2.1. Three-dimensional representation of Class II molecule with helical configuration of "walls" of the antigen presenting site or "groove." "Floor" of groove given critical structural variability based on amino acid sequence #70-74 in third hypervariable region. (Modified after Gregersen PK, Winchester R, Dwyer E, Rose S. The genetic basis of rheumatoid arthritis: the shared epitope hypothesis. *Rheum Dis Clin North Am* 1992;18:761–783, with permission.)

The converse hypothesis is also possible. The specific amino acid–based structure of the binding cleft may prevent a potential pathogenic peptide from binding and being pre-

TABLE 2.3. NOMENCLATURE FOR HLA–DR ALLELES

Old Nomenclature	New Nomenclature (HLA-DRB1* Alleles)	Association with Rheumatoid Arthritis
HLA-DR1	0101	+
HLA-DR4 Dw4	0401	+
HLA-DR4 Dw14	0404/0408	+
HLA-DRw14 Dw16	1402	+
HLA-DR4 Dw10	0402	–
HLA-DR2	1501, 1502, 1601, 1602	–
HLA-DR3	0301, 0302	–
HLA-DR5	1101–1104, 1201, 1202	–
HLA-DR7	0701, 0702	–
HLA-DRw8	0801–0803	–
HLA-DR9	0901	–
HLA-DRw10	1001	–
HLA-DRw13	1301–1304	–
HLA-DRw14 Dw9	1401	–

From Weyand CM et al. (Weyand, CM, Hicok, KC, Conn DL, et al. The influence of HLA-DRB1 genes on disease severity in rheumatoid arthritis. *Ann Intern Med* 1992;117:801–806.)

sented to the T-cell receptor. This might abrogate what, under normal circumstances, would be a mechanism to clear the etiologic agent.

The concept of DR4 subtypes has been expanded to include a role for disease expression. Several investigators have demonstrated that homozygosity for these critical HLA-DRB1 alleles is associated with increased severity of disease expression (25–29,32). For example, individuals with a "double-dose" of HLA-DR4 are much more likely to have major organ involvement and subcutaneous nodules compared to individuals with only one gene. These observations, however, have not been substantiated in large population studies of patients with RA.

Finally, the genotypic distribution of shared epitope DRB1 marker alleles suggests that the mode of inheritance of the DRB-associated disease susceptibility gene must be recessive and not additive (33).

PATHOLOGY

Classically, the pathology of RA comprises serositis, subcutaneous nodules, and vasculitis. Serosal surfaces affected by the rheumatoid process include the pericardium and the pleura as well as synovial lined structures (the diarthrodial joint, tendon sheathes, bursae). Synovitis is the clinical hallmark of RA.

The earliest pathologic lesion in RA appears to be an acute inflammatory reaction within the synovial membrane. In patients with synovitis of less than six weeks' duration, Schumacher (34) demonstrated microvascular injury with increased vascularity and vascular permeability in the synovial membrane. The synovial membrane, normally a thin lacy structure one to three cell layers thick, becomes congested. This acute synovitis is mediated by both lymphocytes and polymorphonuclear leucocytes. Schumacher also identified a variety of virus-like particles in the endothelium and perivascular cells (34). The significance of these particles remains unknown. These changes may take place in patients before the development of symptoms in new cases or in clinically uninvolved joints of patients with established RA (35). Furthermore, edema of periarticular bone appears to be an early pathologic change in RA, as demonstrated by magnetic resonance imaging, and seems to correlate with the degree of synovitis (36).

Subsequent to this acute process, significant pathologic changes develop in the synovial membrane as the initial inflammatory reaction evolves into chronic synovial inflammation. The cellular components that characterize this transformation include synoviocytes, complex dendritic cells, macrophages, T- and B-lymphocytes, fibroblasts, and plasma cells. Neutrophils are less evident in the synovial membrane but become the predominant cell type in the synovial fluid within a few months of the onset of RA (17). The cellular population in the synovial membrane consists of resident cells (fibroblasts, synovial lining cells, mesenchymal cells, and complex dendritic cells), some of which are activated, and cells that derive from the circulation, especially B- and T-lymphocytes, monocytes, plasma cells, and mast cells.

Perhaps the most important cells in this transformation are the synovial lining cells. There are two types: type A synoviocytes (macrophage-like) and type B synoviocytes (fibroblasts-like). The former cell is bone marrow–derived and expresses macrophage surface markers including HLA-DR gene products. The latter cell is immunologically inactive. During the development of rheumatoid synovitis, both type A and type B cells (which in normal synovium exist in equal proportions) increase in number with a slightly higher ratio of type A to type B cells. These type A cells accumulate in the more superficial region of the intimal lining. They are likely responsible, in part, for antigen presentation to T-cells. Increases in both type A and type B cells account for the synovial hyperplasia characteristic of progressive RA (17).

Another important cell in the rheumatoid synovium is the dendritic. DC are potent antigen-presenting cells and can activate resting T-cells (37,38). They are found throughout lymphoid and non-lymphoid tissue in several organs including the lung and the gastrointestinal tract. Recently, they have been identified in rheumatoid synovium and synovial fluid (37,38). Their exact role in the rheumatoid synovium is uncertain, but it is possible that their capacity to present antigen functions uniquely in RA to present endogenous self-peptides to T-cells (39).

The increased vascularity in the synovial membrane is accompanied by the up-regulation of adhesion molecules in the endothelial environment, particularly in the high endothelial venules. Adhesion molecules facilitate the homing of B- and T-cells from the circulation to the synovium under a variety of chemotactic stimuli (see below). In particular, CD4+T-cells that express a memory phenotype are proficient at gaining access to the synovial membrane and are particularly important in the perpetuation of rheumatoid synovitis (40).

As rheumatoid inflammation proceeds, the synovial membrane takes on the appearance of an activated lymphoid organ with follicular hyperplasia and germinal centers. Aggregates of T- or B-cells may predominate in different areas of the synovium. Clusters of these cells occupy different locations within the synovial membrane. However, the cellular distribution within the synovium in RA does not appear to differ between the early and later stages of the disease (41). T-cells, which migrate mainly through high endothelial venules, form perivascular "cuffs" especially in the early stages of synovitis (17,42). These T-cells are primarily of the helper-inducer phenotype. T-cells isolated from the joint tissue and the synovial fluid express CD45 surface-markers characteristic of terminally differentiated memory cells (40). In the synovial fluid of patients with RA, there is a significant increase in the number of CD4-positive helper cells and a significant decrease in CD8 positive cytotoxic suppressor cells compared to the circulating lymphocyte population (43).

B-cells tend to reside in reactive lymphoid follicles or germinal centers, usually with a venule at the center of each cluster (44,45). CD8 positive cells occur in closer proximity to lymphoid centers than do activated CD4 positive cells. Plasma cells, expressing immunoglobulin, form rosettes around the germinal centers and follicles. Macrophage-like cells, accounting for 10% to 20% of the cellular population, are distributed throughout the synovium, typically in the subsynovial layers in proximity to CD4 positive T-cells (17,45).

The microenvironment of the rheumatoid synovium is heterogeneous, suggesting not only variations in function within various synoviocytes, but that ongoing inflammation and ongoing proliferation may not occur in parallel (17). Factors driving immunologically mediated inflammation may be different from those promoting tissue invasion and destruction.

The great majority of cells populating the rheumatoid synovial membrane are mononuclear cells (17). Only about 5% to 10% of cells in the synovial membrane are polymorphonuclear leucocytes (PMN). This is in distinct contrast to the situation in chronic rheumatoid synovial effusions where the predominate cell type is the PMN. Presumably, synovial fluid PMN have arrived there after gaining access to, and traversing, the synovium. Except possibly at the advancing edge of the rheumatoid pannus, the PMN has no clear role in the perpetuation of rheumatoid synovitis. However, it has a major role in the synovial fluid as a phagocytic cell and a reservoir of proteolytic enzymes.

This chronic inflammatory reaction leads to the development of the rheumatoid pannus. The pannus is a mass of granulation tissue with an expanded connective tissue matrix and a population of cells including lymphocytes, plasma cells, macrophages, neutrophils, and fibroblasts. It is not clear whether the rheumatoid pannus is merely an extension of the proliferative synovium or a more specific vascular connective tissue with the unique capacity to invade and destroy bone, cartilage, and connective tissue. (17,46,47). There appear to be more activated synovial lining cells and complex dendritic cells at the pannus interface than are present in the subsynovial immunologic environment (46). At the advancing edge of the pannus, there is a vascular zone of fibroblast-like cells, which extends onto the cartilage surface (marginal transitional zone) (17,46). Before there is an ingrowth of vessels into adjacent cartilage, synovial-derived cells dissect under the layer of fibroblast-like cells. Proteoglycan depletion occurs. In situ localization studies demonstrate the presence of collagenase and other matrix metalloproteinases. Later, neovascularization takes place accompanied by the invasion of fibroblast-like cells and macrophages.

Recently, a population of cells referred to as pannocytes has been identified at pannus-cartilage junctions but also at a distance from the pannus interface (46). These pannocytes resemble small fibroblast-like synoviocytes and may have importance in mediating cartilage destruction either directly or indirectly through interaction with complex dendritic cells.

TABLE 2.4. STAGING OF RA IN THE KNEE

Stage I	■ Visible evidence of pathology only in synovial lining with villi ■ No invasion of meniscus or articular cartilage
Stage II	■ Proliferative pannus extends over meniscus ■ Erosions and fissuring of menisci ■ Articular cartilage normal macroscopically
Stage III	■ Full thickness meniscal tears ■ Erosions of articular cartilage ■ Minimal joint narrowing on X-ray in 25%; Normal X-ray in 75%
Stage IV	■ Severe erosions in articular cartilage ■ Menisci severely thinned or absent ■ Majority with radiographic narrowing

Modified after Salisbury RB, Nottage WM. A new evaluation of gross pathologic changes and concepts of rheumatoid articular cartilage degeneration. *Clin Orthop* 1985;199:242–247.

At the interface between the synovium, the articular cartilage, and marginal bone, the advancing edge of the pannus has a centripetal orientation toward cartilage and bone at the joint margin and has invasive and destructive potential. Cells at the advancing edge, including PMN, macrophages, fibroblast-like cells, and perhaps pannocytes, release neutral and acid proteases, collagenases, and other matrix metalloproteinases. The rheumatoid pannus is directly responsible for the articular and osseous destruction of which RA is capable.

Recently, a staging system for RA has been proposed based on a series of arthroscopic evaluations of knees with rheumatoid synovitis (Table 2.4) (48). This staging system emphasizes that, at least in the knee, meniscal cartilage is eroded with full thickness craters at a time when there is minimal articular damage at least arthroscopically and radiographically.

PATHOGENESIS

The theory that a microbial agent participates in the early lesion of RA in the joint is an attractive one. One hypothesis would require active microbial replication in the joint space and a microbe-specific immune response. As mentioned, the failure to culture infectious agents from the joint of early arthritis patients confound this theory as does the inability to demonstrate microbial genomic material in the synovium or synovial fluid of patients with early arthritis. It is also possible that a nonspecific reaction takes place in the synovial membrane following inoculation with one or more microbial species.

An alternative hypothesis is that a microbial infection at a site distant from the joint results in the release of peptide antigens that are transported to the joint and elicit specific and/or nonspecific inflammation and immune disregulation. Acute synovitis caused by a local or distant infectious agent (or antigen) is apparent in the early stages of RA. This process is mediated by both lymphocytes and neutrophils. In individuals who do not possess an allelic risk for RA, there is prompt healing within the synovium. However, in genetically susceptible individuals, chronic synovitis ensues.

Until recently, there was general agreement that the transformation of acute to chronic synovitis and the perpetuation of the rheumatoid process were antigen driven. The antigen could be the original arthrotropic pathogen or a derivative peptide of this pathogen, which is processed by the antigen-presenting cell. An alternative mechanism would be that the original triggering pathogen is not responsible for the perpetuation process. This theory would hold that other antigens, uncovered or exposed during the acute joint injury, are responsible for perpetuation of arthritis. Candidates for this secondary antigen include type II collagen from articular cartilage or other autoantigens such as autologous IgG (rheumatoid factor).

Type II collagen is the major collagen type found in articular cartilage, comprising 85% to 90% of the supporting framework. Since articular cartilage is an avascular structure and thus a "protected" site, the participation in autoimmune responses of this protein is minimal. However, during cartilage degradation, associated with acute synovitis, it is possible that immune complexes involving type II collagen are sequestered (49,50). Type II collagen may function as an

autoantigen and also may participate in immune complex formation within the rheumatoid joint. Such complexes would be ingested by phagocytic cells with the resultant release of proteolytic enzymes.

IgG 7S rheumatoid factors are produced by B-cell transformation in the synovial membrane and are synthesized by plasma cells. These IgG rheumatoid factors have the capacity to form self-aggregating dimers (immune complexes), but IgG rheumatoid factor may also function as an autoantigen and drive T-cell transformation (17).

The pathogenesis of RA involves several cell types and their secretory products and receptors (Fig. 2.2). The following will be considered: (a) endothelial cells, (b) adhesion molecules, (c) T-cells, (d) B-cells, (e) macrophages, (f) cytokines, (g) arachidonic acid metabolites, and (h) matrix metalloproteinases.

Endothelial Cells

Increased access of immunologically active cells to the sites of synovial inflammation is essential to the development and propagation of the rheumatoid lesion. This access occurs predominately through the endothelial cell. Acute synovial inflammation results in the release of vasoactive peptides that increase vascular permeability. Chemotactic factors are generated

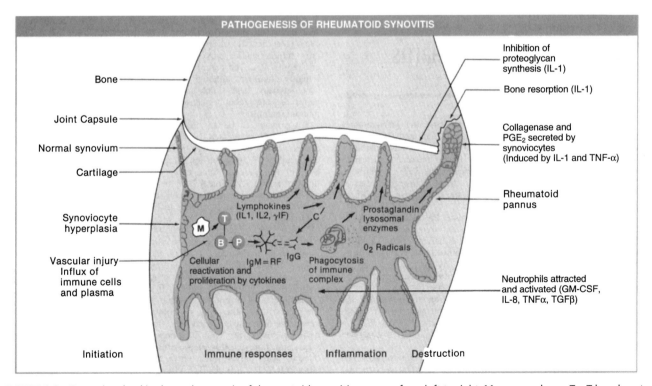

FIGURE 2.2. Events involved in the pathogenesis of rheumatoid synovitis progress from left to right. M = macrophage; T = T lymphocyte; B = B lymphocyte; P = plasma cell; Il = Interleukin; TNFα = tumor necrosis factor alpha; TGFβ = transforming growth factor beta; GM-CSF = granulocyte-macrophage colony stimulating factor; γIF = gamma-interferon; RF = rheumatoid factor; PGE$_2$ = prostaglandin E$_2$; IgM = immunoglobulin M; IgG = immunoglobulin G; C = complement. (From Arnett FC. Rheumatoid arthritis. In: Bennett JC, Plum F, eds. *Cecil textbook of medicine*, 20th ed. Philadelphia: WB Sanders, 1996:1459–1466, with permission.)

through acute inflammatory mechanisms. They also occur as a consequence of T-cell activation and macrophage recruitment. Antigen presentation and subsequent T-cell activation cause the release of cytokines, which activate endothelial cells and up-regulate the expression of adhesion molecules (51,52). These peptides serve to attract and retain cells from the circulation. The capacity of endothelial cells to respond to cytokine stimulation and enhance the recruitment of immunologically active cells is central to the pathogenesis of RA. Propagation of rheumatoid synovitis would not occur in the absence of increased access of inflammatory cells through the endothelium.

Adhesion Molecules

Circulating T-cells gain access to the inflamed synovial membrane via increased vascularity under the influence of cytokines derived from resident synovial cells, in particular synoviocytes and transformed accessory cells. The trafficking of T-cells into the joint and the ultimate distribution of T-cells in the subsynovial layers occur under the influence of adhesion molecules and their receptor ligands (53).

Adhesion molecules are a family of cell-surface receptor peptides that facilitate cell-to-cell binding (54). In conjunction with their associated ligands, they are responsible for control of the trafficking of cells in a variety of tissues. The four major families of adhesion molecules are the integrins, immunoglobulin-super family, cadherins, and selectins (54). Of particular importance in RA are the integrins (53). These are membrane glycoproteins with two subunits, alpha (α) and beta (β); these may exist in active and inactive forms (54). Once cellular activation occurs, the surface conformation of the integrin subunits can be modified, thus, increasing the affinity of the integrin for its ligand.

In RA, the expression of adhesion molecules within the synovial environment reflects the distribution of T-cells in the vicinity of the endothelium (55–57) and of macrophages and other antigen-presenting cells throughout the synovium (58). Both lymphocyte function-associated antigen 3 (LFA-3) and intercellular adhesion molecule 1 (ICAM 1) are widely distributed among several cell types in the synovial membrane (59). In particular, increased expression of adhesion molecule receptors occurs in perivascular cells and matrix proteins and acts as a "glue" to retain T-cells from the circulation. The further distribution of T-cells in the synovial membrane depends on the increased expression of adhesion molecules in various subsynovial sites. Furthermore, a variety of cytokines released by synoviocytes and accessory cells help regulate the expression of adhesion molecules. These cytokines include interleukin-1 beta (IL-1β), tumor necrosis factor-alpha (TNFα), interferon gamma (INFγ), and interleukin-6 (IL-6). The emigration of lymphocytes, particularly T-cells, to the joints under the influence of adhesion molecules is essential to provide a local population of T-cells necessary to perpetuate the inflammatory process.

T-Cells

A large body of information lends support to the central position of T-cells in the rheumatoid synovium (60–64). T-cells comprise about 50% of cells in most RA synovial specimens and are predominately found in perivascular cuffs in the subsynovial sites. They presumably gain access to the synovium via migration through high endothelial venules under the influence of up-regulated adhesion molecules. The majority of these cells express CD4-positive surface markers indicative of a helper-inducer phenotype. The purpose of these cells is presumably to participate in antigen presentation via the T-cell receptor (TCR) and to become activated after stimulation by antigen-TCR interactions. Chronic synovitis in RA is an antigen-driven event and requires presentation of peptide antigens to inducer T-cells or direct activation of T-cells by antigen. Within the synovium, there is also a preferential accumulation of T-cells bearing the CD45 RO surface marker for memory cells.

In the early stages of rheumatoid synovitis, antigen-specific T-cells expand within the synovium and recruit or modulate other cells through the release of cytokines. Autoreactive T-cell clones stimulate macrophages and fibroblastic synoviocytes to release IL-1 and TNF, two of the major

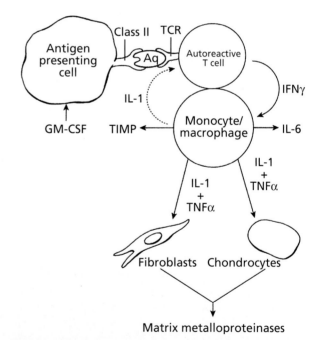

FIGURE 2.3. Antigen presentation to T-cell receptor in context of Class II surface molecule. Subsequent activation of T-cell and monocyte macrophage resulting in release of IL-1 and TNFα and other cytokines. GM-CSF = granulocyte-macrophage colony stimulating factor; TCR = T-cell receptor; IL-1 = Interleukin-1; IFNγ = interferon gamma; IL-6 = Interleukin 6; TNFα = tumor necrosis factor alpha; TIMP = tissue inhibitor of metalloproteinases. (Modified after Arend WP, Dayer JM. Cytokines and cytokine inhibitors or antagonists in rheumatoid arthritis. *Arthritis Rheum* 1990; 33:305–315, with permission.)

cytokines responsible for matrix degradation and joint destruction in RA (Fig. 2.3) (65). During the 1980s, T-cells were considered the central cellular mediator responsible not only for the initiation but also the perpetuation of RA.

Recently, however, the T-cell-centric paradigm has been challenged (61–63). The lack of consistent evidence of T-cell activation, either in the synovial membrane or the synovial fluid, has been problematic regarding this hypothesis. The majority of T-cells in the rheumatoid synovium are not activated even under circumstance of hectic immunologic activity. Levels of interleukin-2 (IL-2) or interleukin-2 receptors (IL-2R) are not generally increased in the joints of RA. Furthermore, the failure to demonstrate significant sustained clinical improvement in RA with therapies directed at T-cell inhibition or depletion (see below) have caused investigators to look elsewhere for cells and/or cytokines that may be more important pathogenetically.

Thus, the primacy of the T-cell paradigm has been debated, and there has been no unanimity about the relative importance of T-cells in RA or where in the hierarchy of effector cells T-cells should be positioned. Based strictly on potential therapeutic intervention, attention has shifted to inhibitors of informational molecules, particularly cytokines. It can be surmised that T-cells may be important in the initiation phase of rheumatoid arthritis (62) and that other effector molecules are more important in the propagation of RA at a later point.

B-Cells

The presence of B-cells in lymphoid follicles and germinal centers is a characteristic finding in the rheumatoid synovium (17). However, only about 5% of the cellular infiltrate in the rheumatoid joint comprise B-cells. The localization of B-cells in intimate association with CD4-postive T-cells suggests T-cell-dependent B-lymphocyte activation. Immunoglobulin-secreting plasma cells are arranged in the periphery of lymphoid follicles but in relative proximity to large clusters of B-cells.

The main role of synovial B-cells is the production of immunoglobulin. Of particular pathogenetic significance is the generation of IgG 7S rheumatoid factors by synovial B-cells. These antiglobulin molecules self-aggregate into dimers and function as immune complexes. They circulate within the joint tissue, activate complement, and are ingested by inflammatory cells in the synovial fluid, in particular PMN, resulting in the release of a variety of proteolytic enzymes.

Although B-cells and their participation in the generation of rheumatoid factors lend credence to the notion that RA is an "autoimmune" disease, B-cell participation is most likely an effector mechanism triggered by antigen interactions with APC and, possibly, T-cells.

Macrophages

As the central role of T-cells in rheumatoid synovitis has been diminished, or at least challenged, the importance of tissue macrophage-like synoviocytes and DC cells has come to the forefront (66). Macrophages in the synovium derive from circulating monocytes. The current hypothesis that macrophage-like cells are of central importance begins with the notion that APC presents peptide antigens to the TCR in the context of the class II molecule. As a consequence of this interaction, macrophage activation and helper-inducer T-cell activation takes place (Fig. 2.3). Cytokines, particularly INFγ, are released and direct stimulation of tissue macrophages ensues. This stimulation results in a release of a variety of potent cytokines with complex biologic activities. The two most important cytokines released by the macrophage are IL-1 and TNFα.

Cytokines

Currently, the major area of investigation in the pathogenesis of RA is the role of cytokines in the rheumatoid joint. Cytokines are informational molecules, which are synthesized and secreted at local sites and which have profound biologic effects carried out through receptor-mediated target cell activation. As a result of T-cell:APC interactions, T-cells and, more importantly, macrophages are activated. Cytokines characteristically released from T-cells or macrophages are listed in Table 2.5. The major T-cell cytokine is INFγ. This effector molecule induces class II surface receptor activity especially on monocyte/macrophages. This observation initially led investigators to consider INFγ as a potent inducer of macrophage activation in RA. However, only very small levels of INFγ could be found in the synovial membrane or synovial fluid of RA joints. INFγ has a number of biological effects including antagonism of TNFα. The relative deficiency of INFγ in the joints of RA patients could be considered as evidence for unchecked TNFα activity in the same joint. This antagonism has been utilized in combination of therapeutic strategies to increase INFγ activity and to inhibit TNF activity. Other T-cell cytokines, including IL-2, IL-4, TNFβ, and IL-3, have either not been detected or detected in only small amounts in the joints of RA patients. These observations provide additional evidence that T-cell cytokines are not of primary importance in RA.

The major effector cytokines in RA appear to be derived from macrophages and fibroblasts (Table 2.5). The two major cytokines are IL-1 and TNF. IL-1 is a ubiquitous family of polypeptides with diverse biologic activities (67,68), some of which are relevant to RA (Table 2.6). IL-1 exists in two forms: IL-1α and IL-1β. Both forms bind to the same IL-1 receptor on target cells. Significant mRNA for IL-1β is contained in nearly half of the rheumatoid synovial macrophages (69). IL-1α and IL-1β are generated from synovial macrophages after activation by antigen triggered inducer T-cell processes. IL-1 can also be generated by immunoglobulin Fc fragments and, to a lesser extent, by immune complexes.

IL-1 exerts both systemic and local effects. Major symptoms of RA, including fever, weight loss, and anorexia, are

TABLE 2.5. SYNOVIAL CYTOKINES IN RA

Cellular Source	Level of Production in RA Synovium
T cells	
Interleukin-2	–
Interleukin-3	–
Interleukin-4	–
Interleukin-6	±
Interferon-γ	–
TNF-α	–
TNF-β	–
GM-CSF	–
Macrophages*/Fibroblasts†	
Interleukin-1	+
IL-1ra	+
Interleukin-6	+
Interleukin-10	+
TNF-α	+
M-CSF (Csf-1)	+
GM-CSF	+
TGF-β	+
Interferon-α	±
Chemokines (IL-8, MCP-1, etc.)	+
Fibroblast growth factor	+

Adapted from Firestein GS, Zuaifler NJ. How important are T cells in chronic rheumatoid synovitis? *Arthritis Rheum* 1990;33:768, with permission.

*Tissue macrophages or type A synoviocytes.
†Tissue fibroblasts or type B synoviocytes.
–, absent or very low concentrations.
+, present.
Abbreviations: M-CSF, macrophage colony-stimulating factor; GM, granulocyte-macrophage; TNF, tumor necrosis factor; TGF: transforming growth factor.

TABLE 2.6. BIOLOGIC EFFECTS OF IL-1 IN RA

Site	Effects
Systemic	Fever
	Decreased appetite
	Increased granulocyte-macrophage colony-stimulating factor production
	Synthesis of acute-phase proteins
Local	Chemotaxis of polymorphonuclear cells lymphocytes, and monocytes
	Adherence of white blood cells to endothelial cells
	Fibroblast proliferation
	Prostaglandin E_2, collagenase, and neutral protease production by fibroblasts and chondrocytes
	Increased production of collagen and an inhibitor of neutral proteases
	Stimulation of T and B lymphocytes

From Arend WP, Dayer JM. Cytokines and cytokine inhibitors or antagonists in rheumatoid arthritis. *Arthritis Rheum* 1990;33:305–315, with permission.

mediated by IL-1; this cytokine is also responsible for acute phase responses in RA. More important are the local effects of IL-1 within the synovial environment. These include augmentation of T- and B-cell functions, chemotaxis for inflammatory cells, adherence of leucocytes to endothelial cells, fibroblast proliferation, and generation of prostaglandin E2. IL-1 also induces synovial fibroblasts and chondrocytes to produce collagenase (Fig. 2.3). Under some circumstances, IL-1 also stimulates synthesis of IL-6 and granulocyte-macrophage-colony stimulating factor (GM-CSF) by synovial cells and enhances collagen production. Each of these effects serves to promote inflammation and helps drive immunologically mediated synovitis. Therapeutic intervention aimed at direct inhibition of IL-1 or its receptor has been utilized and will be discussed below.

The other major cytokine existing in RA is TNF. This cytokine also exists in two forms: TNFα and TNFβ (also called lymphotoxin). TNFα is the most important cytokine for RA, being detectable in rheumatoid synovial effusions. There are two TNF receptors, p55 and p75, on target cells. Both receptor types bind TNFα. TNF and IL-1 have very similar biologic activities and often act synergistically. Important activities of TNF in RA include stimulation of macrophages to release pro-inflammatory cytokines and chemokines, up-regulation by endothelial cells of adhesion molecules, and induction of metalloproteinase synthesis by synoviocytes, fibroblasts, and chondrocytes. Direct inhibition of TNF has been a therapeutic goal in RA and has recently been introduced to the clinical arena (see below).

Other macrophage-derived cytokines are of importance in RA. Interleukin 6 (IL-6) is inducible by IL-1 and is capable of stimulating immunoglobulin synthesis by B-cells. It is also involved in differentiation of cytotoxic T lymphocytes. GM-CSF is the major DR inducing cytokine in RA synovial fluid. It also regulates neutrophil function, enhancing antibody dependant cytotoxicity, phagocytosis, chemotaxis, and production of oxygen radicals. Macrophage activation and the release of IL-1, TNF, and PGE2 are other important functions of GM-CSF. Platelet-derived growth factor (PDGF) is both chemoattractant and mitogenic for fibroblasts and induces collagenase expression. This cytokine plays a major role in the perpetuation of rheumatoid synovitis by generating proliferation of synovial cells.

Taken together, cytokines, derived mainly from macrophages/fibroblasts, appear to fuel the rheumatoid process after T-cell mediated events, including peptide antigen presentation, initiate the process. Since cytokine effector mechanisms are important in perpetuating RA, they have long been recognized as potential therapeutic targets for disease amelioration. It should be emphasized that the effects of cytokines have been analyzed individually mainly using in vitro systems. The complex circuitry achieved by cell-cell communication mainly through the cytokine network may not reflect the sum of the biologic activities of individual molecules. Until we more fully understand the effect of this immunologic milieu in aggregate, we will need to be cautious about interpreting mechanism of individual cytokine components.

Arachidonic Acid Metabolites

Arachidonic acid is generated from plasma membranes under the influence of phospholipase. This substrate is then catalyzed by two different pathways, one utilizing lipoxygenase and leading to leukotriene production and the other utilizing cyclooxygenase and leading to thromboxane, prostacyclin, and other prostaglandins. Both leukotrienes and prostaglandins subserve diverse, biologic, and pathologic functions, including the maintenance of normal homeostasis and acute and chronic inflammation under certain circumstances. Traditional nonsteroidal anti-inflammatory agents (NSAIA) inhibit prostaglandin generation by interacting with the enzyme cyclooxygenase. Many patients treated with NSAIA experience clinical improvement and thus appear to have inflammation at least partially controlled. Yet in many of these same patients progressive joint damage occurs. This highlights the dichotomy in RA of inflammation versus destruction. Under most circumstances, these two pathways follow a parallel course, but it is dangerous to assume that progressive erosive arthritis will not develop in the individual who demonstrates improving or stabilizing clinical parameters.

Arachidonic-acid metabolites are felt to mediate acute and chronic inflammation in RA, although direct evidence for this is still lacking. Pro-inflammatory mediators, including prostaglandins and leukotrienes, are released from synovial fluid PMN as well as synovial macrophages. Increased activities for both of these molecules can be found in situ. However, the best evidence that these mediators are important in rheumatoid arthritis comes from therapeutic data suggesting that clinical improvement takes place in patients receiving inhibitors of prostaglandins.

Matrix Metalloproteinases

The matrix metalloproteinases (MMP) are a family of enzymes that participate in extracellular matrix degradation and remodeling (Table 2.7) (70). Cytokine-mediated stimulation of synoviocytes, fibroblasts, and chondrocytes results in the release of metalloproteinases, which are ultimately responsible for the final pathways of cartilage depletion and connective tissue breakdown. The major cytokines that induce MMP are IL1 and TNFα, and their effect may be additive or synergistic in this regard.

The two major MMP are collagenase and stromolysin. Between them, they have the capacity to degrade all of the major structural proteins within the joint cavity. Genes for these enzymes are expressed in rheumatoid synovial tissue and in chondrocytes (17).

In addition to cytokines that stimulate the activity of MMP, there are factors that serve to inhibit this activity. The cytokine transforming growth-factor beta (TGFβ) inhibits collagenase synthesis and enhances collagen production. Naturally occurring inhibitors of MMP have been discovered, and the first one was designated tissue inhibitor of metallopro-

TABLE 2.7. MATRIX METALLOPROTEINASES (MMP)

Enzyme	Source
Collagenase (MMP-1)	Fibroblasts, Chondrocytes
Gelatinase A (MMP-2)	Fibroblasts, Chondrocytes
Stromelysin (MMP-3)	Fibroblasts, Chondrocytes

teinase (TIMP), but other members of this family of inhibitors have been isolated. These inhibitors are primarily localized to the synovial intimal lining. Furthermore, the production of TIMP is enhanced under the influence of TGFβ (70).

In addition to MMP, acid and neutral proteases are also released by PMN in the synovial fluid (70). This occurs particularly after ingestion by PMN of immune complexes or immunoglobulin fragments. The protease-rich synovial fluid bathes articular cartilage, which is also under attack from the advancing pannus and the synovial derived MMP.

The ultimate integrity (or destruction) of the joint in RA depends on the balance between degradative processes and molecules serving to inhibit enzyme activity and promote matrix repletion. The end result is different in each patient with RA.

The complex milieu of the rheumatoid synovium and synovial fluid represents an accumulation of cells and cytokines, which act in concert to produce degradation of cartilage, bone, and periarticular structures. Individual cells and cytokines have been studied *ex vivo*, but critical information about *in vivo* reactions involving these participants in the joint is still lacking.

It is vital that developments regarding the genetic and immunologic aspects of RA be applied directly to the treatment of patients with this disease. Conventional therapies for RA have been palliative only in the short term, have not been well studied methodologically and have been associated with significant toxicity. Prevailing knowledge of the etiopathogenesis of RA, although imprecise, nonetheless provides the basis for the implementation of unique treatment strategies directed at specific rather than global abnormalities of immune function and regulation in this disorder. As has already been demonstrated, it is possible to apply this knowledge to develop newer pharmacological agents that could potentially replace existing remedies (71).

NONSURGICAL TREATMENT

The management of RA requires a fundamental understanding of the pathophysiologic basis of the disease, its protean clinical manifestations, and its negative impact on functional parameters. Patients with RA have prolonged morning stiffness, diffuse joint pain, and swelling as well as profound fatigue. Destructive arthritis causes structural joint abnormalities and impairment of occupational and recreational activities.

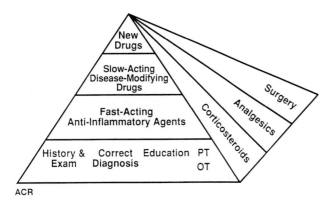

FIGURE 2.4. Rheumatoid arthritis therapeutic pyramid. (From American College of Rheumatology Teaching slide collection, with permission.)

However, each patient with RA is unique. Treatment strategies in RA need to be individualized and approached from a broad therapeutic perspective. Traditional therapy of RA includes both nonpharmacologic and pharmacologic treatment prescribed in parallel (1,72,73). The therapeutic pyramid for RA (Fig. 2.4) comprises a broad base of patient and family education, proper diet, attention to concomitant medical problems, and a physiotherapy program consisting of rest and exercise. Patients with RA require appropriate rest and a balanced nutritional program. Individual joints that are inflamed should be rested and properly positioned with the use of splints or orthotics.

To the broad base of the therapeutic pyramid is added pharmacologic therapy consisting initially of anti-inflammatory medications. Therapy with aspirin and nonaspirin, nonsteroidal anti-inflammatory agents (NSAIA's) is strictly empiric, and appropriate doses of medication need to be administered in sequence for periods of two to three weeks to ascertain whether appropriate reduction in inflamed joints takes place. Many patients will have their disease brought under reasonable control with NSAIA's alone. However, in the majority of cases, active synovitis is accompanied by evidence of ongoing joint damage. It is at this stage in the treatment program that attention is given to disease modifying anti-rheumatic drugs (DMARD) or "second line" therapy (Table 2.8) (74). Traditional drugs in this category include gold, hydroxychloroquine D-penicillamine, sulfasalazine, and immunosuppressive agents such as azathioprine and

TABLE 2.8. TRADITIONAL SECOND LINE DRUGS FOR RA

■ Gold	■ Azathioprine
■ Hydroxychloroquine	■ Methotrexate
■ Sulfasalazine	■ Cyclophosphamide
■ D-penicilliamine	■ Cyclosporine
■ Minocycline	

cyclophosphamide. More recently, minocycline has been added to this list (75,76). These agents were prescribed with the supposition that their administration would result in disease suppression and modification and that the progression of disease (usually measured radiographically) would be ameliorated or retarded. These drugs were studied (with the exception of minocycline) in great detail and utilized between 1950 and 1975 by practicing rheumatologists. Usually second-line therapy was recommended once it was evident that joint damage was present. With most agents in this category, it was recommended continuing the drug for 6 to 12 months before expecting clinical improvement. Although anecdotal "remissions" were achieved in a few patients, long-term studies evaluating the benefit of second-line drugs demonstrated little improvement in outcome and a high degree of patient and physician dissatisfaction (77,78). Only three studies have demonstrated established evidence of disease modification based on X-ray data: one each with gold (79), methylprednisolone (80), and high-dose cyclophosphamide (81). Only a small number of patients in whom second-line therapy is initiated actually remain on the drug due either to lack of efficacy or unacceptable side effects (78).

Two major developments heralded the "modern era" of RA therapy, which began in the late 1970s. The first was the recognition that joint destruction in RA occurred early (often within the first three years) and that control of disease signs and symptoms did not necessarily provide reassurance that joint damage would not take place. It was emphasized that the "window of opportunity" to influence disease progression and outcome was relatively narrow and that therapeutic strategies should be aggressively implemented in the early stages of the disease ("inversion of the pyramid") (82).

The second major development was the introduction of methotrexate as a potent anti-rheumatic drug. Clinical trials began in the late 1970s and extended for periods of 15 to 20 years or longer (83–85). These studies demonstrated major therapeutic benefit, which was relatively rapid in onset and responses that were durable. Once weekly, oral methotrexate administered in doses of between 7.5 and 20 mg was found to provide unequivocal benefit in a large percentage of RA patients with a risk-benefit ratio that was extremely favorable (86). The introduction of MTX as the premier second-line therapy for RA advanced rheumatologic therapeutics. Currently, methotrexate, either alone or in combination with other second-line therapy forms the conventional framework for the treatment of RA. However, there is still debate as to whether or not MTX modifies RA, and studies supporting (87,88) or refuting (89–91) this notion exist. Moreover, the mechanism of action of MTX is incompletely understood (92). It appears that MTX as an antimetabolite inhibits T-cell function in several ways, mainly as an inhibitor of purine nucleotide pathways (92). It also appears to have distinct anti-inflammatory capabilities (92).

Although the mechanisms of action of all of the conventional anti-rheumatic drugs remain incompletely understood, strategies have been implemented to administer these agents in various combinations analogous to chemotherapeutic "cocktails" given for the treatment of malignant disease (93–96). Currently, the majority of patients with RA who are receiving second-line therapy are receiving combinations of at least two, and usually three or more, antirheumatic drugs.

In spite of these recent developments, antirheumatic therapy has been based traditionally on empiricism. For example, the beneficial effects of gold salts in RA was noted initially when this agent was administered as antimicrobial therapy because of its use in tuberculosis and the belief that RA was caused by an infectious agent (97). Methotrexate as an antimetabolite was initially used to treat psoriasis and then, by extension, psoriatic arthritis. The beneficial effect in this latter disease led to its introduction in the treatment of RA. Until recently, drug therapy for RA remained largely empiric and provided symptomatic clinical improvement by reducing inflammation or by "suppressing" the immune system at multiple levels. Thus, anti-inflammatory agents and cytotoxic or immunosuppressive drugs have dominated antirheumatic therapy for many years.

As discussed previously, significant advances in molecular biology and immunogenetics have identified pro-inflammatory mediators in RA as well as informational molecules (cytokines) that amplify the integrated circuit of immune synovitis characteristic of RA. In order for this understanding to translate into clinical benefit, this accumulated knowledge must be applied innovatively to develop more specific means for modulating the immune system in a restricted yet specific and beneficial fashion. This is the challenge that clinicians face in order to advance rheumatologic therapeutics beyond the frontier of methotrexate. Within the past ten years, two major forms of biologic therapy have been developed: anti-T-cell therapy and anti-cytokine therapy.

Anti-T-Cell Therapy

The central role of the T-cell in the initiation and/or propagation of the rheumatoid lesion has been discussed. Even though the primacy of the T-cell paradigm in RA has been debated, a number of strategies have been developed to inhibit T-cell numbers or function. This is based on several observations. In many therapeutic trials, clinical improvement in RA has been associated with preferential reduction or depletion of T-cell subsets by a variety of methods. These include gold (98), D-penicillamine, (99), antimalarial compounds (100), thoracic duct drainage (101), lympha-pheresis (102), and total lymphoid irradiation (103). Also, cyclosporine A, a specific inhibitor of T-cell activity (via inhibition of IL-2 production) has produced clinical improvement (104). Although the specific action of methotrexate is incompletely understood, it does appear to have cellular and subcellular effects on T-cells acting as a purine antimetabolite in this regard (92). It is still not known whether the anti-T-cell activities of MTX explain its clinical efficacy.

Initially, it was felt that monoclonal antibodies directed preferentially against pathogenic CD4 positive helper-inducer T-cells would show clinical benefit without effecting the remainder of the immune system. In animal models, it was possible to abrogate specific immune responses by pretreatment with anti-T-cell antibodies (105). As monoclonal antibody technology was refined, it was possible to consider clinical trials in humans with RA. Pilot studies analyzed the use of murine monoclonal antibodies directed against T-cell surface receptors or target cell receptors in small numbers of patients with RA. These receptors included CD4, CD5, and CD7 T-cell surface receptors and IL2 receptors on target cells (106–109).

Monoclonal antibodies were further developed against specific T-cell receptors. For example, CD52 is a universal lymphocyte surface antigen, which is also present in some monocytes. The humanized monoclonal antibody CAMPATH-1H is an antilymphocyte IgG1 monoclonal antibody directed against CD52. Trials using this agent demonstrated widespread T-cell depletion and clinical benefit (110,111). However, toxic reactions were common. A chimeric monoclonal antibody, cM-T412, was administered to patients with severe RA (112,113). This trial demonstrated significant T-cell depletion but no clinical benefit. Other studies using depleting T-cell monoclonal antibodies did demonstrate clinical improvement. It was then recognized that some anti-T-cell antibodies only coated the receptors while others produced a strong modulation sometimes associated with profound depletion.

Other investigators studied the effects of nondepleting anti-T-cell monoclonal antibodies against CD4-positive helper-inducer cells (114,115). Although side effects with nondepleting anti-T-cell antibodies were much less, consistent clinical benefit was not observed. The variable responses in different trials using anti-CD4-positive monoclonal antibodies have been attributed to many factors including expectation bias (116). However, contemporary biologic treatment strategies have drifted away from monoclonal antibody therapy against T-cells.

Recently the antimetabolite leflunomide was approved for use in RA (Table 2.9). This compound is an antipyrimidine and accomplishes this by inhibiting the enzyme dihydroorotate dehydrogenase. Because of this antipyrimidine effect, it blocks clonal T-cell expansion. Leflunomide has been studied alone (117) and in combination with methotrexate in RA trials (118,119). It has shown striking clinical benefit in both types of protocols. It has even been demonstrated to retard

TABLE 2.9. NEWER SECOND LINE THERAPY FOR RA

- Leflunomide
- Etanercept
- Imfliximab

radiographic progression in RA and function as a true disease-modifying drug. Long-term trials will be necessary to demonstrate a durable effect.

Finally, a novel T-cell therapy was recently proposed by Moreland et al. This involves targeting the T-cell receptor (TCR) by TCR peptide vaccination (120). Although the clinical benefit in this study was modest, it opens the door for unique strategies to target T-cells in novel ways (121).

Anti-cytokine Therapy

A clear understanding of the cellular and cytokine network in RA provides a provocative rationale for more directed biologic therapy in RA. Rather than targeting cellular components of the rheumatoid pannus (and thus risking compromising normal cellular function), it was apparent that therapy designed to block cytokines themselves or their cellular receptors would provide a more directed and potentially more controllable treatment.

As discussed previously, the two major pro-inflammatory cytokines operative in the rheumatoid synovium are TNFα and IL-1. Biologic therapies against each of these have been developed in the last ten years and have been brought to market in the case of anti-TNF therapy (Table 2.9) (122).

In 1993, Elliott, Maini, et al. reported on the administration of a chimeric human-murine monoclonal antibody (cA2) against TNFα administered to patients with RA in small clinical trials (123) and later in larger studies (124–126). Marked benefit was noted in patients, many of whom had advanced disease. This compound has been administered also in combination with MTX, and significant improvement has been noted after a single infusion. This compound, imfliximab, is administered as an intravenous infusion and has been shown to have relatively few of the side effects usually associated with anticytokine therapy. Imfliximab was recently approved by the FDA for use in RA.

TNF inhibition has also been accomplished by the development of a fusion protein consisting of two molecules of p75, a TNF receptor, and an IgG1 construct. This agent, known as etanercept, inhibits both soluble and bound TNF. It has been demonstrated in clinical trials to have significant benefit in RA patients (127,128). This has also been approved by the FDA for the treatment of RA. Other TNF therapies are currently under development.

The other major pro-inflammatory cytokine in RA is IL-1. IL-1α and IL-1β have been discussed above. The third member of the IL-1 gene family is IL-1 receptor antagonist (IL-1Ra). This is a naturally occurring IL-1 inhibitor presumably present to modulate or regulate the effect of IL-1.

Attempts to inhibit IL-1 and its effects have been developed. Administration of IL-1 receptors would be expected to abrogate the local effect of IL1. Recombinant IL-1 receptor has been cloned and administered in a pilot study to patients with RA (129). Four of eight patients in the trial reported clinical benefit. Another approach is to administer IL-1R

antagonist, and this has been carried out using a recombinant IL-1 receptor antagonist (130). Further attempts at IL-1 inhibition are being developed and subjected to clinical trials. Currently, no specific IL-1 inhibitor is approved for the treatment of RA.

It appears at this time that anticytokine therapy will offer better treatment of RA patients then anticellular treatment or nonspecific immunosuppression. However, unforeseen side effects that occur as a result of unfettered manipulation of cytokine channels will have to be carefully monitored. Furthermore, long-term clinical trials will have to be carried out in order to demonstrate a consistent and durable effect.

Future Directions

Advances in the understanding of the immunogenetics and pathogenesis of RA have provided a more refined substrate in which the developed RA therapies can be more directed and targeted at specific pathogenetic pathways (131,132). Currently, monotherapy with anticytokines or anticytokine therapy in combination with traditional antirheumatic therapy is being carried out. It is anticipated that combination therapy with various anticytokines, anti-T-cell therapies and existing antirheumatic therapies will be expanded.

Other investigational drugs under study in RA include mycophenolic mofetil, tacrolimus, rapamycin, amiprilose, azarabine, and thalidamide (133). There has also been renewed interest in the use of inhibitors of metalloproteinases to interrupt the destructive tissue potential of RA (134).

The past two years have seen an explosion of newer and better treatments for RA. However, having the tools available makes it incumbent to develop strategies on how to best utilize them (131,132). Should biologic therapies be introduced at any early stage of disease? Should patients with unfavorable genetic risk factors be identified early and given aggressive therapy? Which combination of antirheumatic drugs is best suited for which patients? Will gene therapy have a future role to play? What about immunization therapy for RA?

As we embark on the twenty-first century, we are presented with unique opportunities to advance the level of therapy for RA to unprecedented heights. This is possible through a better understanding of disease processes in RA. In order for the full impact of these discoveries to be realized, this accumulated knowledge must be applied innovatively to develop more specific means for modulating the immune dysfunction associated with RA, and yet caution must be applied to avoid pitfalls of such therapies.

REFERENCES

1. Arnett FC. Rheumatoid arthritis. In: Bennett JC, Plum F, eds. *Cecil textbook of medicine*, 20th ed. Philadelphia: WB Sanders, 1996:1459–1466.
2. Harris ED. Clinical features of rheumatoid arthritis. In: Kelley WN, Harris ED, Ruddy S, Sledge CB, eds. *Textbook of rheumatology*, 5th ed. Philadelphia: WB Sanders, 1997:898–932.

3. Alaracon GS. Epidemiology of rheumatoid arthritis. *Rheum Dis Clin North Am* 1995;21:589–604.

4. Specter TD. Rheumatoid arthritis. *Rheum Dis Clin North Am* 1990;16:513–536.

5. Abdel-Nasser AM, Rosker JJ, Valkenberg HA. Epidemiological and clinical aspects relating to the variability of rheumatoid arthritis. *Semin Arthritis Rheum* 1997;27:123–140.

6. VanSchaardenburg D, Breedveld FC. Elderly-onset rheumatoid arthritis. *Semin Arthritis Rheum* 1994;23:367–378.

7. Dugowson CE, Koepsell TD, Voigt LF, et al. Rheumatoid arthritis in women: incidence rates in group health cooperative, Seattle, Washington, 1987–1989. *Arthritis Rheum* 1991;34:1502–1507.

8. Jacobsson, LTH, Hanson, RL, Knowler, WC, et al. Decreasing incidence and prevalence of rheumatoid arthritis in Pima Indians over a twenty-five year period. *Arthritis Rheum* 1994;37:1158–1165.

9. Chan KA, Felson DT, Yood RA, et al. Incidence of rheumatoid arthritis in central Massachusetts. *Arthritis Rheum* 1993;36:1691–1696.

10. Cobb S, Anderson F, Bauer W. Length of life and cause of death in rheumatoid arthritis. *N Engl J Med* 1953;249:553–556.

11. Phillips PE. Infectious agents in the pathogenesis of rheumatoid arthritis. *Semin Arthritis Rheum* 1986;16:1–10.

12. Holoshitz J, Drucker I, Yaretzky A, et al. T-lymphocytes of rheumatoid arthritis patients show augmented reactivity to a fraction of mycobacteria cross-reactive with cartilage. *Lancet* 1986;2(8502):305–309 .

13. Ottehnhoff THM. DeLasAguas JT, van Eden W. et al. Evidence for an HLA-DR4-associated immune-response gene for mycobacterium tuberculosis: a clue to the pathogenesis of rheumatoid arthritis? *Lancet* 1986;2(8502):310–312.

14. Rook G, Lydyard P, Stanford J. Mycobacteria and rheumatoid arthritis. *Arthritis Rheum* 1990;33:431–436.

15. Depper JM, Zvaifler NJ. Epstein-Barr virus: its relationship to the pathogenesis of rheumatoid arthritis. *Arthritis Rheum* 1981;24:755–760.

16. Tosato G, Steinberg AD, Blaese RM. Defective EBV-specific suppressor T-cell function in rheumatoid arthritis. *N Engl J Med* 1981;305:1238–1243.

17. Firestein GS. Etiology and pathogenesis of rheumatoid arthritis. In: Kelley WM, Harris ED, Ruddy S, Sledge CB, eds. *Textbook of rheumatology*, 5th ed. Philadelphia: WB Sanders, 1997:851–897.

18. Newkirk MM, Watanabe-Duffy KN, Paleckova A, et al. Herpes viruses in multicase families with rheumatoid arthritis. *J Rheumatol* 1995;22:2055–2060.

19. Cohen BJ, Buckley MM, Crewley JP, et al. Human parvovirus infection in early rheumatoid and inflammatory arthritis. *Ann Rheum Dis* 1986;45:832–838.

20. Hajeer AH, MacGregor AJ, Rigby AS, et al. Influence of previous exposure to human parvovirus B19 infection in explaining susceptibility to rheumatoid arthritis: an analysis of disease discordant twin pairs. *Ann Rheum Dis* 1994;53:137–139.

21. Harrison B, Silman A, Barrett E, et al. Low frequency of recent parvovirus infection in a population-based cohort of patients with early inflammatory polyarthritis. *Ann Rheum Dis* 1998;57:375–377.

22. Zhang D, Nikkari S, Vainonpaa R, et al. Detection of rubella, mumps, and measles virus genomic RNA in cells from synovial fluid and peripheral blood in early rheumatoid arthritis. *J Rheumatol* 1997;24:1260–1264.

23. Stastny P. Association of the B-cell alloantigen DRw4 with rheumatoid arthritis. *N Engl J Med* 1978;298:869–872.

24. Wordsworth BP, Stedeford J, Rosenberg, WMC, et al. Limited heterogeneity of the HLA class II contribution to susceptibility to rheumatoid arthritis is suggested by positive associations with HLA-DR4, DR1 and DRw10. *Br J Rheumatol* 1991;30:178–180.

25. Weyand, CM, Hicok, KC, Conn DL, et al. The influence of HLA-DRB1 genes on disease severity in rheumatoid arthritis. *Ann Intern Med* 1992;117:801–806.

26. MacGregor A, Ollier W, Thompson W, et al. HLA-DRB1 *0401/0404 genotype and rheumatoid arthritis: increased association in men, young age at onset, and disease severity. *J Rheumatol* 1995;22:1032–1036.

27. Meyer JM, Evans TI, Small RE, et al. HLA-DRB1 genotype influences risk for and severity of rheumatoid arthritis. *J Rheumatol* 1999;26:1024–1034.

28. Reveille JD, Alarcon, GS, Fowler SE, et al. HLA-DRB1 genes and disease severity in rheumatoid arthritis. *Arthritis Rheum* 1996;39:1802–1807.

29. Seldin MF, Amos CI, Ward A, et al. The genetics revolution and the assault on rheumatoid arthritis. *Arthritis Rheum* 1999;42:1071–1079.

30. Gregersen PK, Silver J, Winchester RJ. The shared epitope hypothesis: an approach to understanding the molecular genetics of susceptibility to rheumatoid arthritis. *Arthritis Rheum* 1987;30:1205–1212.

31. Winchester R, Dwyer E, Rose S. The genetic basis of rheumatoid arthritis: the shared epitope hypothesis. *Rheum Dis Clin North Am* 1992;18:761–783.

32. Calin A, Elswood J, Klouda P. Destructive arthritis, rheumatoid factor and HLA-DR4: susceptibility versus severity, a case-control study. *Arthritis Rheum* 1989;32:1221–1225.

33. Evans TI, Han J, Singh R, et al. The genotypic distribution of shard-epitope DRB1 alleles suggests a recessive mode of inheritance of the rheumatoid arthritis disease-susceptibility gene. *Arthritis Rheum* 1995;38:1754–1761.

34. Schumacher HR. Synovial membrane and fluid morphologic alterations in early rheumatoid arthritis: microvascular injury and virus-like particles. *Ann NY Acad Sci* 1975;256:39–64.

35. Kraan MC, Versendaal H, Jonker M, et al. Asymptomatic synovitis precedes clinically manifest arthritis. *Arthritis Rheum* 1998;41:1481–1488.

36. McGonagle D, Conaghan PG, O'Connor P, et al. The relationship between synovitis and bone changes in early untreated rheumatoid arthritis: controlled magnetic resonance imaging study. *Arthritis Rheum* 1999;42:1706–1711.

37. Zvaifler NJ, Steinman RM, Kaplan G, et al. Identification of immunostimulatory dendritic cells in the synovial effusion of patients with rheumatoid arthritis. *J Clin Invest* 1985;76:789–800.

38. Thomas R, Daris LS, Lipsky PE. Rheumatoid synovium is enriched in mature antigen presenting dendritic cells. *J Immunol* 1994;152:2613–2633.

39. Thomas R, Lipsky P. Presentation of self peptides by dendritic cells: possible implications for the pathogenesis of rheumatoid arthritis. *Arthritis Rheum* 1996;39:183–190.

40. Cush JJ, Pietschmann P, Oppenheimer-Marks N, et al. The intrinsic migratory capacity of memory T cells contributes to their accumulation in rheumatoid synovium. *Arthritis Rheum* 1992;35:1434–1444.

41. Tak PP, Smeets TJM, Daha MR, et al. Analysis of the synovial cell infiltrate in early rheumatoid synovial tissue in relation to local disease activity. *Arthritis Rheum* 1997;40:217–225.

42. Kurosaka M, Ziff M. Immunoelectron microscopic study of the distribution of T-cell subset in rheumatoid synovium. *J Exp Med* 1983;158:1191–1210.

43. Lasky HP, Bauer K, Pope RM. Increased helper inducer and decreased suppressor inducer phenotypes in the rheumatoid joint. *Arthritis Rheum* 1988;31:52–58.

44. Konttinen YT, Reitamo S, Ranki A, et al. Characterization of the immunocompetent cells of rheumatoid synovium from tissue sections and eluates. *Arthritis Rheum* 1981;24:71–78.

45. Yanni G, Whelan A, Feighery C, et al. Analysis of cell populations in rheumatoid arthritis synovial tissues. *Semin Arthritis Rheum* 1992;21:393–399.

46. Zvaifler NJ, Firestein GS, Pannus and pannocytes: alternative models of joint destruction in rheumatoid arthritis. *Arthritis Rheum* 1994;37:783–789.
47. Woolley DE, Tetlow LC. Observations on the microenvironmental nature of cartilage degradation in rheumatoid arthritis. *Ann Rheum Dis* 1997;56:151–161.
48. Salisbury RB, Nottage WM. A new evaluation of gross pathologic changes and concepts of rheumatoid articular cartilage degeneration. *Clin Orthop* 1985;199:242–247.
49. Noyori K, Jasin H. Repair characteristics of the articular cartilage surface following acute inflammatory arthritis. *J Rheumatol* 1994; 21:1731–1734.
50. Jasin HE. Autoantibody specificities of immune complexes sequestered in articular cartilage of patients with rheumatoid arthritis and osteoarthritis. *Arthritis Rheum* 1985;28:241–248.
51. Ziff M. Role of the endothelium of chronic inflammatory synovitis. *Arthritis Rheum* 1991;34:1345–1352.
52. Kaul A, Blake DR, Pearson JD. Vascular endothelium, cytokines, and the pathogenesis of inflammatory synovitis. *Ann Rheum Dis* 1991;50:828–832.
53. Liao HX. Haynes BF. Role of adhesion molecules in the pathogenesis of rheumatoid arthritis. *Rheum Dis Clin North Am* 1995;21: 715–740.
54. Frenette PS, Wagner DD. Molecular medicine: adhesion molecules—Part I. *N Engl J Med* 1996;334:1526–1530.
55. Krzesicki RF, Fleming WE, Winterrowd GR, et al. T lymphocyte adhesion to human synovial fibroblasts: role of cytokines and the interaction between intercellular adhesion molecule 1 and CD11a/ CD18. *Arthritis Rheum* 1991;34:1245–1252.
56. Johnson BA, Haines GK, Harlow LA, et al. Adhesion molecule expressions in human synovial tissue. *Arthritis Rheum* 1993;36: 137–146.
57. Gerritsen ME, Kelley KA, Ligon G. Regulation of the expression of intercellular adhesion molecule 1 in cultured human endothelial cells derived from rheumatoid synovium. *Arthritis Rheum* 1993; 36:593–602.
58. Mojcik CF, Shevach EM. Adhesion molecules: a rheumatologic perspective. *Arthritis Rheum* 1997;40:991–1004.
59. Hale LP, Martin ME, McCollum DE, et al. Immunohistologic analysis of the distribution of cell adhesion molecules within the inflammatory synovial microenvironment. *Arthritis Rheum* 1989; 32:22–30.
60. Klarekog L, Forsum U, Scheynius A, et al. Evidence in support of a self-perpetuating HLA-DR-dependent delayed-type cell reaction in rheumatoid arthritis. *Proc Natl Acad Sci USA* 1982;79: 3632–3636.
61. Firestein GS. Zvaifler NJ. How important are T cells in chronic rheumatoid synovitis? *Arthritis Rheum* 1990;33:768–772.
62. Panayi GS, Lanchbury JS, Kingsley GH. The importance of the T cell in initiating and maintaining the chronic synovitis of rheumatoid arthritis. *Arthritis Rheum* 1992;35:729–734.
63. Fox, DA. The role of T cells in the immunopathogenesis of rheumatoid arthritis. *Arthritis Rheum* 1997;40:598–609.
64. Goronzy JJ, Weyand CM. T Cells in rheumatoid arthritis: paradigms and facts. *Rheum Dis Clin North Am* 1995;21:655–674.
65. Arend WP, Dayer JM. Cytokines and cytokine inhibitors or antagonists in rheumatoid arthritis. *Arthritis Rheum* 1990;33:305–315.
66. Burmester GR, Stuhlmuller B, Keyszer G, et al. Mononuclear phagocytes and rheumatoid synovitis: mastermind or workhorse in arthritis? *Arthritis Rheum* 1997;40:5–18.
67. Platanias LC, Vogelzang NJ. Interleukin-1: biology, pathophysiology and clinical prospects. *Am J Med* 1990;89;621–630.
68. Dinarello CA, Wolff SM. The role of Interleukin-1 in disease. *N Engl J Med* 1993;328:106–114.

69. Firestein GS, Alvaro-Gracia JM, Maki R. Quantitative analysis of cytokine gene expression in rheumatoid arthritis. *J Immunol* 1990; 144:3347–3353.
70. Nagase H, Okada Y. Proteinases and matrix degradation. In: Kelley WN, Harris ED, Ruddy S, Sledge CB, eds. *Textbook of rheumatology*, 5th ed. Philadelphia: WB Sanders, 1997.
71. Arend WP. The pathophysiology and treatment of rheumatoid arthritis. *Arthritis Rheum* 1997;49:595–597.
72. Brooks PM. Clinical management of rheumatoid arthritis. *Lancet* 1993;341:286–290.
73. American College of Rheumatology Ad Hoc Committee on Clinical Guidelines. Guidelines for the management of Rheumatoid Arthritis. *Arthritis Rheum* 1996;39:713–722.
74. Cash JM, Klippel JH. Second-line drug therapy for rheumatoid arthritis. *N Engl J Med* 1994;330:1368–1376.
75. Tilley BC, Alarcon GS, Heyse SP, et al. Minocycline in rheumatoid arthritis. *Ann Intern Med* 1995;122:81–90.
76. O'Dell, JR, Paulsen G, Haire CE, et al. Treatment of early seropositive rheumatoid arthritis with minocycline. *Arthritis Rheum* 1999;42:1691–169.
77. Iannuzzi L. Dawson N, Zein N, et al. Does drug therapy slow radiographic deterioration in rheumatoid arthritis. *N Engl J Med* 1983; 309;1023–1028.
78. Gabriel SE, Luthra HS. Rheumatoid arthritis: can the long-term outcome be altered? *Mayo Clin Proc*, 1988;63:58–68.
79. Sigler JW, Bluhn GB, Duncan H, et al. Gold salts in the treatment of rheumatoid arthritis: a double-blind study. *Ann Intern Med* 1974;80:21–26.
80. Joint Committee of the Medical Research Council and Nuffield Foundation. A comparison of prenisolone with aspirin or other analgesics in the treatment of rheumatoid arthritis. *Ann Rheum Dis* 1959;18:173–188.
81. Cooperating Clinics Committee of the American Rheumatism Association. A controlled trial of cyclophosphamide in rheumatoid arthritis. *N Engl J Med* 1970;283;883–889.
82. Van der Heide A, Jacobs JWG. Bijlsma WJ, et al. The effectiveness of early treatment with second-line antirheumatic drugs. *Ann Intern Med* 1996;124:699–708.
83. Weinblatt, ME, Coblyn JS, Fox DA, et al. Efficacy of low-dose methotrexate in rheumatoid arthritis. *N Engl J Med* 1985;312: 818–822.
84. Kremer JM, Phelps CT. Long-term prospective study of the use of methotrexate in the treatment of rheumatoid arthritis: update after a mean of 90 months. *Arthritis Rheum* 1992;35:138–146.
85. Weinblatt, ME, Maier AL, Fraser PA. et al. Long-term prospective study of methotrexate in rheumatoid arthritis: conclusion after 132 months of therapy. *J Rheumatol* 1998;25:238–242.
86. O'Dell JR, Methotrexate use in rheumatoid arthritis. *Rheum Dis Clin North Am* 1997;779–796.
87. Rau R, Herborn G, Karger T, et al. Retardation of radiologic progression in rheumatoid arthritis with methotrexate therapy: a controlled study. *Arthritis Rheum* 1991;34:1236–1244.
88. Rich E, Moreland LW, Alarcon G. Paucity of radiographic progression in rheumatoid arthritis treated with methotrexate as the first disease modifying antirheumatic drug. *J Rheumatol* 1999;26: 259–262.
89. Nordstrom DM, West SG, Andersen PA, et al. Pulse methotrexate therapy in rheumatoid arthritis: a controlled prospective roentgenographic study. *Ann Intern Med* 1987;107:797–801.
90. Alarcon GS, Lopex-Mendez A, Walter J, et al. Radiographic evidence of disease progression in methotrexate treated and non-methotrexate disease modifying antirheumatic drug treated rheumatoid arthritis patients: a meta-analysis. *J Rheumatol* 1992;19: 1868–1872.

91. Maravic M, Bologna C, Daures JP, et al. Radiologic progression in early rheumatoid arthritis treated with methotrexate. *J Rheumatol* 1999;26:262–267.

92. Cronstein BN, The mechanism of action of methotrexate. *Rheum Dis Clin North Am* 1997;23:739–755.

93. Tugwell P, Pincus T, Yocum D, et al. Combination therapy with cyclosporine and methotrexate in severe rheumatoid arthritis. *N Engl J Med* 1995;333:137–141.

94. Willkens RF, Sharp JT, Stablein D, et al. Comparison of azathioprine, methotrexate and the combination of the two in the treatment of rheumatoid arthritis: a forty-eight-week controlled clinical trial with radiologic outcome assessment. *Arthritis Rheum* 1995;38:1799–1806.

95. O'Dell JR, Haire CE, Erikson N, et al. Treatment of rheumatoid arthritis with methotrexate alone, sulfasalazine and hydroxychloroquine, or a combination of all three medications. *N Engl J Med* 1996;334:1287–1292.

96. Rau R, Schleusser B, Herborn G, et al. Long-term combination therapy of refractory and destructive rheumatoid arthritis with methotrexate (MTX) and intramuscular gold or other disease modifying antirheumatic drugs compared to MTX monotherapy. *J Rheumatol* 1998;25:1485–1492.

97. Forestier J. Rheumatoid arthritis and its treatment by gold salts. The results of six years' experience. *J Lab Clin Med* 1935;20:827–840.

98. Griswold DW, Lee J. Modulation of macrophage-lymphocyte interactions by the antirheumatic gold compound, auranofin. *J Rheumatol* 1985;12:490–497.

99. Lipsky PE. Immunosuppression by D-penicillamine in vitro. Inhibition of human T Lymphocyte proliferation in copper or ceruloplasmin-dependant generation of hydrogen peroxide and protection by monocytes. *J Clin Invest* 1984;73:53–65.

100. Karlsson-Parra A, Svenson K, Hollgren R, et al. Peripheral blood T-lymphocytes subsets in active rheumatoid arthritis—effects of different therapies on previously untreated patients. *J Rheumatol* 1986;13:263–268.

101. Veo T, Tanaka S, Tominaga Y et al. The effect of thoracic duct drainage on lymphocyte dynamics and clinical symptoms in patients with rheumatoid arthritis. *Arthritis Rheum* 1979;22:1405–1412.

102. Karsh J, Klippel JH, Plotz PH, et al. Lymphapheresis in rheumatoid arthritis. A randomized trial. *Arthritis Rheum* 1981;24:867–873.

103. Field EH, Strober S, Hoppe RT, et al. Sustained improvement of intractable rheumatoid arthritis after total lymphoid irradiation. *Arthritis Rheum* 1983;26:937–946.

104. Yocum DE, Torley H. Cyclosporine in rheumatoid arthritis. *Rheum Dis Clin North Am* 1995;21:835–844.

105. Wofsy D. Administration of monoclonal anti-T-cell antibodies retards murine lupus in BXSB mice. *J Immunol* 1986;136:4554–4560.

106. Herzog C, Walker C, Pichler W, et al. Monoclonal anti-CD4 in arthritis. *Lancet* 1987;2:1461–1462.

107. Caperton E, Byers V, Shepard J, et al. Treatment of refractory rheumatoid arthritis (RA) with anti-lymphocyte immunotoxin (abstract). *Arthritis Rheum* 1989;32(suppl.):5130.

108. Kirkham BW, Thien F, Pelton BK, et al. Chimeric CD7 monoclonal antibody therapy in rheumatoid arthritis. *J Rheumatol* 1992;19:1348–1352.

109. Kyle V, Coughlin RJ, Tighe H, et al. Beneficial effect of monoclonal antibody to Interleukin 2 receptor or activated T-cells in rheumatoid arthritis. *Ann Rheum Dis* 1989;48:428–429.

110. Matteson EL, Yocum DE, St. Clair EW, et al. Treatment of active refractory rheumatoid arthritis with humanized monoclonal antibody CAMPATH-1H administered by daily subcutaneous injection. *Arthritis Rheum* 1995;38:1187–1193.

111. Weinblatt ME, Maddison, PJ, Bulpitt KJ, et al. CAMPATH-1H, a humanized monoclonal antibody, in refractory rheumatoid arthritis. *Arthritis Rheum* 1995;38:1589–1594.

112. Moreland LW, Pratt PW, Mayes MD, et al. Double-blind, placebo-controlled multicenter trial using chimeric monoclonal anti-CD4 antibody, cM-T412, in rheumatoid arthritis patients receiving concomitant methotrexate. *Arthritis Rheum* 1995;38:1581–1588.

113. Van der Lubbe PA, Dijkmans BAC, Markusse HM, et al. A randomized, double-blind, placebo-controlled study of CD4 monoclonal antibody therapy in early rheumatoid arthritis. *Arthritis Rheum* 1995;38:1097–1106.

114. Wendling D, Racadot E, Wijdenes J, et al. A randomized, double-blind, placebo controlled multicenter trial of murine anti-CD4 monoclonal antibody therapy in rheumatoid arthritis. *J Rheumatol* 1998;25:1457–1461.

115. Moreland LW, Haverty TP, Wacholtz MC, et al. Non-depleting humanized anti-CD4 monoclonal antibody in patients with refractory rheumatoid arthritis. *J Rheumatol* 1998;25:221–228.

116. Epstein WV. Expectation bias in rheumatoid arthritis clinical trials. *Arthritis Rheum* 39:1996:1773–1780.

117. Mladenovic V, Domljan Z, Rozman B, et al. Safety and effectiveness of leflunomide in the treatment of patients with active rheumatoid arthritis. *Arthritis Rheum* 1995;38:1595–1603.

118. Weinblatt ME, Kremer JM, Coblyn JS. Pharmacokinetics, safety, and efficacy of combination treatment with methotrexate and leflunomide in patients with active rheumatoid arthritis. *Arthritis Rheum* 1999;42:1322–1328.

119. Kremer JM. Methotrexate and leflunomide: biochemical basis for combination therapy in the treatment of rheumatoid arthritis. *Semin Arthritis Rheum* 1999;29:14–26.

120. Moreland, LW, Morgan EE, Adamson III TC, et al. T-cell receptor peptide vaccination in rheumatoid arthritis. *Arthritis Rheum* 1998;41:1919–1929.

121. Kotzin BL, Kappler J. Targeting the T-cell receptor in rheumatoid arthritis. *Arthritis Rheum* 1998;41:1906–1910.

122. Arend WP, Dayer JM. Inhibition of the production and effects of Interleukin-1 and tumor necrosis factor α in rheumatoid arthritis. *Arthritis Rheum* 1995;38:151–160.

123. Elliott MJ, Maini RN, Feldman M, et al. Treatment of rheumatoid arthritis with chimeric monoclonal antibodies to tumor necrosis factor α. *Arthritis Rheum* 1993;36:1681–1690.

124. Elliott NJ, Maini RN, Feldmann M, et al. Randomized double-blind comparison of chimeric monoclonal antibody to tumour necrosis factor α (cA2) versus placebo in rheumatoid arthritis. *Lancet* 1994;344:1105–1109.

125. Elliott NJ, Maini RN, Feldmann M, et al. Repeated therapy with monoclonal antibody to tumournecrosis factor α (cA2) in patients with rheumatoid arthritis. *Lancet* 1994;344:1125–1127.

126. Maini FN, Breedveld FC, Kalden JR, et al. Therapeutic efficacy of multiple intravenous infusions of anti-tumor necrosis factor α monoclonal antibody combined with low-dose weekly methotrexate in rheumatoid arthritis. *Arthritis Rheum* 1998;41:1552–1563.

127. Moreland LW, Baumgartner SW, Schiff MH, et al. Treatment of rheumatoid arthritis with a recombinant human tumor necrosis factor receptor (p75)-Fc fusion protein. *N Engl J Med* 1997;337:141–146.

128. Weinblatt ME, Kremer JM, Bankhurst AD, et al. A trial of etanercept, a recombinant tumor necrosis factor Fc fusion protein, in patients with rheumatoid arthritis receiving methotrexate. *N Engl J Med* 1999;340:253–260.

129. Drelow BE, Lovis R, Haag MA, et al. Recombinant human inter-leukin-1 receptor type in the treatment of patients with active rheumatoid arthritis. *Arthritis Rheum* 1996;39:257–265.

130. Bresnihan B, Alvaro-Garcia JM, Cobby M, et al. Treatment of rheumatoid arthritis with combinant human interleukin-1 recep-tor antagonist. *Arthritis Rheum* 1998;41:2196–2204.

131. Moreland LW, Heck LW, Koopman WJ. Biologic agents for treat-ing rheumatoid arthritis: concepts and progress. *Arthritis Rheum* 1997;49:397–409.

132. Cush JJ, Kavanaugh AF. Biologic interventions in rheumatoid arthritis. *Rheum Dis Clin North Am* 1995;21:797–816.

133. Merkel PA, Letourneau EN, Polisson RP. Investigational agents for rheumatoid arthritis. *Rheum Dis Clin North Am* 1995;21:779–796.

134. Vincenti MP, Clark IM, Brinckerhoff, CE. Using inhibitors of metalloproteinases to treat arthritis: easier said than done? *Arthritis Rheum* 1994;8:1115–1126.

GENERAL CLINICAL CONSIDERATIONS IN RHEUMATOID SURGERY

JOHN A. MCAULIFFE

The term *rheumatoid arthritis* does not begin to describe the essential nature of this potentially devastating affliction (1,2). Rheumatoid *disease* is a process with protean manifestations that is capable of affecting almost every organ system in the body (3,4).

Even if we limit our concerns to the musculoskeletal system, the impact of rheumatoid disease on extremity function often reaches far beyond the mere destruction of articular surfaces. This is particularly true when one considers the effects of rheumatoid involvement on the hand and wrist. Being primarily a disorder of synovium, rheumatoid effects on the abundant tenosynovium in the distal upper extremity are both obvious and manifold. In fact, some of our most striking surgical successes occur not in the treatment of the arthritis itself, but in the management of such proliferative tenosynovitis (4–7). Although we often operate on destroyed joints that articulate on subchondral bone, the greatest technical challenge is clearly posed not by the absence of articular cartilage, but by the loss of soft tissue support and normal tendon function (4).

GOALS AND LIMITATIONS

The goals of surgery on the rheumatoid hand and wrist have been enumerated by various authors (3,5,6,8–10). As is the case when any arthritic condition is treated surgically, relief of pain and restoration of function are usually of primary importance. Closely associated objectives include the correction or prevention of deformity, which will also serve to improve the appearance of the hand. Although it is unusual to operate on the rheumatoid hand solely for cosmetic reasons, it must be remembered that, in advanced stages, typical rheumatoid hand deformities can be the source of much unwelcome attention. A hand that goes unnoticed in a social situation can sometimes be of just as much value as a hand with greater functional capability.

Frequently, many of these goals will overlap, as it is often impossible to achieve one without the other. It is also true that one or the other of these goals may assume paramount importance in a given situation and for a particular patient. Our surgical efforts are most likely to be judged successful when we appreciate and strive to achieve our patients' goals, not our own. It is important to realize that what we consider to be the "best" surgical procedure in a specific circumstance may not suit the needs and desires of a certain individual.

We must also acknowledge, and make our patients aware of, the very definite limitations of surgery on the rheumatoid hand (3,5). Younger patients, in particular, may find strength deficits especially troublesome, but it is unlikely that surgery of any kind will significantly improve power. Similarly, normal dexterity cannot be restored, despite our best efforts. Surgery on affected joints may place the arc of motion in a more functional range, but is unlikely to achieve a greater total range of motion, or a range that approaches normal.

GENERAL PRINCIPLES

There are genuine controversies regarding when, or even in some cases, whether to operate on the rheumatoid hand or wrist. Certain guidelines do, however, meet with fairly general acceptance.

The presence of a deformity does not necessarily constitute an impairment, and is not, in itself, an indication for surgery (5,6). Patients can compensate admirably for deformities that occur gradually over time. For example, moderate degrees of metacarpophalangeal (MP) joint ulnar deviation are not incompatible with functional grip and pinch, and may be observed in selected patients. Conversely, we do not want to carefully monitor and document a deformity as it progresses over time to the point at which only salvage surgery is possible.

It is not necessary to wait until the disease is quiescent, as was once thought, before performing surgery (11). In fact, it is the inflamed joint or active tenosynovitis not responsive to appropriate medical management that may reap the greatest benefit from surgical intervention (3,12,13).

Whatever the magnitude of deformity or dysfunction, it is imperative that the surgical plan be tailored to the individual patient, and that options are discussed fairly and realistically

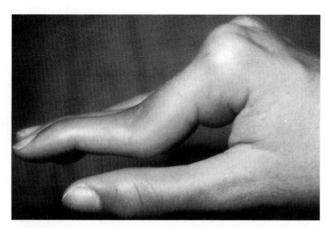

FIGURE. 3.1. This digit with a rigid swan neck deformity displays the typical zig-zag pattern of collapse seen in rheumatoid arthritis. Hyperextension at the proximal interphalangeal joint is associated with flexion of the distal interphalangeal joint.

(5,6). Patients with very specific needs, such as musicians and certain hobbyists, should be approached with particular caution. What would be a clear functional improvement to the average person performing routine activities of daily living may only complicate the one activity these individuals have as their goal. We must endeavor to understand specifically what the patient hopes to gain from the surgery. It may sometimes be helpful to arrange for a patient to speak with another who has undergone similar surgery.

An experienced hand therapist can also be an excellent source of information and advice for the patient contemplating surgery (14). Certain procedures will necessitate significant periods of postoperative therapy, splint wear, and limited use of the hand. Patients must be prepared for this eventuality and understand that lack of compliance with the prescribed therapy regimen will jeopardize the results of even the most well-executed surgery. In this era of managed health care, the surgeon must see to it that approval is obtained not only for the proposed surgery, but for the requisite splinting and therapy as well.

Some of the greatest challenges in evaluating and treating the rheumatoid hand and wrist arise from the fact that deformities are often interrelated. At times this is a causative relationship, as when angular deformity at a given joint leads to the reciprocal deformity at the next most distal joint, resulting in the well-known pattern of collapse or zig-zag deformity described by Landsmeer (Fig. 3.1) (15). In these cases, proximal alignment and stability must be achieved before the distal joint can be treated with any reasonable hope of success (16,17). At other times, deformity may arise as a compensatory mechanism in the face of adjacent joint derangement. Losing sight of this possibility may have unfortunate consequences, as when the markedly angulated wrist of a patient with limited elbow flexion is fused in a neutral position, correcting the obvious deformity, while leaving the patient unable to reach his face or head with this hand (18).

Rheumatoid disease is an ongoing process that occurs over time, and this can make planning particularly difficult. Subsequent involvement of a currently unaffected joint, or progression of disease in a previously treated joint, may negate prior surgical accomplishments. Patients must be made aware that certain benefits of surgery are, by their very nature, temporary (3,5,6).

Conventional wisdom suggests that surgical reconstruction of an extremity should proceed from proximal to distal (7). Although this is sometimes necessary in the treatment of adjacent joints, as noted above, it is not an inviolable rule. For example, a patient with both shoulder and hand involvement may elect to have either surgery performed first, depending upon which area is most symptomatic, so long as dysfunction at one level would not adversely impact the necessary postoperative care at the other site. Similarly, the decision as to whether upper or lower extremity surgery should be performed first can usually be left to the patient. Ambulatory aids will usually require adaptation no matter what order of upper and lower extremity surgery is chosen. I do not favor the use of conventional crutches by rheumatoid patients under any circumstances out of concern for the significant deforming forces placed across the wrist (3). Platform devices can be safely used whether hand and wrist surgery has been performed or is pending. At times, carefully selected upper and lower extremity procedures can be accomplished simultaneously by surgical teams working concurrently, avoiding the need for multiple anesthetics and hospitalizations.

I believe strongly that surgery of the hand and wrist should be restricted to that which can be safely accomplished in a single tourniquet time (9). It is advantageous to combine appropriate surgical procedures on the hand and wrist, provided they can be accomplished in a timely fashion. Prolonged procedures tend to cause unnecessary edema, potential wound healing problems, secondary stiffness, and may create debility and the need for ongoing therapy that would not otherwise be required. Remember that these patients will probably undergo numerous surgical procedures in the course of a lifetime. We should strive not only to control potential complications, but to limit the incursion of any single procedure on the patients everyday life, insofar as this is possible.

Many of the characteristic deformities seen in the rheumatoid hand and wrist result from the destruction of moment arms. Successful treatment requires that we appreciate the abnormal forces acting to perpetuate the deformity and that we diminish these forces and restore a state of stable equilibrium by restoring the moment arms that will allow for normal tendon function (16). Deformity will recur if proper soft tissue balance is not reestablished (4,16).

Stanley has reminded us of the importance of establishing surgical priorities in the treatment of rheumatoid disease, commenting that the generally accepted surgical dictum of progressing from proximal to distal in the limb tends to draw attention to the joints, but often leads the clinician to ignore the soft tissues (7). He emphasizes the importance of

TABLE 3.1. SURGICAL PROCEDURES AS RANKED BY SOUTER

	Most Reliable
Group I	Thumb MP joint fusion
	Extensor tenosynovectomy and ulnar head excision
Group II	Flexor tenosynovectomy
	MP joint arthroplasty
Group III	PIP joint fusion
	Wrist stabilization
Group IV	Correction of swan neck deformity
	MP and PIP joint synovectomy
	Thumb IP joint fusion
Group V	PIP joint arthroplasty
	Correction of boutonniere deformity
	Least Predictable

early nerve decompression and tenosynovectomy. Although these procedures may not result in the same obvious and impressive correction of deformity as is accomplished by operating on affected joints, they can provide significant, and potentially long-lasting, preventative, and functional benefits (4).

Souter has presented an impressive review of the relative merits of the surgical procedures commonly performed on the rheumatoid hand and wrist (6). He analyzed these from his personal perspective based upon their ability to relieve pain, restore function, improve cosmesis, and prevent further damage, while doing no further harm to an already impaired hand. Five groups are then established to categorize our surgical options, beginning with those that are most reliable, and progressing to those that can be frankly unpredictable (Table 3.1).

He very wisely suggests that we begin any proposed reconstruction with those relatively straightforward procedures that have the highest chance of success. This will place the patient at ease, build confidence, and, hopefully, achieve the greatest functional improvement with the least effort. More complex secondary reconstruction can then be contemplated depending upon the patients' needs and desires. Adherence to Souter's principles is one of the surest ways of achieving success and creating the strong physician-patient relationship that is a necessity in the ongoing treatment of this chronic progressive disease.

CLASSIFICATION AND STAGING

Rheumatoid disease may pursue a highly variable course, both anatomically and temporally. There are numerous descriptions of the natural history of rheumatoid disease in selected groups of patients, but these are seldom of assistance in making a clinical judgment regarding a particular individual (19–24).

Three general patterns of disease progression have been described (3,9,25).

■ Monocyclic: A single bout of disease, which may, however, involve multiple anatomic areas, is followed by permanent remission.
■ Polycyclic: Manifestations of disease occur for varying periods of time and with varying degrees of severity at unpredictable intervals.
■ Progressive: Signs and symptoms pursue an unrelenting course.

The reported incidence of each of these patterns varies widely, with my personal experience most closely approximating that of Lister who states that only 10% of patients exhibit the monocyclic pattern of disease, and the remaining 90% of patients are fairly evenly distributed between the other two categories (9). This is a purely descriptive classification in which we can all recognize manifestations of disease that we have encountered in various patients, but these patterns can generally be appreciated only retrospectively. It is interesting to note that perhaps the most prevalent, polycyclic pattern of disease is, by definition, said to be unpredictable.

Various classifications of joint deformities have been proposed, most notably by Nalebuff and Zancolli (26,27). Details may vary depending on the specific joint under consideration, but these classifications can be summarized by the following four general stages of joint involvement (10).

■ I.   Synovitis without deformity
■ II. Passively correctable deformity
■ III. Fixed deformity
■ IV. Articular destruction

Rates of progression between stages vary widely among individuals and even among corresponding joints in the same hand. A given joint may not necessarily pass through every stage, and it is possible for joint destruction to occur at any stage. Nalebuff has also popularized a classification of patterns of deformity in the rheumatoid thumb that is in general use (28).

Radiographic classifications of rheumatoid disease, some utilizing templates and some standard descriptors, have been proposed, although none are in widespread use (29,30). A recent evaluation of one such radiographic classification of wrist destruction found significant limitations. This particular scheme could be applied to only 50% of patients with early disease for whom we are most concerned with the likelihood of progression, and demonstrated limited consistency over time (29).

Each of these systems allows us to associate surgical alternatives with various degrees of joint involvement or specific patterns of disease. Unfortunately, none of them are predictive. The essential questions of whether and when deformity will progress in a given joint remain unanswered by any classification of rheumatoid disease of which I am aware.

A very promising recent report suggests that by following measures of carpal height, ulnar translocation, and scapholunate dissociation over time, those wrists likely to exhibit progressive destruction and collapse could be identified (31). Despite the limitations of this study and the fact that these findings need to be further refined and replicated in a prospective fashion, it is an excellent first step. This is the type of information needed to enable us to be proactive in our treatment of rheumatoid disease.

NONOPERATIVE TREATMENT

The hand therapist is a critical component of the team caring for the rheumatoid patient. Even in the postoperative period, when actively engaged in a program of splinting and exercise, to my mind the most important role of the therapist is that of being an educator. A properly designed and fabricated splint is of little value if the patient does not understand when and how to wear it. A carefully delineated and properly monitored home exercise program is necessary if progress is going to be made, whereas a single hour of therapy per day performed on a passive recipient of such ministrations is unlikely to produce much long-lasting effect.

Patients in the early stages of rheumatoid disease must be instructed in joint protection measures and the proper balance of rest and exercise (14,32). Resting splints can be a valuable adjunct in the treatment of an acutely inflamed or symptomatic joint, and have been shown to control pain without negatively affecting recovery of motion (33–35). Patients report that static wrist splints are useful during activities requiring strength, but do not improve dexterity (36).

A hand-based orthosis has been shown to be capable of remarkable correction of deformity for MP joints without fixed contracture, however, hand function, pain, gross grip strength, and lateral pinch were not improved (37). Splint wear has never been shown to have any value in the prevention or correction of deformity (14,37). Splints should be worn if the patient finds them to be of benefit (38) or to protect or mobilize healing tissue in the postoperative period, not for the potential of long-term benefit or prophylaxis.

Local corticosteroid injections can prove helpful in the control of synovitis or tenosynovitis that is not responsive to systemic medications (3,9). Such therapy should be used judiciously and sparingly, as the catabolic effects of the steroid combined with the invasive and erosive character of rheumatoid synovium can result in marked soft tissue destruction, potentially complicating subsequent surgical reconstruction.

PERIOPERATIVE CONSIDERATIONS

A thorough preoperative evaluation is designed to avoid complications and assure patient safety by identifying conditions that can be treated and corrected prior to surgery or that require special attention perioperatively. Such evaluation is particularly important for the rheumatoid patient in whom a host of comorbidities or iatrogenic factors may conspire to complicate care.

A complete history should include an assessment of responses to previous surgery and anesthesia and inquire about symptoms indicating obvious defects in hemostasis or immune function. Neurologic signs and symptoms, particularly those indicative of cord compression or cervical spine instability should be sought. These patients may, of course, experience the same disorders that could potentially complicate surgery for anyone, as well as the particular involvement of cardiac, pulmonary, and other organ systems peculiar to their underlying disease.

Laboratory evaluation should include determination of hematologic indices. Rheumatoid patients frequently suffer from anemia of chronic disease and may experience occult blood loss due to gastrointestinal side effects of long-term salicylates or other anti-inflammatory agents (39). Although significant blood loss is unusual during hand or wrist surgery, even relatively minor bleeding can sometimes render these marginally compensated patients symptomatic. Rare but potentially devastating manifestations of rheumatoid disease, such as Felty's syndrome, will display characteristic neutropenia and thrombocytopenia. The need for additional laboratory evaluation is variable, depending on the patient's age, medication regimen, and other historical factors.

Regional anesthesia is preferred for the rheumatoid patient, as it obviates the need to cope with a host of potentially complex and dangerous airway management issues (40). Conversion to general anesthesia may always prove necessary, and cervical spine radiographs, including flexion/extension views, are required to assess possible unrecognized instability (9,39). Uncontrolled manipulation of the unstable cervical spine during intubation can prove catastrophic. Temporomandibular joint dysfunction can further complicate airway management if intubation is required (3,39).

Glucocorticoid use is common in these patients, and will result in suppression of the native pituitary-adrenal axis, necessitating supplemental corticosteroid administration in the perioperative period. Aspirin has an effect on platelet function that lasts the life of the platelet, and should, therefore, be withheld approximately one week prior to surgery to avoid bleeding complications. In contrast, platelet effects of nonsteroidal anti-inflammatory agents are reversible. It is recommended that these drugs be withheld for a period equal to five times the customary dose interval schedule (39).

Penicillamine and gold may cause neutropenia or thrombocytopenia. The administration and dosing schedule of these agents does not need to be altered in the face of normal hematologic indices. Methotrexate can affect both hepatic and marrow function, necessitating preoperative determination of liver function in addition to cell counts (39).

There are conflicting reports concerning increased infection rates in patients receiving methotrexate therapy, leading some authors to suggest that the drug be discontinued peri-operatively (41,42). Corticosteroid usage is associated with increased rates of postoperative infection, although this effect is difficult to quantify (43). Since steroid administration cannot be discontinued or tapered abruptly in the perioperative period, our only recourse is the judicious use of short-term prophylactic antibiotics combined with atraumatic tissue handling and meticulous technique. The latter technical considerations should, of course, be observed an all surgical circumstances, but especially in the care of rheumatoid patients who demonstrate some degree of delayed or impaired wound healing even in the absence of medication effects or wound infection (43).

SYNOVECTOMY

There are five basic surgical procedures performed on the rheumatoid hand and wrist: synovectomy, tenosynovectomy, tendon surgery, arthroplasty, and arthrodesis (1). A sixth, nerve decompression, is usually performed in concert with one of the others. These procedures can be utilized in one of three ways, as prevention, reconstruction, or salvage (3,9,10). Certain procedures may serve more than one purpose depending upon their specific application. For example, I would consider a limited wrist arthrodesis to be a reconstructive procedure, whereas few would argue that MP joint arthrodesis of a central digit would rightfully be deemed a salvage procedure.

The greatest controversies in rheumatoid hand surgery center around the indications for and efficacy of preventive surgery, particularly synovectomy (4,13). Compression neuropathy is frequently encountered even in the general population, and surgical treatment of this problem is commonplace and undisputed. Tenosynovectomy, especially on the dorsum of the hand and wrist, has gained widespread acceptance, however similar surgery on the flexor surface sometimes prompts a good deal more deliberation and delay and is viewed with some suspicion.

Despite acceptance in northern Europe, endorsement by multiple surgeons with decades of experience caring for rheumatoid patients, and many positive reports in the literature, the value of synovectomy is still questioned (3,13,44). Concern is expressed as to whether synovectomy can truly alter the natural history of the disease process, while widely prescribed medical regimens in daily use have never been shown to be capable of this (13,45,46). It is said that rheumatoid disease is so unpredictable that there is no way of knowing when to perform synovectomy, or on which joint. Flatt has admitted that we cannot accurately predict the rate or precise mechanism of deterioration of the rheumatoid hand, but we do know that the ultimate result is so crippling that there is no justification for a prolonged "wait and see" attitude (3).

Numerous reports have detailed the success of extensor tenosynovectomy, which is usually accompanied by distal

ulnar resection or, in some cases, the Sauve-Kapandji procedure. Recurrent tenosynovitis or tendon ruptures are rarely seen, pain relief is good, and function is quickly recovered (47–49). Souter, in fact, considers this surgery to be among the most successful and reliable performed on the rheumatoid hand, giving it his highest rating (Table 3.1) (6).

Flexor tenosynovectomy, either at the level of the wrist, digits, or both, is a bit more challenging technically and certainly demands more of the patient in terms of postoperative therapy. Flexor tenosynovitis is not as readily apparent as that on the extensor surface, but careful examination will reveal the characteristic bogginess along the digital flexor sheaths and throughout the distal forearm and base of the palm, sometimes accompanied by frank triggering. The hallmark of this process is the finding that active digital motion is significantly less than passive motion (50). Dexterity, grip, and power are limited, digital joint deformities are fostered by tendon imbalance, and, if the process is left unchecked, the resultant tendon ruptures are much more difficult and less satisfying to treat than their counterparts on the dorsum of the hand. Success equivalent to that seen on the extensor surface has been reported by numerous authors following flexor tenosynovectomy (13,51,52). Active range of motion has been reported to double, and recurrent tenosynovitis is seen in fewer than 5% of patients with average follow-up approaching six years in one large series (51).

Synovectomy of the proximal interphalangeal (PIP) joints seems to effectively retard the effects of joint destruction for approximately 5 years (12,53). Loss of motion is rarely greater than 10 degrees, and 70% of 98 cases obtained complete pain relief at an average follow-up of 3 years in one series (54). Recurrent synovitis is seen in 20% to 30% of cases, but persists in a very small minority (54,55). MP synovectomy yields similar results, with recurrences being perhaps even less likely at this articulation than at the PIP joint (56). Although it would seem that soft tissue support would benefit by control of synovial proliferation, the effect of synovectomy on angular or collapse deformities of the digital joints has not been adequately studied. Attempts at pharmacologic synovectomy of the small joints of the hand have proven unpredictable and have largely been abandoned (57).

Results of synovectomy of the wrist are a bit more challenging to interpret as this surgery is usually performed in concert with extensor tenosynovectomy and distal radioulnar joint reconstruction, and the effects of the various procedures are difficult to isolate. There is little effect on motion and pain relief is good; however, radiographic progression of disease does continue (47–49). Arthroscopic synovectomy of the rheumatoid wrist has been described with short-term follow-up; however, since wrist synovectomy almost always accompanies other dorsal surgery, I expect that the need for the isolated arthroscopic procedure will be limited (58). There is need for a study comparing wrist synovectomy to limited radiocarpal arthrodesis in an effort to determine which is most effective in controlling progression of disease, while maintaining wrist posture and some degree of functional motion over the long term.

In the absence of any widely accepted predictive classification or staging system, we are left with what seems obvious: "If this joint doesn't get better, it will do poorly." A joint or tendon bed with proliferative synovial involvement that does not respond to medical management over three to six months and exhibits signs of deformity or dysfunction is most unlikely to improve over time (3,13,59). Joints that are radiographically normal at the time of synovectomy seem to enjoy the most complete and longest lasting relief, attesting to the importance of early treatment (45). Rheumatoid patients are ideally evaluated and followed by a medical team that includes the rheumatologist, orthopaedic and hand surgeons, and therapists, so that the opportunity for early treatment is not lost, leaving only reconstructive and salvage surgical options. Synovectomy does not cure rheumatoid disease, nor does any available medical therapy. It can, however, delay the process of relentless destruction and provide several years of improved function (4,13,53).

Hagglund et al. have reported that persistent joint swelling was the only measure of disease activity to influence pain and function scores (60). As many clinicians with great experience treating rheumatoid patients have pointed out, it seems that surgical treatment of persistent synovitis is appropriate and justified on symptomatic and functional grounds, although long-term success may not be assured (3,9,13). I believe that a good deal of the mistrust concerning preventive surgery and synovectomy in particular has been generated by circumstances in which these procedures have been performed too late in the course of the disease to have any hope of being effective. For preventive surgery to achieve its goals, it must, by definition, be performed early (4,13,53).

SURGICAL CONSIDERATIONS

There are a host of surgical options available to us in the treatment of the rheumatoid hand and wrist. Specific surgical indications and techniques are discussed throughout this text. I would like to briefly outline a few pertinent details of the treatment of the various soft tissues and joints that highlight the important principles of rheumatoid surgery.

Nerves

Patients with rheumatoid disease do not often complain of symptoms of nerve compression (3,9). Sensory disturbance is perhaps perceived as a minor annoyance compared to the other hardships these individuals endure, while weakness and atrophy are attributed to or masked by the underlying disease process. Progressive neural dysfunction is so insidious that it is easily overlooked. It is our duty to elicit signs and symptoms of compression neuropathy which, if neglected, can lead to irreversible neural damage. Although the immediate effects of

nerve decompression are not as dramatic as are surgical efforts to correct an obvious finger or wrist deformity, the long-term benefits to the patient are potentially far greater (4).

Remember that extrinsic extensor dysfunction is not always a result of tendon rupture or subluxation. Posterior interosseous nerve compression, usually caused by hypertrophic elbow synovitis, can result in the loss of active MP joint extension. Surgical decompression of the nerve, accompanied by elbow synovectomy, is usually quite effective in restoring function (61).

Tendons

I firmly believe that we should not intentionally sacrifice supporting soft tissue structures in the treatment of a disease whose major manifestations often stem from the attritional loss of such structures (16). When performing flexor tenosynovectomy, the first annular pulley should be retained. Triggering in the rheumatoid hand is treated by tenosynovectomy combined with excision of one slip of the flexor digitorum sublimis, not by incision of the pulley (62). There are numerous deforming forces that contribute to MP joint angulation and subluxation (63), and the precise role of those forces emanating from the flexor tendons may be debated (64). Nonetheless, I believe we tempt fate unnecessarily if we disrupt the function of this important pulley, thereby increasing flexion and ulnar deviation forces across the MP joint.

The importance of the extensor retinaculum as a pulley, which prevents bowstringing of the long extensor tendons, is often neglected in our zeal to protect these tendons following dorsal wrist surgery. Absence of the extensor retinaculum limits simultaneous wrist and MP joint extension (16). In the rheumatoid patient with a mobile wrist, I think it best to retain a strip of retinaculum in order to maintain a dorsal

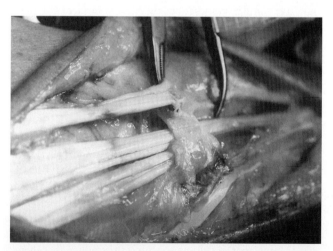

FIGURE 3.2. Operative photograph following extensor tenosynovectomy. The hand is to the left. The clamps hold proximal and distal stumps of ruptured tendons. Note that a strip of retinaculum over the fourth compartment has been retained.

restraint for the extensor tendons (Fig. 3.2). The majority of the retinacular tissue can be placed deep to the tendons in an effort to prevent erosion from underlying osseous prominences and to reinforce the dorsal wrist capsule as is customarily suggested (4).

Rheumatoid Nodules

The presence of rheumatoid nodules is generally considered to be an ominous sign, and is usually associated with highly aggressive underlying disease. These subcutaneous lesions tend to appear in areas of high mechanical or contact stress including the subcutaneous border of the ulna, the dorsum of the MP and PIP joints, and sometimes even in the pulps of the digits. Occasionally they may ulcerate and become secondarily infected, further complicating treatment (3,65).

Intralesional steroid injections are of questionable benefit, and have been implicated in promoting ulceration. Rheumatoid nodules have a reputation for rapid recurrence following surgical excision, but I would agree with Flatt that this reputation seems undeserved, at least in the upper extremity (3). Nodules can be excised on an elective basis depending on symptomatology and the patient's wishes, unless, of course, ulceration or infection necessitate treatment. Limiting mechanical stress to the healing wound will help to avoid recurrence, although lesions may occur in adjacent areas.

Wrist and Distal Radioulnar Joint

The rheumatoid wrist deteriorates over time in a characteristic pattern of combined deformities including radial deviation, ulnar translocation, and carpal supination. Early control of this cascade of deformities may, in some cases, be accomplished by tendon transfer and joint synovectomy (4,48,66,67) or in others may necessitate partial fusion (20,68,69). Taleisnik has pointed out that the midcarpal joint

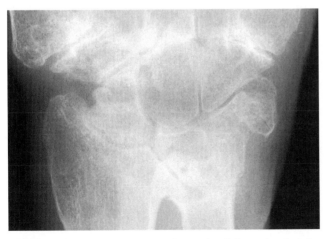

FIGURE 3.3. Anteroposterior radiograph of the wrist. Despite marked destruction of the radiocarpal joint, the midcarpal articulation is nearly intact.

is often relatively well preserved (Fig. 3.3) (68). In these instances, stability can be achieved by radiolunate arthrodesis, while midcarpal motion is maintained.

One of the criticisms of wrist synovectomy is that it does not halt the typical pattern of carpal collapse (47–49). Although this concern is not without basis in fact, analysis of this issue is complicated by the fact that distal ulnar excision often accompanied wrist synovectomy in reported series. The resultant loss of ulnar support may help to explain some degree of ongoing deformation in wrists so treated. Vincent and coauthors have found that retaining the ulnar head by substituting the Sauve-Kapandji procedure for the more traditional Darrach excision eliminates ulnar translocation over the medium term (70). For these reasons, I am loathe to resect the ulnar head in a rheumatoid patient with a mobile wrist.

Metacarpophalangeal Joints

Although there are many influences that help to create the typical MP joint deformity (4,63,71–73), carpal collapse is one factor that has been strongly implicated (17,74). Maintenance of MP joint correction is unpredictable in the face of uncorrected wrist deformity, and MP joint surgery should not be attempted prior to stabilizing the wrist. With respect to the MP joints, the wrist is most certainly the "key to the hand" (Fig. 3.4) (16,75).

Many reports have documented the efficacy of early soft tissue reconstruction or later silastic arthroplasty in correcting MP joint alignment (76–82). When necessitated by the presence of joint destruction, the implant functions largely as a spacer, providing only a minimal degree of positioning capability. Obtaining and maintaining alignment of the MP joints is solely dependent on expert soft tissue reconstruction (4). I favor re-creating radial collateral ligament function in all digits, not just the index as is usually recommended. In selected younger patients who will place relatively greater demands on their reconstructed hands, arthrodesis of the index MP joint may help to re-create excellent pinch strength and serve to protect the arthroplasties on the ulnar side of the hand.

It is impossible to effectively rehabilitate mobile MP and PIP joints at the same time (83). Patients with well-preserved PIP joints will develop far greater MP joint motion following arthroplasty if the PIP joints are temporarily stabilized with static digital splints.

Proximal Interphalangeal Joints

Silastic arthroplasty of the rheumatoid PIP joint often yields disappointing results. Correction of preoperative deformity is unpredictable, range of motion is often quite limited despite prolonged therapy and salvage by conversion to arthrodesis is problematic because of diminished bone stock (84,85). In general, there is no reason to recommend arthroplasty of both the MP and PIP joints in the same digit, as both joints usually achieve suboptimal motion in this circumstance.

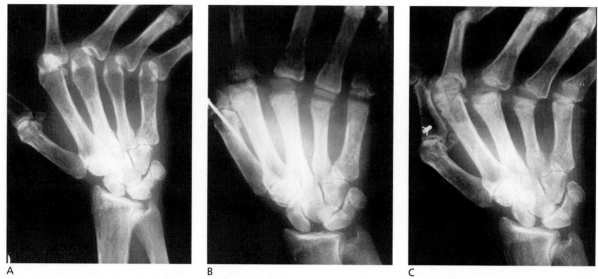

FIGURE 3.4. Anteroposterior radiographs of the wrist and hand. **A.** This patient displays the typical deformities of radial deviation of the wrist and ulnar deviation of the metacarpophalangeal joints. **B.** Metacarpophalangeal joint deformity is reasonably corrected following silastic arthroplasty. Note that the wrist deformity has not been addressed. **C.** One year postoperatively, there is recurrence of metacarpophalangeal joint ulnar deviation deformity.

Swan neck deformity is by far the most functionally limiting of PIP joint derangements, as grasp is severely limited. Conversely, the digit with a boutonniere deformity often retains excellent function (Fig. 3.5), and loss of distal interphalangeal joint flexion may pose the greatest limitation for these patients (4). When supple, both deformities can be treated with reasonable expectation of success. Both deformities arise from primary joint synovitis destroying the integrity of the extensor tendon apparatus with additional secondary joint deformity from altered tendon pull and subsequent mechanics (Fig. 3.6). Treatment of the rigid swan neck defor-

mity will, at worst, result in a joint in a more functional degree of flexion, even if motion is negligible. Attempted reconstruction of a fixed boutonniere deformity can actually diminish function by creating a joint that is stiff in extension and should be undertaken with caution. Any degree of instability in the coronal plane is probably an indication for arthrodesis.

Early procedures to correct PIP joint deformity may need to be accompanied by flexor tenosynovectomy as tendon dysfunction may be a significant contributing cause of lost mobility (52,55). PIP joint function is so dependent upon the status of the MP joint that efforts to salvage a mobile PIP

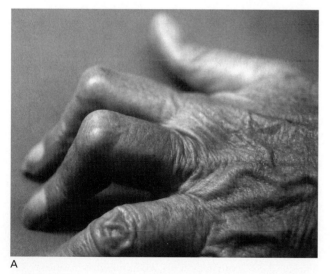
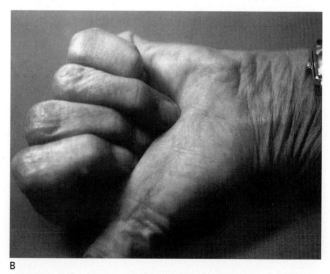

FIGURE 3.5. **A.** Boutonniere deformity in a patient with rheumatoid arthritis. **B.** The patient retains excellent functional grip.

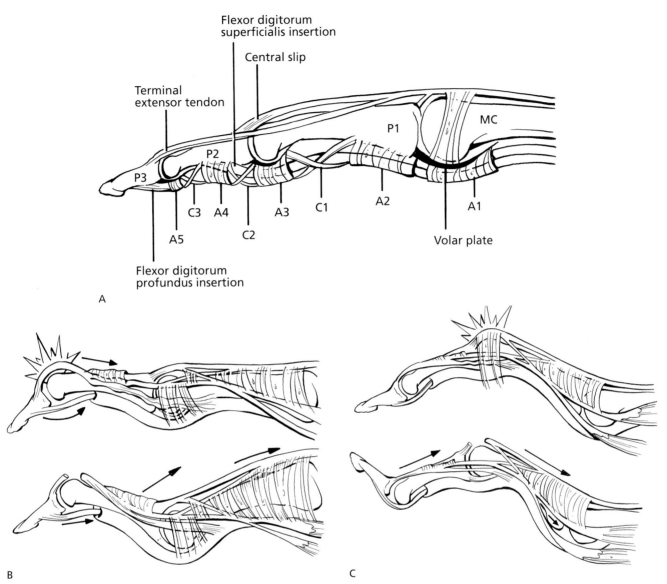

FIGURE 3.6. **A.** An illustration of the normal tendon anatomy of the finger. Note the relationship of the extensor tendons to the axis of joint rotation. **B.** Disruption of the terminal extensor tendon due to DIP joint synovitis leads to DIP joint flexion and secondary PIP joint hyperextension from overpull of the remaining intact extensor apparatus resulting in a Swan Neck deformity. **C.** With PIP joint synovitis, disruption of the central slip occurs with resulting flexion of the PIP joint and hyperextension of the DIP joint due to overpull of the lateral bands on the terminal tendon causing a boutonniere deformity.

joint should almost always be delayed pending reconstruction and rehabilitation of the MP joint (83). PIP arthrodesis can reasonably be combined with MP arthroplasty if the combined procedures can be accomplished in a single tourniquet time.

CONCLUSION

The available evidence suggests that there is a definite place for preventive surgery in the treatment of rheumatoid disease involving the hand and wrist. This conclusion is certainly not universally accepted by our medical colleagues and even the most ardent surgical believers among us may have their confidence shaken by the inexorable progression of this relentless disease. There is work to be done in more clearly defining the role of early surgery and consensus building across the range of medical specialists that care for rheumatoid patients. Prospective studies utilizing the tools of outcome research will enable our patients to express what works for them, helping us to more appropriately match the specifics of our treatment to the stage of disease.

4

DISTAL INTERPHALANGEAL JOINT

SCOTT H. KOZIN

HISTORICAL PERSPECTIVE

The distal interphalangeal (DIP) joint can be affected by osteoarthritis, inflammatory arthritis, and posttraumatic arthritis. Osteoarthritis is an ancient disease with evidence of its existence detected in skeletons of prehistoric man (two million years ago) and Egyptian mummies (1). Signs of osteoarthritis have also been observed in ancient dinosaurs, amphibians, mammals, and certain species of birds. In humans, the prevalence and severity of osteoarthritis rises steeply with age and has a particular affinity for the DIP joint. Interphalangeal arthritis occurs in 70% of individuals greater than 70 years of age, and history has commented on the "gnarled hands of the octogenerian" (2). In fact, osteoarthritis is regarded as a sign of aging and the two conditions are considered synonymous and comorbid (1). The gross and microscopic pathology of osteoarthritis reveals fibrillation and disintegration of cartilage along with new bone formation causing subchondral sclerosis and osteophyte formation (1). The progressive loss of joint cartilage results in "bone on bone contact," diminished joint motion, loss of strength, and decreased function.

Irregular bone spur formation and the development of articular osteophyte nodules is a consequence of cartilage destruction. In 1802, Dr. William Heberden, a Welsh rheumatologist, distinguished the osteoarthritic nodules about the DIP joint from inflammatory nodules (3). This clinical categorization was one of the first attempts to differentiate between the various arthritides. In 1887, Bouchard described comparable nodules (Bouchard's nodes) at the proximal interphalangeal (PIP) joint level attributed to osteoarthritis (4). This bone formation is identical to normal bone structure and no different than osteophytes that form elsewhere (e.g., hip and knee).

Osteoarthritis is a major cause of chronic disability and has considerable economic and social ramifications. Osteoarthritis is actually a heterogenous group of diseases with different heritability, etiology, distribution, clinical findings, and natural histories. All types have in common the progressive degeneration of articular cartilage, compensatory subchondral bone sclerosis, osteophyte formation, joint space narrowing, and alterations in the periarticular structures. The exact cause of osteoarthritis remains undefined but appears to be an interplay of genetic, biochemical, and mechanical factors.

The primary and erosive types of osteoarthritis have a high predilection for the DIP joint. Primary generalized osteoarthritis is the most common form of osteoarthritis and is characterized by symmetric involvement of the DIP, PIP, trapeziometacarpal, hip, and knee joints (Fig. 4.1) (5). Primary osteoarthritis is often seen in families, and epidemiological data support a role for hereditary and genetic factors (6). In the hand, the DIP joint is most frequently effected (85%), followed by trapeziometacarpal joint involvement (65%) and proximal interphalangeal joint disease (45%) (5,7). The metacarpophalangeal (MP) joints are relatively spared in contrast to inflammatory arthritis. The onset of primary osteoarthritis is usually in the third to fourth decade of life with an initial inflammatory phase indicative of cartilage destruction followed by exuberant osteophyte formation (Heberden's and Bouchard's nodes). This irregular bone formation represents the subchondral bone's response to increased load. These nodes can further interfere with joint motion and produce disfigurement about the DIP joint. A gradual diminution in pain is characteristic of primary osteoarthritis.

Although osteoarthritis is considered a noninflammatory disease, there is a variable inflammatory component. In erosive osteoarthritis, the inflammatory constituent dominates with soft tissue swelling, warmth, and erythema (8–11). Painful inflammatory episodes with the eventual development of bony erosions, joint deformity, and ankylosis is the typical course. This type of osteoarthritis tends to occur in middle-aged females and has a relatively abrupt onset with rapid progression of deformity. The DIP joint is again most frequently affected (75%), followed by PIP joint involvement (50%), and trapeziometacarpal disease (40%). Erosive osteoarthritis is more aggressive and destructive than primary osteoarthritis and simulates inflammatory arthritis. This condition is often misdiagnosed as inflammatory or crystalline-induced (e.g., gout) arthritis.

Inflammatory arthritis also encompasses numerous disease subsets with a principle autoimmune etiology (12,13). The distribution of hand joint involvement is primarily proximal with the greatest impact at the intercarpal, MP, and PIP joints and relative sparing of the DIP joints. In contradistinction,

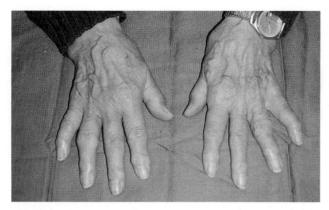

FIGURE 4.1. 65-year-old female with primary generalized osteo-arthritis. Symmetric enlargement of the interphalangeal joints (Heberden's and Bouchard's nodes) with associated trapezio-metacarpal joint arthritis.

psoriatic arthritis is an inflammatory arthritis that is seroneg-ative for rheumatoid factor and has a predilection for the DIP joint. Most psoriatic patients have a relatively benign arthritic course, but a subset develops recalcitrant synovial inflamma-tion, bony erosions, deformity, instability, and pain. In severe cases, destructive arthritis mutilans can involve all the digits with marked digital shortening and ankylosis (Fig. 4.2).

Deposition diseases (e.g., gout, calcium pyrophosphate, and hemochromatosis) are secondary causes of osteoarthritis and present similar to erosive osteoarthritis. These diseases alter the structural properties of cartilage by crystal deposi-tion, induce inflammation, and promote joint degradation. Gout commonly affects the DIP joint and causes consider-able subchondral cyst formation and progressive joint destruction.

Posttraumatic arthritis can occur after fractures and dislo-cations of the DIP joint. The presence of persistent articular incongruity or subluxation will increase articular wear and degeneration. In addition, continual radial or ulnar collateral ligament instability causes shear across the articular cartilage

and deterioration. Posttraumatic DIP joint arthritis tends to affect young laborers because of their susceptibility to digital trauma. Repeated microtrauma, ligament laxity, or altered proprioception can also accelerate the development of arthri-tis. Occupational tasks and repetitive motion appear to be risk factors for arthritis of the hand (14–16).

This chapter will concentrate on the management of the osteoarthritic DIP joint. This disease affects the DIP joint most commonly, and the vast majority of patients with DIP joint symptomatology will have underlying osteoarthritis. The principles of treatment discussed for osteoarthritis are appli-cable to DIP joint derangement from other arthritides, such as inflammatory, crystalline-induced, and posttraumatic.

INDICATIONS/CONTRAINDICATIONS

Osteoarthritis is a clinical diagnosis based on a careful history and physical examination. There are no specific serologic abnormalities. The history should cover onset of symptoms, progression of deformity, previous trauma, specific painful activities, and family history. The indications for treatment of DIP joint arthritis are based upon the patient's complaints. Asymptomatic deformities of the DIP joint are common and do not require intervention. These deformities range from a "mass" to a "crooked finger." The mass represents a mucous cyst and/or a protruding osteophyte. The patient's underlying concern is often the potential for malignancy or the appear-ance of their crooked fingers. Additional concerns about progression similar to a friend or family member are often expressed. Patient education and reassurance that they are not afflicted with rheumatoid arthritis is the only treatment nec-essary in these instances (1,17). The patient should be edu-cated on the pathophysiology of arthritis with a comment on articular wear, joint space degradation, and osteophyte formation. The favorable response to treatment should be highlighted.

Physical examination of the DIP joint begins with obser-vation. Soft-tissue swelling indicative of inflammation may be readily apparent. The amount of soft tissue reaction varies with the type of arthritis (osteoarthritis versus inflammatory) and stage (early versus late) of presentation. Angular joint deformities from irregular joint destruction or ligamentous instability should be noted. Active and passive ranges of motion are recorded with a goniometer. Gentle axial loading and concomitant flexion/extension may illicit crepitation from bone on bone contact (grind test) (1).

X-rays are useful to confirm the diagnosis, although symp-toms do not always correlate with findings on plain film. Anteroposterior, lateral, and oblique x-rays are included in the initial evaluation (Fig. 4.3). Significant disease must be present to detect changes on plain x-rays. Early x-ray findings are osteophyte formation and compensatory subchondral sclerosis prior to joint space narrowing. Advanced findings include joint space reduction, subchondral cysts, and abun-

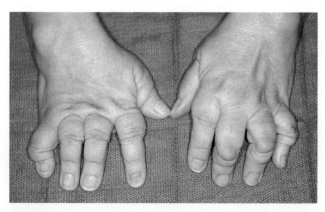

FIGURE 4.2. 50-year-old female with combination of psoriatic and rheumatoid inflammatory arthritis resulting in arthritis mutilans of the hands. Marked digital shortening, instability, and ankylosis.

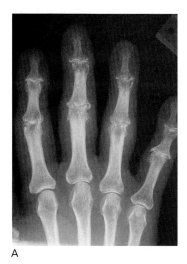

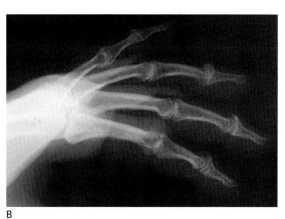

A   B

FIGURE 4.3. Anteroposterior and lateral finger x-rays of 65-year-old female depicted in Fig. 4.1 with primary osteoarthritis. DIP changes with subchondral sclerosis, joint space reduction, and osteophyte formation.

dant osteophyte formation. Early methods of disease detection are evolving with imaging modalities and biochemical analysis as potential sources. Scintigraphy with technetium 99-m-labeled phosphates has been shown to be a sensitive indicator of osteoarthritis with increased uptake in the early and delayed phases. In addition, delayed image abnormalities indicate bone remodeling and are predictive of subsequent joint narrowing (18,19). Biochemical research for markers indicative of abnormal cartilage metabolism offers promise for earlier detection and therapeutic intervention prior to the onset of joint space narrowing (20).

Nonoperative Treatment

The symptoms of DIP joint arthritis can range from mild, intermittent discomfort and minimal functional disability to severe continuous pain and considerable impairment. For patients with mild to moderate symptoms, the initial treatment is nonoperative and aimed at patient education and relief of symptoms. The hallmark symptoms of osteoarthritis are joint pain and stiffness related to joints involved. The joint pain is usually gradual in onset, mild in intensity, worse with heavy joint use, and improved with periods of rest. The stiffness occurs in the morning and following prolonged inactivity of the involved joints. Patients complain of pain that interferes with daily activities that involve fine motor skills (e.g., tying, buttoning, and pulling). The pain and stiffness increases with cool, damp, rainy weather, which is attributed to alterations in intra-articular pressure that occur with changes in atmospheric and barometric pressure (21).

Therapeutic Modalities

The goal of nonoperative treatment is to obtain pain relief by reduction of joint inflammation. The management program consists of patient education, splints, activity modification, and medication. An educated patient can avoid overuse of the affected joint(s) and modify functional use patterns to reduce the stress across the arthritic joint(s). Adaptive equipment can increase independence and allow completion of certain daily living tasks that are particularly painful (e.g., buttoning). These joint protection techniques and ergonomic modifications are an important part of the nonoperative regimen. Heat application can provide symptomatic relief using warm soaks, diathermy, or paraffin baths. Intermittent periods of joint inactivity can be beneficial to reduce joint inflammation. Nighttime static splinting is the most convenient manner to accomplish this task. The splint can be a piece of aluminofoam or fabricated from a lightweight plastic material. Full-time splinting should be avoided as joint motion promotes normal metabolism and nutrition of the remaining cartilage via diffusion from the synovial fluid. Prolonged splinting will actually cause deterioration in the cellular milieu and further decline in joint motion with concurrent periarticular stiffness. Elastic gloves worn at night may also be helpful to reduce any swelling (10).

Medical Management

Pharmaceutical interventions for osteoarthritis of the hand are predominately analgesics to control the symptoms. Some subsets with a substantial inflammatory component (e.g., erosive osteoarthritis) or other inflammatory arthritides (e.g., psoriatic arthritis) will benefit from medications that modulate inflammation. Nonsteroidal anti-inflammatory medications (NSAIDs) and corticosteroid preparations are most commonly prescribed. These medications are effective in the reduction of symptoms, but do not retard the progression of disease.

The benefits of drug therapy must be weighed against the potential risks of treatment. The drug of first choice is acetaminophen because of its safety profile and because studies have indicated comparable efficacy as NSAIDs for pain relief (22). Topical analgesics (e.g., capsaicin and methylsalicylate creams) can also be used as adjunctive treatment (23). The use of NSAIDs is based on the concept of at least some degree of inflammation present in osteoarthritis (1,17). Despite the numerous NSAIDs available, no single compound has been found to be more efficacious (24). In addition, chronic use of NSAIDs or oral corticosteroids for isolated DIP joint arthritis is not recommended as the long-term side effects far outweigh the potential benefits. Gastric mucosal ulcers have been endoscopically visualized in 20% of patients using NSAIDs for six months and 1% to 2% of these patients will develop hemorrhage or perforation. Fortunately, 90% of these lesions heal after discontinuation of the NSAID and use of acid-reducing medication (22,25,26). The recent introduction of COX-2 inhibitors that target specific prostaglandins may diminish these side effects, although their long-term efficacy and safety profile remains to be determined. For patients with polyarticular erosive or inflammatory arthritis, NSAIDs or other more potent modulators of inflammation (e.g., hydroxychloroquine) are indicated (27).

Corticosteroid injections are utilized in the treatment of DIP joint arthritis. This technique avoids the sequelae of oral steroid use and is clinically efficacious, although relief may only be temporary. There is controversy as to whether the corticosteroid injection has a protective or deleterious effect on the remaining cartilage (28). Under aseptic conditions, a small amount (0.25 cc) of corticosteroid can be introduced with a 25 or 27 gauge needle (Fig. 4.4). A water-soluble preparation (e.g., betamethasone) is preferred because of its high potency and decreased incidence of skin depigmentation and fat atrophy. The injection can also contain a similar amount of lidocaine to ameliorate some of the discomfort. The patient should be warned the injection can be painful,

an increase in discomfort can occur for a few days, and the medication will not take effect until three to seven days later.

Operative Treatment

Surgery for DIP joint arthritis is performed for soft tissue and/or bony indications. The soft tissue pathology is the mucous cyst, which represents a ganglion that emanates from an arthritic DIP joint between the extensor tendon and collateral ligament (Fig. 4.5). This eccentrically located cyst can range in size from 1 to 12 mm and can be located proximal or distal to the joint (29). The cavity is filled with a viscid gel or mucoid material (30,31). Some degree of arthritis and a marginal osteophyte is always present underlying the cyst. This bony spur is best seen on the oblique x-ray projection (29). Longitudinal grooving of the nail can also occur with a mucous cyst secondary to pressure applied to the germinal matrix. This grooving may precede the appearance of the cyst and be the primary reason for the patient to seek medical attention.

A small cyst without a nail bed deformity is best managed by observation. In contrast, an enlarging cyst with thinning of the skin and nail bed deformity is treated by surgical excision and osteophyte debridement (29). Cyst rupture either intentional (e.g., needle) or accidental (e.g., trauma) can lead to bacterial inoculation and septic arthritis. In addition, persistent pressure on the nail bed may result in permanent abnormalities of the nail plate (32). Therefore, elective excision is recommended for the majority of large mucous cysts.

The bony indications for treatment of DIP joint arthritis are persistent pain, deformity, and instability that result in functional disability. Persistent pain implies discomfort that

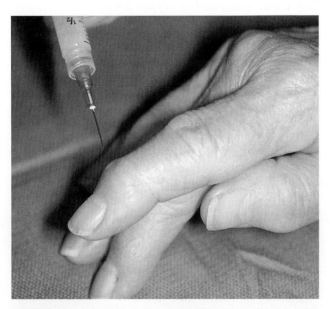

FIGURE 4.4. Technique for corticosteroid injection into the DIP joint. Needle inserted just dorsal to collateral ligament.

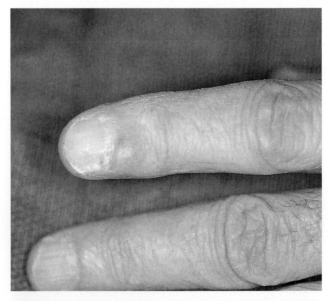

FIGURE 4.5. 66-year-old male with left index mucous cyst and longitudinal grooving of the nail plate.

interferes with activities of daily living despite nonoperative measures. An unstable or painful DIP joint can severely hamper ones ability to perform self-care (buttoning, grasping toothbrush), leisure (needlepoint, gardening), housework (cooking, cleaning), and work (typing, writing). Deformity secondary to osteoarthritis is primarily in the coronal plane with progressive ulnar deviation of the distal phalanx. A subtle rotational deformity is often present and should be considered during surgical correction. Sagittal plane deformity is usually associated with inflammatory arthritis (e.g., psoriatic arthritis) or trauma (e.g., fracture or mallet finger) and may require treatment depending on the pain and degree of disability.

Arthrodesis is the standard operative procedure for DIP joint arthritis, and the DIP joint is the most common site of fusion in the hand. A successful fusion produces a painless, stable joint that is durable without considerable impairment in function (33). However, certain patients may benefit from a motion-preserving procedure (i.e., DIP joint arthroplasty). Patients with involvement of multiple joints and digits or those individuals that require DIP joint flexion for fine manipulative activities are viable candidates. Silicone hinge arthroplasty remains an option to retain a limited arc of flexion, although the long-term outcome of arthroplasty remains indeterminate (34–36). Symptomatic arthritis of successive PIP and DIP joints should not be treated with arthroplasties at both levels. Since 85% of digital flexion occurs at the PIP joint compared to 15% at the DIP joint, arthroplasty is favored at the PIP joint level and fusion at the DIP joint (37). Currently, arthroplasty should be considered in hands with isolated DIP joint disease that requires exceptional mobility (e.g., musician) (38,39).

The main contraindication for reconstructive DIP joint surgery is active infection. The infection should be treated by formal debridement and antibiotics prior to the definitive surgical procedure. DIP joint arthroplasty is contraindicated in these instances and fusion is the recommended treatment. Relative contraindications to surgery are inadequate bone stock (e.g., opera glass hand) or an insensate digit (e.g., Charcot joint or diabetic neuropathy) (33).

PREOPERATIVE PLANNING

Preoperative planning is based on a careful history, physical examination, and x-ray analysis. Any patient with a mucous cyst should be specifically questioned regarding episodes of drainage. Thick gelatinous drainage implies cyst decompression while purulence indicates previous infection and the possibility of latent disease. Infection often requires a staged reconstruction with initial debridement and removal of any sequestrum prior to formal arthrodesis.

The status of the skin overlying the DIP joint should be assessed. Scarred adherent skin from previous surgery or trauma may require initial resurfacing or alternative coverage at the time of surgery. Thin skin from a large mucous cyst may require a rotational flap for sufficient coverage.

The degree of coronal and sagittal DIP joint deformity should be measured with a goniometer. The amount of passive correction should also be determined. Incomplete passive correction is secondary to soft tissue contracture and/or bony deformity. This pathology must be corrected at the time of surgery and incorporated into the preoperative plan. Soft tissue release of the contracted side and/or differential bony resection is required to realign the digit.

X-rays do not correlate with degree of symptoms, but are an important part of the preoperative plan (Fig. 4.3). The X-rays are assessed for joint space narrowing, bone loss, angular deformity, and osteophyte burden. These bony changes will influence the operative plan. Scrutiny of the X-rays will also delineate the altered anatomy and prevent confusion during surgical reconstruction. For example, substantial dorsal osteophyte formation may prohibit joint exposure until this irregular bone is removed. In addition, bone loss from osteopenia or severe erosions may require alternate plans for internal fixation and even obligate supplemental bone graft.

Preoperative planning for DIP joint arthrodesis requires a determination of the position of fusion. The exact angle should provide the best function for the patient rather than applying a predetermined arbitrary value (40). No coronal or frontal plane angulation should be incorporated into the fusion position, as this will yield digital crossover or malalignment during fist formation. The desired sagittal position ranges from 0 to 25 degrees of flexion and depends on the patient, the finger involved, and the status of the surrounding joints (41,42). The arthrodesis position should be discussed with the patient prior to surgery, along with the potential advantages and disadvantages. The occupational and recreational expectations of the patient should be part of the decision-making process. Certain activities require a specific amount of DIP joint flexion (e.g., rowing or playing an instrument) and influence the selected fusion position. A temporary splint can be used to simulate the position of fusion. A position of slight flexion (10 to 20 degrees) allows adequate grasp and will not interfere with release of objects. However, patients with concerns about appearance tend to prefer an extended position to produce a more normal finger alignment in extension (43). This posture will sacrifice hook grip but the deleterious functional effect of an extended DIP joint is minimal (Fig. 4.6).

When planning a DIP joint arthrodesis, the finger involved is another factor to consider. The ring and small fingers are instrumental during grasp, and a flexed DIP joint position will facilitate power grip. In contrast, the index and long digits are more contributory in oppositional pinch, which requires a more extended posture. Therefore, the angle of fusion often increases from index to small digit. Last, the status of the surrounding joints should be considered in the decision-making process. For example, a patient with diseased MP and PIP joints and limited flexion may not be able

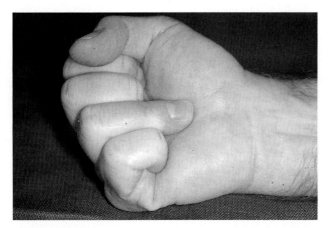

FIGURE 4.6. 60-year-old male status following isolated right ring DIP joint arthrodesis positioned in extension. Grasp reveals lack of DIP joint flexion, but minimal functional consequences.

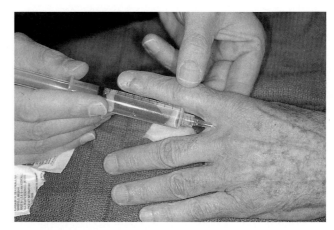

FIGURE 4.7. Digital block anesthesia performed in preparation for mucous cyst excision.

to adapt to a DIP joint fused in full extension. In this case, the DIP joint is fused in flexion to facilitate grasp (40).

Techniques

Debridement

Debridement of Heberdens nodes for reasons of appearance is not recommended. Patients are unlikely to be satisfied with surgical removal of these nodules. The DIP joint still appears enlarged, can develop chronic swelling, and has a surgical scar. In addition, debridement of large dorsal osteophytes can yield an extension lag, which further dissatisfies the patient (32). The surgeon should not succumb to the patient adamant about removal of these nodules for cosmesis.

Mucous cyst excision

Mucous cyst excision is a common procedure employed for the soft tissue component of DIP joint arthritis. The cyst represents a ganglion that originates from the arthritic joint between the extensor tendon and collateral ligament. The goals of the procedure are cyst excision and debridement of the underlying osteophyte. Loupe magnification is required to visualize the stalk originating from the joint. The operation is performed as an outpatient in the operating room using digital block anesthesia (Fig. 4.7). Tourniquet control is required and can be accomplished by a penrose drain or a tournicot (Mar-Med, Grand Rapids, Michigan) placed at the base of the finger (Fig. 4.8) (44). The tournicot exsanguinates upon insertion, maintains a low profile, and avoids the use of a hemostat, which can interfere with the procedure.

The mucous cyst is always eccentric, located between the extensor tendon and collateral ligament. A variety of incisions can be used for cyst excision. Complicated cysts with extremely thin skin coverage may require the development of a rotational flap for coverage. This strategy must be incorpo-

rated into the design of the skin incision. An uncomplicated cyst is approached via a longitudinal incision beginning proximal to the DIP joint and angled along the dorsal or volar border of the cyst (Fig. 4.9). A skin flap is elevated over the cyst by sharp dissection. The lateral margin of the extensor tendon is gently retracted (Fig. 4.10). The skin can be extremely thin at the cyst apex and a small buttonhole can occur. This skin defect is irrelevant and will granulate over time. The borders of the cyst are mobilized and its origin carefully traced to the DIP joint margin. The germinal matrix is avoided and the collateral ligament not disturbed. The cyst and stalk are excised from the joint and the underlying osteophyte removed with a rongeur (Fig. 4.11). The osteophyte may arise from either the condylar margin of the middle phalanx or the distal articular margin of the distal phalanx (29). The wound is closed by interrupted skin sutures and a compressive dressing is applied (Fig. 4.12).

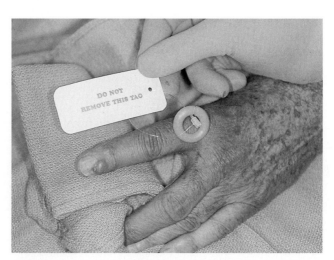

FIGURE 4.8. A finger tournicot (Mar-Med, Grand Rapids, Michigan) is applied for exsanguination and hemostasis.

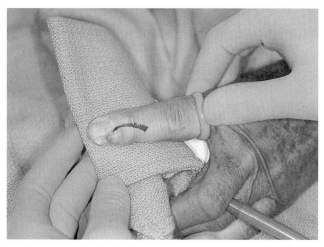

FIGURE 4.9. A longitudinal incision beginning proximal to the DIP joint and angled along the dorsal border of the cyst.

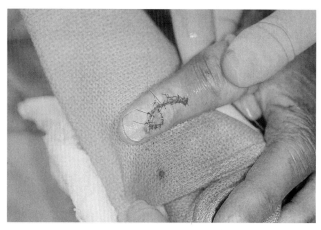

FIGURE 4.12. Skin closure after mucous cyst excision and debridement of osteophytes with interrupted skin sutures. Thin skin is present over area of cyst excision.

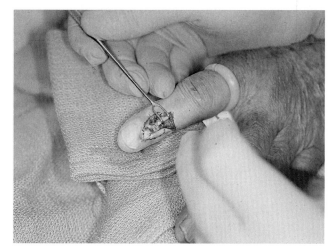

FIGURE 4.10. Elevation of skin flap over mucous cyst and retraction of extensor tendon. (See Color Fig. 4.10.)

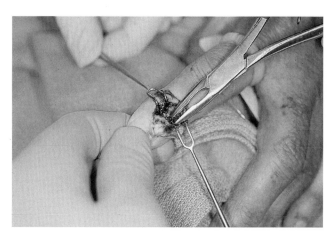

FIGURE 4.11. Debridement of marginal osteophytes along the joint line with a rongeur. (See Color Fig. 4.11.)

Arthrodesis

Arthrodesis is the "gold standard" operation for DIP joint arthritis. Moberg and Hendrickson (33) in 1959 stated that "the prime requisites of good digital arthrodesis are a painless and stable union in proper position and in a reasonable space of time." This accurately defines the goals of DIP joint arthrodesis and remains the ultimate objective. The recent emphasis in DIP joint arthrodesis has been device-oriented with a goal of rigid internal fixation to promote immediate stability and achieve consistent bony union. However, the basic principles of fusion are more important than the choice of internal fixation device (42,45).

The surgery is performed as an outpatient procedure in the operating room. Digital block anesthesia is usually sufficient although supplemental sedation is offered as an option. A long-acting anesthetic agent (e.g., carbocaine or mepivicaine) is preferred to provide postoperative analgesia. Regional anesthesia (e.g., wrist, Bier, or axillary block) is another option for DIP joint surgery, although regional is usually reserved for more extensive procedures combined with DIP joint arthrodesis.

Tourniquet control is required and can be accomplished by a one-quarter inch Penrose drain or a tournicot placed at the base of the finger (44). A tournicot is low profile and also exsanguinates the digit upon insertion. The tournicot also avoids the use of a hemostat clamped to the Penrose, which can interfere with the procedure.

Joint Exposure

Multiple incisions have been described for dorsal exposure of the DIP joint with a Y- or H-shaped configuration most common (Fig. 4.13). The incision may have to be modified in cases with previous surgery (e.g., mucous cyst excision). The exposure must use sizable skin flaps that include the subdermal

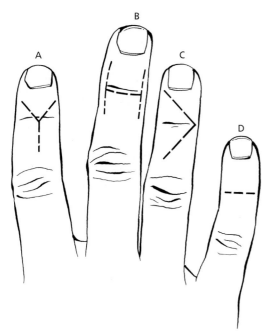

FIGURE 4.13. Skin incisions for exposure of the DIP joint (**A.** "Y" incision, **B.** "H" incision, **C.** Brunner incision, **D.** transverse incision).

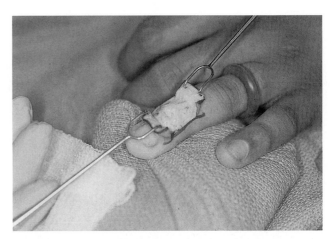

FIGURE 4.15. Full thickness flaps skin flaps elevated from the extensor tendon epitenon during DIP joint exposure. (See Color Fig. 4.15.)

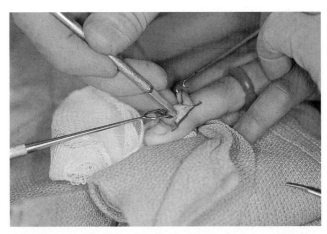

FIGURE 4.16. Technique for "back-cutting" origin of the collateral ligament. Beaver blade is placed between the collateral ligament and head of the middle phalanx. Rotation of the blade releases the collateral ligament from its origin. (See Color Fig. 4.16.)

plexus to preserve the vascularity and avoid skin slough. The flap design must also avoid injury to the germinal matrix, which is located 1 mm distal to the extensor tendon insertion (31).

The H-shaped incision requires the radial and ulnar limbs to be located in the midlateral lines and the crosshatch centered over the DIP joint (Fig. 4.14). The incision is performed sharply to the extensor tendon and full thickness flaps skin flaps elevated from the epitenon (Fig. 4.15). Hemostasis

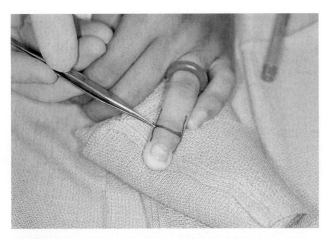

FIGURE 4.14. H-shaped incision used for dorsal DIP joint exposure with limbs located in the midlateral lines.

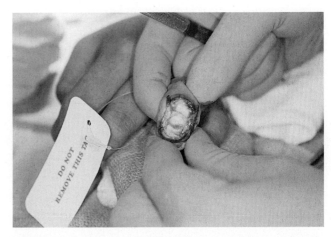

FIGURE 4.17. Flexion of the DIP joint exposes the head of the middle phalanx and the base of the distal phalanx. (See Color Fig. 4.17.)

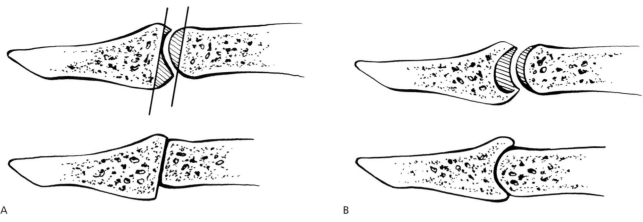

FIGURE 4.18. Types of joint resection for DIP arthrodesis. **A.** Straight angled cuts. **B.** "Cup-and-cone" cuts.

is obtained with a bipolar electrocautery. The extensor mechanism tendon and underlying dorsal capsule are incised transversely to expose the arthritic DIP joint. Dorsal osteophytes are removed with a rongeur to facilitate joint exposure. The origins of the collateral ligaments are released from the middle phalanx by using a Beaver blade and "back-cutting" their origin (Fig. 4.16). This maneuver begins with placement of the blade between the collateral ligament and middle phalanx. Rotation of the blade along the middle phalanx releases the collateral ligament from its origin. The DIP joint is flexed as much as possible (60 to 90 degrees) to expose the head of the middle phalanx and the base of the distal phalanx (Fig. 4.17) (40). Inability to adequately flex the joint implies incomplete collateral ligament release, excessive osteophyte formation, or thickened volar plate. The volar plate may have to be teased from the base of the middle phalanx using a Freer elevator to increase joint exposure.

Bony Preparation

Bony preparation is the most important part of the surgery to obtain a solid arthrodesis. The remaining osteophytes are removed with a rongeur to fully expose the base of the distal phalanx and the head of the middle phalanx. This debridement will remove any Heberdens nodes and improve the postoperative appearance following arthrodesis. Any remaining articular cartilage and subchondral bone needs to be resected to obtain a solid arthrodesis. In preparation for fusion, the head of the middle phalanx and base of the distal phalanx can be fashioned into a variety of configurations for arthrodesis (Fig. 4.18). The bony resection can resemble a straight cut, cup-and-cone (a.k.a. cup-and-spike), convex-concave (a.k.a. cup-and-saucer or ball-and-socket), chevron, and even a mortise and tenon (peg) (40,41,46,47). The bone resection can be accomplished with a rongeur, osteotome, burr, small oscillating saw, or trephine.

The bony configuration of a mortise and tenon or the use of a bone peg is designed to create a stable construct by bony

interface (33,47). The bone peg or dowel is shaped to fit into a square hole to obtain "exact fixation" (Fig. 4.19) (33). The square holed design is to prevent rotation and provide fixation. On occasion, the bone peg is supplemented with a Kirschner wire. Currently, internal fixation devices are used to provide stable fixation and obviate the need for such meticulous bone modeling (37).

The convex-concave method for DIP joint arthrodesis requires minimal bone removal, maintains the normal contour of the articular surfaces, and is easily adjustable. In contrast, cutting parallel surfaces has less room for error and relies on the angulation of the saw cut for fusion position in both the sagittal and coronal planes. Incorrect DIP joint posi-

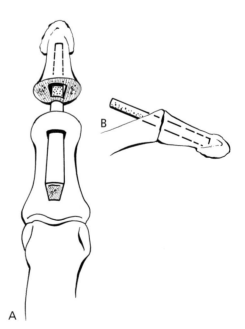

FIGURE 4.19. Schematic of the use of a bone peg shaped to fit into a square hole to prevent rotation and create a stable construct by bony interface.

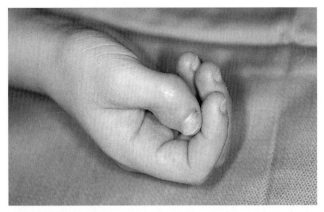

FIGURE 4.20. 10 year-old male with an unstable, angulated, and stiff thumb interphalangeal joint after excision of duplicated thumb as an infant. Convex-concave method of arthrodesis (chondrodesis) planned.

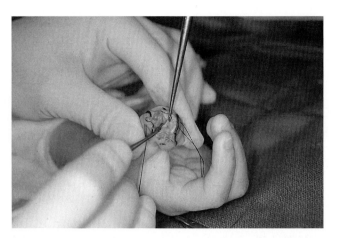

FIGURE 4.22. A curette is utilized to remove any remaining cartilage from the distal phalanx base and create a reciprocal convex surface. (See Color Fig. 4.22.)

tion requires re-cutting of the bone and additional digital shortening. The convex-concave method creates a convex middle phalanx and reciprocal concave distal phalanx similar to a cup-and-saucer or ball-and-socket (Fig. 4.20). A rongeur or burr is used to fashion the convex curvature of the middle phalanx (Fig. 4.21). A curette or burr is utilized to remove any remaining cartilage from the distal phalanx base and create a reciprocal convex surface (Fig. 4.22). Any angulatory deformity from uneven bone wear should be corrected by appropriate resection. The bony preparation should result in two spherical shaped cancellous surfaces that are easily positioned into the desired angle of arthrodesis. The dense subchondral bone must be removed while a circumferential cortical rim can be preserved for bony contact. The cortical surfaces should accurately abut without any considerable step-off or irregularities. Imperfect contact requires repeat assessment of the bony preparation or the addition of bone graft (42). Accurate apposition of the DIP joint surfaces can

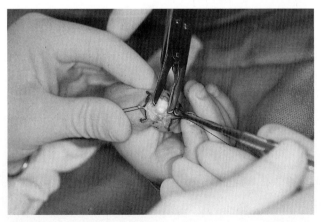

FIGURE 4.21. Following joint exposure, a rongeur is used to fashion the convex curvature of the middle phalanx. (See Color Fig. 4.21.)

also be inhibited by interposition of the volar plate, which tends to buckle into the joint. Additional volar plate release and/or palmar translation of the plate during bony coaptation is required. The sharp portion of the Kleinert elevator is especially useful to depress the volar plate and prevent this interposition.

Fixation

Consolidation of the arthrodesis site requires similar principles of fracture union, including bony contact, immobilization, and time. Static and compressive methods of internal fixation have been used for arthrodesis fixation. Static fixation maintains the DIP joint alignment until union occurs across the fusion site. Compressive devices prevent gap formation and eliminate the shearing strain, which encourages direct or primary union (45). The ideal internal fixation device should be easy to insert, obtain rigid fixation, avoid postoperative immobilization, obviate secondary removal, and minimize complication rate. No currently available device satisfies all of these requirements, and the selection is dependent on the surgeon preference and patient factors, including bone stock, expectations, and compliance.

Kirschner wires and bone dowels have been recommended as static internal fixation devices (48,49). A bone dowel is placed in a hole bored down the long axis of the distal phalanx, across the DIP joint, into the middle phalanx, and out the dorsal cortex of the middle phalanx. A unicortical bone dowel can be fashioned from the iliac crest, proximal ulna, or middle phalanx, placed across the DIP joint to provide stability and promote union (33,50). The bone carpentry to perform this technique is meticulous, labor intensive, and uncommonly employed (37). Currently, multiple percutaneous Kirschner wires (0.35 to 0.45 inches) are the preferred static device (Fig. 4.23). Recently, biodegradable pins have been used for arthrodesis to eliminate some of the inherent

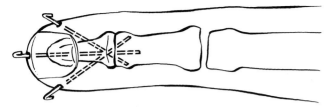

FIGURE 4.23. Multiple K-wires provide excellent DIP joint fixation following joint fusion.

problems associated with K-wires (51). However, these biodegradable implants can incite a foreign body reaction during absorption creating additional problems.

The K-wires can be passed across the DIP joint in either a longitudinal or crossed configuration (40). The K-wires can be driven retrograde from the tip of the finger across the joint or initially drilled antegrade from the joint surface through the distal phalanx. The antegrade wires should be double-ended and driven from the distal phalanx articular surface antegrade across the distal phalanx and tip of the finger just volar to the hyponychium (Fig. 4.24). These K-wires should be passed through the distal phalanx at different starting points to ensure the wires cross in the distal phalanx and not at the arthrodesis site (Fig. 4.25). This configuration provides greater stability (42,46,52). The wires are then withdrawn until their tips are just within the distal phalanx. The fusion surfaces are reduced and the wires drilled retrograde across the joint while maintaining joint compression and axial alignment (Fig. 4.26). Manual compression is required to prevent joint distraction during K-wire insertion. A specialized bone compression clamp has been designed to maximize compression across the arthrodesis during crossed Kirschner wire insertion (53). However, manual compression during K-wire insertion will usually suffice. The wires can be cut beneath the skin or retained in a percutaneous position. The

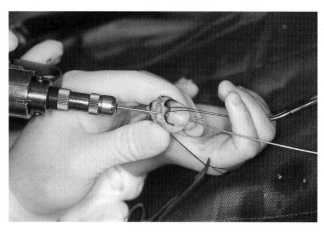

FIGURE 4.25. The first Kirschner wire is withdrawn with wire driver until the tip is just within the distal phalanx and a second K-wire inserted through the distal phalanx at a different starting point to ensure the wires cross in the distal phalanx and not at the arthrodesis site.

advantages of static K-wires are ease of insertion, avoidance of retained hardware, and ability to adjust angle of fusion. The disadvantages are lack of compression, minimal rigidity, and potential for pin track infection.

The compressive devices used for DIP joint arthrodesis include interosseous wiring, tension band wiring, and screw fixation (standard and differential pitch screws). A less commonly employed method is external fixation, which is usually reserved for difficult soft tissue problems. These compressive techniques are more technically demanding than Kirschner wires, but offer the advantages of rigid fixation and compression. Screw placement also requires the DIP joint to be placed in almost full extension and prohibits any considerable flexion posture (54). DIP joint arthrodesis in flexion with a compression screw is possible, but is a particularly difficult technique.

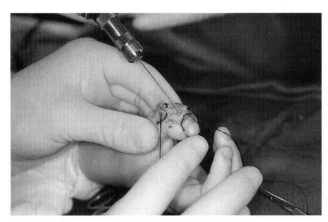

FIGURE 4.24. Antegrade K-wire driven from the distal phalanx articular surface antegrade across the distal phalanx and tip of the finger just volar to the hyponychium.

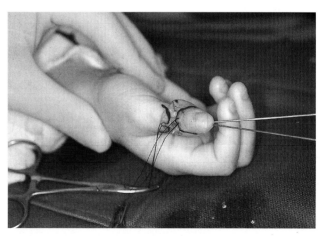

FIGURE 4.26. The fusion surface is reduced and the wires drilled retrograde across the reduced joint to secure position.

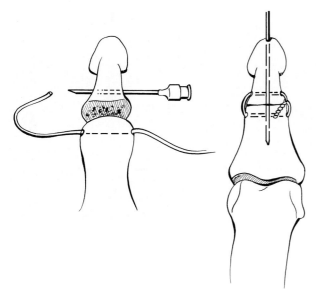

FIGURE 4.27. Schematic of interosseous wiring for DIP joint fusion using a single stainless steel wire supplemented by a Kirschner wire.

Interosseous Wiring

Interosseous wiring was described by Robertson (55) and popularized by Lister (56). This technique requires matching drill holes in the base of the distal phalanx and the head of the middle phalanx coupled by a monofilament stainless steel wire (Fig. 4.27). One or two sets of stainless steel wire can be used for interosseous wiring. If a single loop of wire is utilized, sufficient angulatory stability is not achieved and a sup-

plemental Kirschner wire (0.035 in.) is necessary (56). When using two loops of wire, the parallel drill holes can be oriented 180 degrees (one vertical and the other horizontal) or both can be placed in the vertical direction. The drill holes for wire placements are made with a 0.035-in. Kirschner wire and are located approximately 0.5 mm from the arthrodesis site (56).

A 26- or 28-gauge monofilament stainless steel wire is passed through each pair of holes prior to DIP joint coaptation. A 20-gauge needle can be passed through the hole and the wire threaded into the needle to facilitate passage. The prepared DIP joint surfaces are then manually approximated and held in position. If a single interosseous wire is used, a longitudinal Kirschner is drilled to secure the position. The interosseous wire is then twisted with a needle holder to achieve compression. The needle holder must initially pull the wire from the bone to take up the slack and then rotate the wire into a twist. When two interosseous wires are used, the longitudinal K-wire is not required and both wires are similarly tightened (Fig. 4.28). The twisted ends of the wire are cut short (approximately 1 cm) and bent downward. The cut end of interosseous wire loops oriented in a vertical orientation is placed under the extensor mechanism. If a horizontal wire orientation is selected, the twist of the wire should be placed on the noncontact side of the finger, that is, the ulnar side of the index, long, and ring digit, and the radial side of the small finger. The cut end of the wire can also be bent into an adjacent unicortical hole to bury the wire end (56).

Standard Screw Insertion

A standard screw can be used for DIP joint arthrodesis (Fig. 4.29) (57). The screw diameter must be small (2.0 to 2.4 mm) and the technique carefully followed. A self-tapping

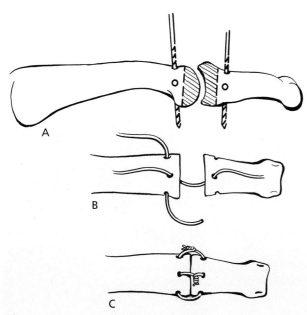

FIGURE 4.28. Technique for 90-90 interosseous wiring. **A.** Drill holes placed close to the arthrodesis site at 90 degree angles. **B.** Wire suture is passed through the holes. **C.** Wires are tightened in a rigid construct.

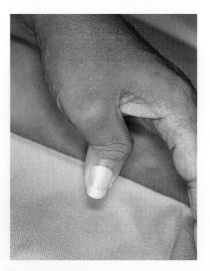

FIGURE 4.29. 50-year-old female with inflammatory arthritis and progressive pain, deformity and instability left thumb interphalangeal joint prior to arthrodesis.

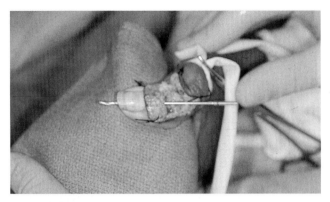

FIGURE 4.30. Drill passed from the distal phalanx articular surface antegrade across the distal phalanx and tip of the finger just volar to the hyponychium.

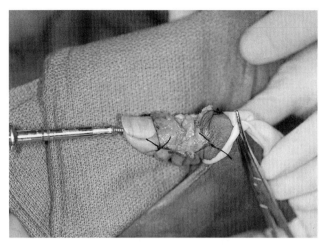

FIGURE 4.32. A self-tapping screw inserted retrograde through the finger pulp and across the reduced DIP joint. (See Color Fig. 4.32.)

screw eliminates the necessity of tapping. The drill can be driven by hand or power depending on the bone quality. The drill (1.5 or 1.8 mm) is passed from the distal phalanx articular surface antegrade across the distal phalanx and tip of the finger just volar to the hyponychium (Fig. 4.30). The drill is then removed, reversed, and passed retrograde through the same hole in the distal phalanx and into the joint space. The DIP joint is held in the planned position of fusion and the drill advanced into the middle phalanx (Fig. 4.31). The drill hole in the distal phalanx can be enlarged with the appropriate drill (2.0 or 2.4 mm) to achieve maximum compression as long as the bone quality is adequate. A depth gauge can be inserted retrograde across the reduced DIP joint to measure the appropriate screw length. A self-tapping screw is then inserted through the finger pulp, into the distal phalanx, and across the reduced DIP joint (Fig. 4.32). A mini-fluoroscopy unit is used to verify intramedullary screw position, check proper screw depth, and ensure coaptation of the fusion surfaces.

The screw can also be inserted in an oblique direction using a lag technique to attain compression (58). A 1.5-mm or 2.0-mm screw is inserted at an angle of 45 to 60 degrees from proximal to distal. The screw head is countersunk into the middle phalanx to increase the surface area of head contact and to minimize soft tissue interference. The proximal hole is overdrilled to allow compression across the arthrodesis site during screw insertion.

Herbert Screw Insertion

The Herbert (Zimmer, Warsaw, IN) screw is a double-threaded, headless, titanium alloy screw. The leading threads are separated from the trailing thread by a smooth 1.75-mm shaft, designed to cross the arthrodesis site. The leading threads have a greater pitch than the trailing threads, which creates compression across the DIP joint during insertion. The thread diameters also differ with the leading threads measuring 3.0 mm compared to the trailing diameter of 3.9 mm. The available screw length is from 12 mm to 30 mm in 2-mm increments. There is a Herbert mini-bone screw version that has an outer leading thread diameter of 2.5 mm and a trailing diameter of 3.2 mm. However, the maximum length available is 18 mm and the smaller diameter decreases fixation rigidity (59).

The small or main Herbert drill, which drills to the core diameter of the leading screw thread, is passed from the distal phalanx articular surface antegrade across the distal phalanx and tip of the finger just volar to the hyponychium. The drill is then removed, reversed, and passed retrograde through the same hole in the distal phalanx and into the joint space. The DIP joint is held in the planned position of fusion and the drill advanced into the middle phalanx. A mini-fluoroscopy unit can be used to verify the position of the drill and joint alignment. The smaller drill is removed, and the larger pilot drill, which drills to the core diameter of the trailing screw

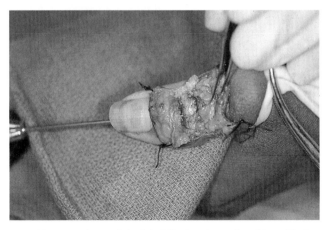

FIGURE 4.31. The DIP joint is held in the planned position of fusion and the drill reversed and passed retrograde through the same hole in the distal phalanx across the joint and into middle phalanx.

thread, is passed antegrade to enlarge the hole in the distal phalanx. The tap is also placed antegrade across the DIP joint and into the middle phalanx (Fig. 4.33).

The screw length is selected by choosing an appropriate length that will attain good purchase in the distal and middle phalanx, usually 22 to 26 mm. The Herbert screw is placed on the hex screwdriver and driven retrograde through the distal phalanx, across the DIP joint, and into the middle phalanx. The screw should be inserted until the trailing threads are completely engaged within the distal phalanx (Fig. 4.34). The DIP joint should be stabilized during screw insertion to prevent rotation of the distal phalanx. A mini-fluoroscopy unit is used to confirm screw position and coaptation of the fusion surfaces.

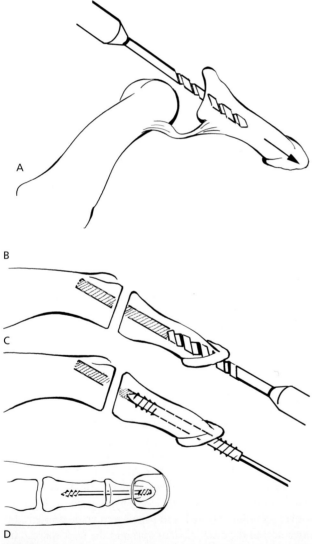

FIGURE 4.33. The sequence for use of a Herbert screw for DIP joint fusion. **A.** Anterograde drilling of the distal phalanx, **B.** retrograde drilling through the distal phalanx into the middle phalanx after joint reduction, **C.** advancement of the chosen screw across the fusion site, **D.** final placement of the screw with subsequent fusion site compression

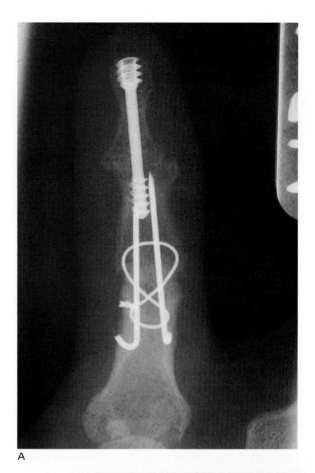

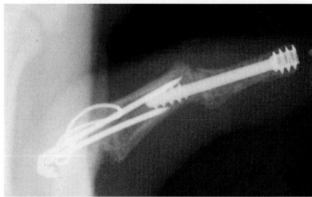

FIGURE 4.34. Anteroposterior (**A**) and lateral (**B**) X-rays of a 40-year-old male who underwent PIP and DIP joint arthrodesis after failed staged tendon reconstruction. Herbert screw fixation of DIP joint fusion and tension band fixation of PIP joint arthrodesis.

Acutrak Screw Insertion

The Acutrak (Acumed, Beaverton, OR) screw is a tapered, fully treaded, cannulated, headless screw. The thread pitch varies at a constant rate along the length of the screw to achieve compression across the fusion site. The mini-Acutrak screw is used for DIP joint arthrodesis and is available from

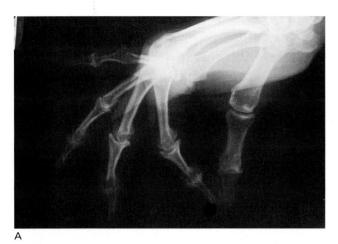

A

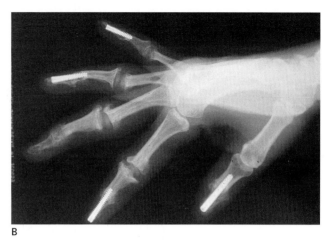

B

FIGURE 4.35. A. Preoperative X-ray of a 50-year-old female with primary osteoarthritis and progressive PIP and DIP joint pain and disability. **B.** Postoperative X-ray one year after DIP joint fusions (index, ring, and small) and thumb interphalangeal joint arthrodesis using Acutrak screws. Subsequent PIP joint arthroplasties performed with silicone implants.

10 mm to 26 mm in 2-mm increments. The leading outer diameter is 2.8 mm and increases to 3.2 to 3.6 mm depending upon the length of screw selected.

The guide wire is passed from the distal phalanx articular surface antegrade across the distal phalanx and tip of the finger just volar to the hyponychium. The guide wire is withdrawn from the end of the finger until flush with the distal phalanx. The DIP joint is held in the planned position of fusion and the guide wire is passed retrograde to secure the reduction. The screw length is selected by placing the drill as a guide along the dorsum of the finger and choosing an appropriate length that will attain good purchase in the distal and middle phalanx. The selected screw length is marked on the drill to gauge the depth of insertion. The drill is hand driven to the proper depth. The DIP joint should be stabilized during drilling to prevent rotation of the distal phalanx.

The drill is removed with care to retain the guide wire. The selected screw is advanced over the guide wire and across the arthrodesis site. The trailing threads should be buried within the distal phalanx. The Acutrak screw enlarges proximally and can expand or even fragment the distal phalanx upon insertion (Fig. 4.35). A mini-fluoroscopy unit is useful to verify appropriate screw position, assess distal phalanx fixation, and evaluate bony coaptation across the fusion site.

Tension Band Fixation

Tension band or wire fixation can be applied to the DIP joint using Kirschner wires and monofilament stainless steel wire. The concept of tension band fixation is to construct an internal fixation device that stabilizes the DIP joint and converts the flexion force from the flexor digitorum profundus into compressive forces at the arthrodesis site (60–62). Kirschner wires placed longitudinally act to neutralize the shear forces

while a dorsal tension band converts the tensile forces into compressive loads across the fusion site. The technique begins with the creation of a transverse hole in the dorsal aspect of the distal phalanx 8 to 10 mm from the joint surface. The hole is made with a 0.035-in. Kirschner wire and must be parallel to the joint line. A 26- or 28-gauge monofilament stainless steel wire is passed through this hole.

Two parallel 0.035-in. K-wires are placed across the DIP joint in the desired angle of fusion. The wires can be drilled in either an antegrade or retrograde direction. K-wires passed antegrade enter from the dorsal aspect of the middle phalanx, traverse the arthrodesis site, and engage the palmar cortex of the distal phalanx. Retrograde wires should be double-ended and are passed from the joint space through the middle phalanx and dorsal cortex. The K-wires are withdrawn until they are just within the medullary canal of the middle phalanx. The arthrodesis site is then reduced and held in the planned position while the K-wires are advanced antegrade across the fusion site into the palmar aspect of the distal phalanx. Manual compression is required to prevent joint distraction during K-wire insertion.

The 26- or 28-gauge wire is passed in a figure-eight fashion over the dorsal aspect of the DIP joint fusion site and around the Kirschner wires. The wire is tightened using a twisting motion, which compresses the dorsal part of the fusion site. The twisted ends of the wire are cut short (approximately 1 cm) and bent downward. The K-wires are withdrawn slightly, bent 180 degrees, and taped into the middle phalanx while capturing the tension band wire.

Minor modifications of this technique have been described including different Kirschner wire configuration or drilling of the tension band through transverse holes on both sides of the fusion site (59,63). However, the concept of tension band fixation still applies to these technical alterations.

Absorbable Screws or Implants

Biodegradable implants manufactured from synthetic polymers can be used for internal fixation of fractures, osteotomies, and arthrodeses (51,64). Polydioxanone (i.e., PDS) and polyglycolide are the most common compositions of these materials. The implants are designed to prevent the problems of stress shielding, pin migration, and prominent hardware associated with internal fixation. These materials have been constructed into rods, pins, and screws. The pins have been utilized for interphalangeal arthrodesis in a limited fashion (51). The pins provide static fixation and are inserted by tapping into predrilled channels across the fusion site. The size of the drill to create the channel varies with the diameter of the implant. The excessive pin length is sharply cut or removed by electrocautery beneath the skin level.

External Fixation

Dynamic compression and external fixation have been described for interphalangeal joint arthrodesis (65,66). Braun's technique (65) uses three 0.045-in. Kirschner wires and methyl methacrylate bone cement. A longitudinal K-wire wire provides sagittal plane stability and is driven retrograde across the joint or initially drilled antegrade through the distal phalanx. The retrograde wire is initially passed from the distal phalanx articular surface across the distal phalanx and tip of the finger just volar to the hyponychium. The surfaces are then reduced and the wire drilled retrograde across the joint while maintaining joint compression and axial alignment.

A second Kirschner wire in passed transversely through the base of the distal phalanx parallel to the joint line. A third wire is drilled parallel to the joint line across the middle phalanx. The distance between the wires should be 2.5 to 3.0 cm. A clamp is applied to each side of the joint to produce a bow in the wires and compress the joint surfaces. Methyl methacrylate is placed around the K-wires on each side of the joint to maintain the dynamic compression. After the bone cement hardens, the clamps are removed and the protruding K-wires cut short.

Tupper (66) described an alternative technique to provide external fixation at the time of DIP joint fusion. This method used an orthodontic traction device obtained from a dental supply house fashioned to the DIP joint. Wexler et al. (67) reported on the use of external fixation using dorsoventral Kirschner wires and rubber bands to maintain dynamic compression. These constructs provide compression across the fusion site similar to the Kirschner wire and bone cement technique (65).

Closure

The extensor mechanism is repaired using a 3-0 or 4-0 nonabsorbable suture to provide coverage over the arthrodesis site

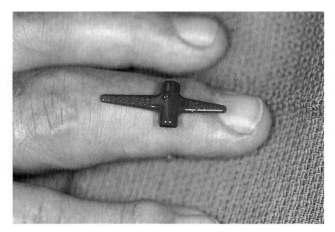

FIGURE 4.36. DIP joint implant arthroplasty is an option for patients that require exceptional mobility (e.g., musician).

and to increase the soft tissue stability. Failure to repair the extensor tendon can result in a swan-neck deformity (68). The skin is approximated with a 4-0 or 5-0 nonabsorbable interrupted suture.

Arthroplasty

Although the indications for arthroplasty are limited, silicone arthroplasty is an option for DIP joint arthritis (Fig. 4.36) (35,36). Tourniquet control is required and can be accomplished by an arm, forearm, or digital method. Anesthesia can be regional or digital block, depending on the patient, surgeon, and ancillary procedures performed at the time of DIP joint arthroplasty.

Joint Exposure

Similar to arthrodesis, multiple incisions have been described for dorsal DIP joint exposure and implant insertion. The incision must follow the same principles described for arthrodesis to avoid skin slough, wound problems, and injury to the germinal matrix. Full thickness skin flaps must be elevated from the epitenon to preserve vascularity. Hemostasis is obtained with a bipolar electrocautery. The terminal tendon is divided sharply 5 mm proximal to its insertion to expose the arthritic DIP joint. Dorsal osteophytes are removed with a rongeur to facilitate joint exposure.

Bony Preparation and Implant Insertion

The head of the middle phalanx is removed distal to the collateral ligament origin with a sagittal saw and osteotome. The saw blade must have a narrow kerf and small excursion to preserve the integrity of the collateral ligaments (36). Any angulatory deformity from uneven wear should be corrected by appropriate bone resection. The intramedullary canals of the middle and distal phalanx are opened with an awl. The canals are sequentially broached to accept the appropriately sized silicone implant. Side cutting burs are helpful in preparation of the medullary canals, but care must be taken to avoid penetration of the cortex. A trial implant is inserted to gauge motion and stability. The hinge portion should be flush with the bone ends and the stems seated within the medullary canals (31). Passive DIP joint motion should be smooth and unimpeded. Buckling of the implant indicates a mismatch between joint resection and implant volume. Additional bony resection and/or soft tissue release is required to accommodate the implant. Once the trial implant fit is acceptable, the definitive prosthesis is carefully inserted with smooth forceps to prevent damage to the implant.

Closure

The extensor tendon is repaired with a 4-0 or 5-0 suture. The DIP joint must be immobilized in full extension. A dorsal splint can be applied or a Kirschner wire can be inserted retrograde through the distal phalanx and into the palmar aspect of the flexor sheath (35). The K-wire must avoid piercing the implant, which would cause damage and particulate debris.

RESULTS/OUTCOMES FOR EACH TECHNIQUE

Mucous Cyst Excision

The initial surgical treatment for a mucous cyst was simple excision of the mass with a reported recurrence rate between 25% and 50% (29). The addition of osteophyte debridement along with cyst excision resulted in a marked decrease in the recurrence rate (29,32). Eaton reported on 45 patients (50 mucous cysts) treated by excision and debridement of osteophytes at the joint margin. There was only one recurrence and all preoperative nail deformities resolved within six months of surgery. No further diminution in DIP joint range of motion was noted.

Fritz et al. (32) reported on 86 mucous cyst excisions in 79 patients with an average follow-up of 2.6 years. The resolution rate was 97% with only 3 digits developing a recurrence. Preoperative nail deformities resolved in 15 out of 25 digits (60%). However, 4 digits developed a nail deformity that was not present prior to surgery. Additional problems included decreased range of motion (extension lag), persistent swelling, infection, numbness, and angulatory deformity.

Overall, mucous cyst excision and osteophyte debridement is an extremely efficacious procedure. However, the underlying joint arthritis may progress and additional treatment may be required.

Arthrodesis

The results following surgical procedures for arthrodesis are based on the success of fusion and rate of complication. A

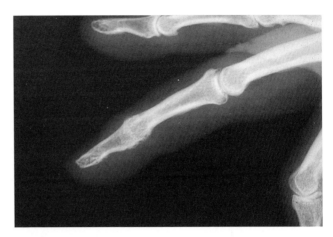

FIGURE 4.37. Lateral X-ray with crossing trabeculae indicative of successful fusion.

solid fusion is best defined by both clinical and x-ray criteria. Clinical union will always precede the radiological findings (33). A DIP joint that is not tender to firm pressure, not painful to stress, and stable is clinically united. An X-ray with trabeculae crossing the DIP joint is radiologically fused (Fig. 4.37) (42). The presence of both findings is designative of a successful arthrodesis. Many series report time to union, although this represents a "nebulous end point" (33).

Static Techniques

Multiple reports of static techniques for DIP joint fusion have been reported with varying efficacy. Moberg and Hendrickson (33) reported a series of digital arthrodesis performed using a square-sectioned bone graft harvested from the proximal ulna. Their study group included 150 arthrodeses with 21 cases of "distal joints." A few cases required supplemental Kirschner wire fixation to enhance stability. Seventeen cases healed by osseous union (81% union rate) and three by stable fibrous ankylosis. Potenza (50) used a corticocancellous bone dowel supplemented by Kirschner wire fixation in nine DIP joints. The dowel was harvested from the middle phalanx and inserted across the DIP joint along with three Kirschner wires. Union was achieved in all instances and immobilization was confined to only the DIP joint. However, there was no mention of extensor mechanism scarring or loss of PIP joint motion, which is likely after dowel harvest from the middle phalanx.

Lewis (47) used the tenon peg method supplemented by longitudinal Kirschner wire fixation for DIP joint arthrodesis. Union was accomplished in 40 out of 41 fingers (97% union rate). This technique requires extensive bone carpentry and can lead to digital shortening. However, shortening of the finger was not "excessive" in any case and not considered a problem.

Carroll and Hill (41) described the cup-and-cone technique for bone preparation secured by a single Kirschner wire in a large series of small joint arthrodesis. The DIP joint underwent fusion in 79 instances and successful arthrodesis was achieved in 72 (91%). An increased rate of pseudoarthrosis occurred in the spastic paralytic population.

McGlynn et al. (40) reported a series of arthrodeses in the hands of 76 patients (103 joints). The technique was a modified version described by Carroll and Hill (41). A dome-shaped middle phalanx and reciprocal distal phalanx were constructed using a high-speed bur. Internal fixation was obtained by a longitudinal and two crossing K-wires. The DIP joint comprised 14 cases and fusion was successful in all instances (100% union rate).

Burton et al. (42) reported on 171 consecutive small-joint arthrodesis in the hand. Bony preparation was performed by cutting parallel surfaces at the desired angle of fusion with an osteotome or power saw. Fixation was accomplished by crossed Kirschner wires and postoperative immobilization. Thirty-two cases of DIP joint fusion were included and all united (100% union rate). These authors stress the principles of small joint fusion, including minimal disruption of blood supply to the fusion site, accurate bony coaptation, circumferential cortical abutment, fusion site fixation, and external immobilization.

Watson and Shaffer (46) described a variation of the cup-and-cone technique to create concave-convex surfaces. Stabilization was accomplished with crossed Kirschner wires. Fifty-one patients who underwent 75 joint arthrodeses were reported. Thirty-four of the joints were interphalangeal without subcategory into specific level (DIP or PIP joint). All interphalangeal fusions united without complication. The author asserts this concentric fusion method is uncomplicated and provides a larger surface area for fusion with less digital shortening than the parallel cutting technique.

A limited number of studies have been reported using bioabsorbable implants in hand surgery. Jensen and Jensen (51) compared biodegradable PDS pins and Kirschner wire fixation for fractures, arthrodeses, and osteotomies in the hand. Fourteen patients underwent fusion of the MP or interphalangeal joints in the hand. Unfortunately, the specific joints fused are not detailed in their report. Five patients had biodegradable pin implantation and nine, K-wire fixation. Two biodegradable patients developed nonunions (60% union rate) as did two patients in the Kirschner wire group (78% union rate). The small numbers in this report prohibit definitive conclusions regarding the use of bioabsorbable implants.

Compression Techniques

Robertson (55) described the technique of "wire-loop fixation" for 64 interphalangeal joints in 52 patients. The DIP joint accounted for "most" of the cases and there were no failures. Lister (56) popularized the technique of interosseous wiring for arthrodesis in the digital skeleton. Twenty-eight DIP joint arthrodeses were included in his study and union

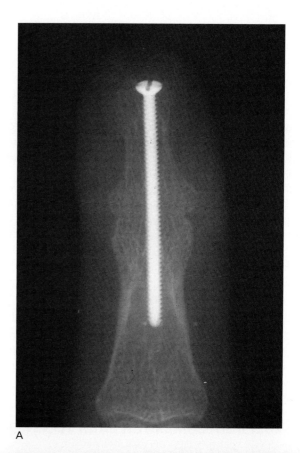

A

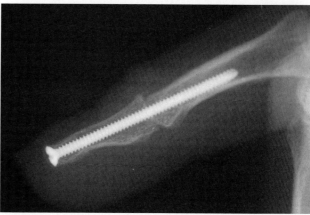

B

FIGURE 4.38. Anteroposterior and lateral X-rays of 60-year-old male depicted in Fig. 4.6 confirming solid DIP joint fusion with retrograde standard screw fixation.

was achieved in 25 (91% union rate). The three failures were attributed to premature accidental Kirschner wire removal. Lister (56) also noted a diminished composite digital motion with a mean of 167 degrees compared to a maximum attainable of 190 degrees.

Teoh et al. (58) reported standard screw insertion as an effective method for DIP joint arthrodesis (Fig. 4.38). A lag screw was used in 14 joints (eight thumb interphalangeal and six finger DIP joints) and union was achieved in all instances (100% union rate). There was one case of delayed union attributed to insufficient bone stock that healed after nine months. No fixation failures were reported although a slight bend of the screw was noted in a few instances.

Faithfull and Herbert (43) reported a series of fusions in the hand using the Herbert screw. Ten fusions involved the DIP joint and all united (100% union rate). No postoperative immobilization was used.

External fixation with dynamic compression has been reported in only a few series (65–67). Braun's series (65) included 19 interphalangeal joints of the thumb and fingers. All arthrodesis sites healed (100% union rate) without failure of fixation or angular deformity. The author cites multiple advantages of this technique including readily available materials in the operating room, ease of the procedure, wire removal accomplished in office, and compression fixation achieved. Tupper (66) reported on the use of an orthodontic traction device for external fixation across the DIP joint at the time of fusion. Twenty patients (23 joints) underwent this procedure with union obtained in 20 joints (87% union rate) with an average fusion time of 2.9 months. Wexler et al. (67) reported on the use of dynamic external compression using dorsoventral Kirschner wires and rubber bands in 46 joints, including nine DIP joints. Fusion was successful in 42 instances for an overall union rate of 91%.

Comparison Studies

Ijsselstein et al. (63) compared Kirschner wire fixation against tension band wire technique for small joint arthrodesis in the hand. Seventy-five cases of DIP joint fusion were included in their study population of 203 fusions. The Kirschner wire group included K-wire fixation alone and K-wire plus interosseous wiring. This group totaled 143 cases and 62 DIP joint fusions. The tension band fixation included 13 DIP joint fusions from a total of 60 cases. The results were reported for the whole study population and not subdivided for each joint. The incidence of repeat arthrodesis (15% versus 5%) and infection rate (18% versus 2%) were significantly higher in the K-wire group compared to the tension band population.

Stern and Fulton (69) reported on 139 patients who underwent 144 DIP and 37 thumb interphalangeal joint fusions. Techniques included crossed Kirschner wires (111 joints), interosseous wire and Kirschner wire (43 joints), and Herbert screw fixation (27 joints). The nonunion rates were similar in all groups (11% to 12%) and attributed more to the condition of the bone prior to surgery rather than the fixation technique.

Engel et al. (54) compared Kirschner wire and compression screw fixation for DIP joint arthrodesis in 30 consecutive patients. Compression screw fixation was used in 15 patients and inserted in either an antegrade or retrograde direction. Kirschner wires were placed in a crossed configuration in 15 patients. In each cohort, three cases of nonunion developed (80% union rate). The only notable difference was an earlier return to work in the compression screw fixation group, which was attributed to lack of immobilization.

Arthroplasty

There are limited follow-up studies after DIP joint arthroplasties (35,36). Brown (36) reported on 21 implants in 13 female patients with an average follow-up of 26 months. All patients achieved pain relief and the range of motion averaged 30 degrees with a 12-degree extensor lag. Zimmerman et al. (35) reported on 38 implants in 23 female patients followed for an average of six years. Osteoarthritis was the underlying process in 22 of the patients. All patients rated their pain as "much better" and motion averaged 33 degrees with a 13-degree extension lag. Only one implant was grossly unstable, but 12 joints demonstrated some increased laxity to lateral deviation.

In general, DIP joint arthroplasty offers retention of limited motion with a stable flexion arc of 30 degrees. Collateral ligament retention appears important to preserve lateral stability and prevent excessive wear of the implant. However, the long-term durability of these flexible implants remains questionable and no study has directly compared arthroplasty against arthrodesis (70–72).

REHABILITATION

Mucous Cyst Postoperative Regimen

The extent of postoperative immobilization varies with the skin condition, degree of extensor tendon mobilization, and extent of osteophyte debridement. A splint is applied across the DIP joint at the time of the procedure. Active PIP and MP joint motion is encouraged immediately after surgery. The dressings and sutures are removed 10 to 14 days after surgery. When there is adequate skin coverage and minimal debridement has been performed, unrestricted DIP joint motion is allowed. In contrast, tenuous skin coverage or extensive osteophyte debridement requires continued splint protection. Range of motion is almost always instituted by four weeks, although intermittent splinting can be continued for six weeks. Formal therapy is usually not necessary after uncomplicated cyst excision.

Arthrodesis Postoperative Regimen

The extent of postoperative immobilization varies with the rigidity of fixation. A splint is applied across the DIP joint at the time of the procedure. Active PIP and MP joint motion is encouraged immediately after surgery. Active motion is aimed at tendon gliding and restoration of joint motion. The splint and sutures are removed 10 to 14 days after surgery. Local wound care consisting of scar massage and desensitization is started after suture removal. The subsequent degree of immobilization varies with the fixation technique. A static fixation device (e.g., K-wires) usually requires continued external immobilization of the DIP joint until fusion is obtained. A compressive device (e.g., screw) provides sufficient rigid fixation to allow proximal finger joint motion without DIP splint immobilization.

Forceful grasp or resisted DIP flexion is postponed until bony consolidation is apparent on x-ray, usually six to eight weeks after surgery. Resistive exercises (e.g., putty fisting and flexion scraping) are initiated following successful fusion.

Arthroplasty Postoperative Regimen

Active PIP and MP joint motions are encouraged immediately after surgery. The splint and sutures are removed 10 to 14 days after surgery. The DIP joint is immobilized for six to eight weeks in extension. Supervised therapy is then prescribed with a gradual increase in active DIP flexion. DIP joint blocking exercises to isolate the flexor digitorum profundus action are emphasized (39). Additional modalities include edema reduction techniques, scar desensitization, and tendon gliding. A DIP joint splint in full extension is applied between exercises until 10 weeks from surgery. Resistive exercises (e.g., putty fisting and flexion scraping) are initiated at that time. Nighttime splinting is continued through the third and fourth postoperative months.

Following DIP joint arthroplasty, lateral pinch against the effected distal phalanx should be avoided (31). The patient should be instructed to either shift lateral pinch to a nonoperated digit, pinch opposing the middle phalanx, or pinch against all the fingers simultaneously for lateral support.

COMPLICATIONS

Complications will occur from DIP joint surgery. Many complications can be traced to the preoperative condition of the digit(s). The principle factors that regulate the incidence of complications are the status of the soft tissue and bone. Adherence to the established principles for soft tissue handling, the tenets of bony preparation (resection, coaptation, alignment), and the conditions necessary for bony healing (immobilization) will maximize the outcome and minimize difficulties. Failure to comply with these principles or disregard for the soft tissue envelope will increase the complication rate.

Stern and Fulton (69) divided DIP joint arthrodesis complications into major and minor groups (Table 4.1). Major problems were defined as problems that had a negative effect on outcome and occurred in 20%. Minor complications had no long-term sequelae and occurred in 16%.

TABLE 4.1. COMPLICATIONS FROM DIP JOINT ARTHRODESIS

Major	Minor
Nonunion	Dorsal skin necrosis
Malunion	Cold intolerance
Deep infection	PIP joint stiffness
Osteomyelitis	Paresthesias
	Superficial wound infection
	Prominent hardware

Adapted from Stern PJ, Fulton DB. Distal interphalangeal joint arthrodesis: an analysis of complications. *J Hand Surg [Am]* 1992;17:1139–1145, with permission.

Soft Tissue

Soft tissue complications can involve the nail, extensor mechanism, and integument. The germinal nail matrix is in close proximity to the DIP joint (1 mm distal to extensor tendon insertion) and can be affected by a mucous cyst, surgical dissection, or prominent hardware (especially tension band fixation) (31). Fritz et al. (32) reported the postoperative development of a nail deformity following mucous cyst excision, presumably from incautious dissection. A screw inserted dorsal in the distal phalanx can also disturb the sterile and/or germinal nail matrix. Wyrsch et al. (59) studied Herbert screw fixation in a cadaver model for DIP arthrodesis. The average palmar to dorsal height of the distal phalanx (3.55 mm) was less than the trailing thread diameter (3.9 mm) of the Herbert screw. The trailing threads penetrated the dorsal cortex in 10 of 15 male fingers and all 15 female digits. This cortical violation can lead to a delayed nail bed deformity.

Wound dehiscence can range from a minor incisional separation to an entire skin slough. Atraumatic handling of the tissues at the time of surgery will minimize wound difficulties. Local care is usually adequate for small areas of breakdown while complete wound dehiscence requires debridement of all nonviable tissue and secondary coverage. Fritz et al. (32) reported dorsal skin necrosis in 4% (4 of 181 joints) and all resolved with local wound care. Prolonged fingertip sensitivity or paresthesias can also occur and is related to the technique, dissection, and fixation device (52). The finger pulp can remain sensitive after placement of fixation devices through the fingertip and a residual area of numbness can result. A prominent screw head or fibrous scarring around Kirschner wires can also be precipitating causes.

The extensor mechanism can be altered by DIP joint fusion surgery. Failure to repair the extensor mechanism after arthrodesis can cause a force imbalance across the PIP joint with subsequent swan-neck deformity (68). Scarring of the extensor apparatus can limit PIP joint motion. Lister (56) reported a diminished composite motion after DIP joint fusion with a mean of 167 degrees compared to a maximum attainable of 190 degrees. Stern and Fulton (69) noted stiffness in 5% (5 of 181 fingers) and all occurred following Kirschner wire fixation. Immediate postoperative active motion of the MP and PIP joints is the mainstay of prevention. Early stiffness requires therapy with treatment aimed at edema reduction, tendon gliding, and PIP joint mobilization. Established stiffness is very difficult to treat and may result from extrinsic tendon adhesions and/or intrinsic PIP joint problems.

Infection

Infection can either be either a superficial cellulitis or deep seeded. Pin track infections are common after percutaneous K-wire fixation, occurring in 18% in one series (63). Instability and skin movements around pins promote inflammatory soft tissue reactions that can become infected (73). Superficial pin tract infections often respond to local wound care and antibiotics (69). Deep infections can result in nonunion, progress to osteomyelitis, and even systemic complications from hematogenous spread. Aggressive management of deep infections with multiple debridements and intravenous antibiotics is necessary to salvage the finger.

Bone and Joint

Bony complications are related to the bone quality and technique. Deficient bone stock can be secondary to resorptive arthropathy, trauma, or previous infection. The bony deficit must be addressed at the time of fusion with supplemental bone graft (42). Failure to address these issues will increase the incidence of nonunion, which has been defined as absent crossing trabecular bone six months following surgery (69). Other causes of nonunion include insufficient bone resection, technical error, premature pin removal, and infection (55,69).

Malunion can also occur from a DIP joint fused in poor position at the time of the primary procedure. Malunion has been defined as fusion greater than 35 degrees of flexion, coronal angulation greater than 5 degrees, or malrotation (69). Treatment of an established malunion depends upon the functional impairment. Corrective osteotomy is reserved for malposition that interferes with function (67).

Shortening of the digit can occur following arthrodesis. A mild reduction in digital length is inconsequential and expected during joint resection. A preoperative coronal deformity often requires more aggressive bony resection to realign the finger and may increase the amount of shortening. When extensive bone resection is required or considerable bone resorption is present, corticocancellous inlay grafting is preferred to avert substantial digital shortening.

Hardware

Hardware complications can occur from inaccurate placement of the internal fixation device, which can act as a cata-lyst for further complications. A wire or screw can violate the cortical bone, impale soft tissues, or disrupt the nail matrix (67). This misdirected internal fixation can cause nail plate deformities and increase the incidence of nonunion secondary to suboptimal fixation.

Premature Kirschner wire removal is another hardware complication associated with arthrodesis. A protruding K-wire can accidentally snare on clothing and be removed from the digit. Lister reported three failures of DIP joint fusions attributed to premature accidental Kirschner wire extraction (56). Careful pin protection is required to prevent this avoidable complication. Hardware prominence is a potential problem after screw insertion across the DIP joint. The screw can be protruding from the tip of the finger or outside the confines of the medullary canal. Tip prominence can lead to finger pad hypersensitivity and may require removal while violation of the cortex can irritate the nail bed or surrounding soft tissues (tendons or skin).

Biodegradable pins can incite an inflammatory foreign body reaction resulting in osteolysis and sinus formation. This complication is more common with implants manufactured from polyglycolide than the slower absorbing PDS polymer (64). This complication occurs during the degradation of the polymer about three months after insertion. The patient presents with fluctuant swelling at the implantation site, which represents an accumulation of the liquid remnants of the degrading implant. Histologic analysis reveals an inflammatory response with an abundance of macrophages phagocytosing the implant particles. Treatment requires prompt drainage to prevent secondary infection.

Implant failure is uncommon after DIP joint arthrodesis. Biomechanical test data has evaluated the stiffness and strength of a variety of internal fixation devices. Wyrsch et al. (59) compared Kirschner wire fixation and Herbert screw fixation in a cadaver model. The Herbert screw demonstrated superior strength and torsional rigidity in anteroposterior bending and axial torsion testing. Breibart et al. (53) employed an *in vivo* rabbit model to compare compression clamp arthrodesis with crossed Kirschner wire fixation and tension band wiring. At two-week testing, the compression group was stiffer and possessed a higher load to failure in extension. In contrast, the flexion failure data favored the tension band group with respect to load, stiffness, and energy to failure. Mechanical testing of the arthrodesis site was performed after hardware removal at eight weeks and equivalent values in load, stiffness, displacement, and energy to failure were obtained in both groups.

Implant

Complications specific to silicone implants for DIP arthritis are implant fracture, instability, and silicone synovitis. Implant failure is a major concern, which could result in particulate synovitis and bone erosion. At this time, the limited number of studies and duration of follow-up preclude

65. Braun RM. Dynamic compression for small bone arthrodesis. *J Hand Surg [Am]* 1985;10:340–343.

66. Tupper JW. A compression arthrodesis device for small joints of the hands. *Hand* 1972;4:62–64.

67. Wexler MR, Rousso M, Weinberg H. Arthrodesis of finger joints by dynamic external compression using dorsoventral Kirschner wires and rubber bands. *Plast Reconstr Surg* 1977;60:882–885.

68. Beltran JE. A complication of distal interphalangeal joint arthrodesis. *Hand* 1976;8:36–38.

69. Stern PJ, Fulton DB. Distal interphalangeal joint arthrodesis: an analysis of complications. *J Hand Surg [Am]* 1992;17:1139–1145.

70. Kozin SH. Arthroplasty of the hand and wrist. *J Hand Ther* 1999; 12:123–132.

71. Murray PM. The results of treatment of synovitis of the wrist induced by particles of silicone debris. *J Bone Joint Surg [Am]* 1998; 80:397–406.

72. Hirakawa K. Isolation and quantitation of debris particles around failed silicone orthopedic implants. *J Hand Surg [Am]* 1996;21: 819–827.

73. Branemark PI, Albrektsson T. Titanium implants permanently penetrating human skin. *Scand J Plast Reconstr Surg* 1982;16:17–21.

5

PROXIMAL INTERPHALANGEAL JOINT

MICHAEL SAUERBIER AND RONALD L. LINSCHEID

HISTORICAL PERSPECTIVE

The mobility of the fingers is very important to achieve a sufficient grasp of the hand. It is the hand surgeon's aim to restore or preserve motion as much as possible in the diseased or injured hand. Loss of motion in the PIP joint caused from arthrosis, however, eliminates the ability to make a tight fist. Osteoarthrosis, posttraumatic arthrosis, and rheumatoid arthritis can all affect the PIP joint and lead to a painful joint with loss of motion and grip strength.

The proximal interphalangeal joint (PIP) is a bicondylar diarthrodial hinge-like joint that normally has a range of motion (ROM) of 0 to 100 degrees with individual variations both in increased and decreased motion, depending on the patient's body type and other factors. Littler (1) has suggested that an equiangular spiral is produced by the tip of the finger as it sweeps through its normal flexion arc from full extension to full flexion and that 34% of the arc is accounted for by the proximal interphalangeal joint. The joint is considered a pin-axis joint. It has 1 degree of freedom, with constraints to rotation and radial-ulnar deviation; only a few degrees of motion are allowed in the frontal or coronal planes as accommodation to externally applied forces. During normal grasping, the closing motions of the metacarpophalangeal, proximal interphalangeal, and distal interphalangeal joints are virtually synchronous. During manipulative functions, the PIP and DIP joint motions are often desynchronous or reciprocal to the direction of angulation of the metacarpophalangeal joint.

The stability of this joint is based primarily on the bicondylar geometric configuration and the collateral ligaments, with secondary support from the lateral bands of the extensor system, the transverse and oblique retinacula, the digital fascia, and the soft tissue envelope (2–4). The lateral capsular structures surrounding the PIP joint are tight. The capsule is rather thin dorsally to accommodate the considerable amount of flexion of which the joint is capable. It is reinforced by the central slip, which is an integral part of the dorsal portion of the capsule. It inserts into the dorsal tubercle at the base of the middle phalanx. The collateral ligaments on either side of the joint are nearly symmetrical and consist of two parts. The first is the phalangophalangeal ligament, which arises from the dorsolateral tubercle on the head of the

proximal phalanx and attaches to the palmar lateral tubercle of the base of the middle phalanx. The ligament is taut on both sides throughout any position of the PIP joint but most taut at 0–15°. The second is the ligamentous stabilizer, the phalangoglenoidal ligament or accessory collateral ligament, which arises just proximal and palmar to the aforementioned ligament and inserts onto the palmar plate and annular ligament of the flexor tendon sheath. The sheath helps to hold the flexor tendons in close approximation to the undersurface of the joint so that the flexor moment arm does not vary appreciably during the complete flexion-extension cycle with reference to the center of rotation in the proximal phalangeal head.

Secondary stabilization of the PIP joint is obtained through the contributions of (a) the lateral bands of the extensor mechanisms that migrate in a lateral palmar direction over the sloping shoulders of the proximal phalangeal head during proximal interphalangeal joint flexion, (b) the transverse retinacular system, which helps to restrain the motion of the lateral bands, and (c) the digital fascia and overlying skin (3–5).

Pain, weakness, malalignment, and loss of motion can have a debilitative effect on hand function and joint motion to the point that surgical treatment is needed. Although conservative treatment with medication, physiotherapy and splinting and operative procedures such as synovectomy and debridement may help occasionally, arthrodesis and arthroplasty of the PIP joint are the definitive surgical options.

The alternatives for the arthrotic PIP joint depend on the severity of symptoms, the nature of deformity, the "patient's" personal profile, and the particular finger involved. As an example, fusion of the index PIP often is well-tolerated, but in the fourth finger, the quadregia effect from the incomplete separation of the origin of the profundi to the three ulnar fingers can reduce motion of the fingers adjacent to the involved digit (5).

INDICATIONS/CONTRAINDICATIONS

Conservative treatment of arthrosis or rheumatoid arthritis of the PIP joint has been limited to the use of systemic anti-inflammatory agents, splinting, and occasionally intra-articular steroid injections (5,6). These measures give limited symptomatic pain relief, but many patients have further progression of their symptoms, often until joint autoankylosis limits motion and relieves pain a little.

The general indications for fusion of any joint are pain, instability, deformity, and loss of associated neuromuscular control. Arthrodesis of the PIP joint is an accepted and well-tolerated procedure and can be used in patients with a traumatic unstable destroyed joint, posttraumatic arthrosis, degenerative osteoarthrosis, and rheumatoid arthritis (7–10).

Arthroplasty of the PIP joint is a well-known and attractive alternative option for hand surgeons dealing with that joint (11–15). It should ideally relieve pain, provide stability, and allow a normal range of motion of the joint. Arthroplasty can be indicated in posttraumatic arthrosis, degenerative joint disease, and rheumatoid arthritis. These diseases present with morphologic differences. Posttraumatic arthrosis and degenerative arthrosis are more likely to present as single problems at the PIP. Displacement and contracture from joint erosion is mostly limited, the cortical thickness is usually well-preserved, and the peri-articular soft tissue complex is largely intact. Rheumatoid arthritis leads into attenuation of the capsular and tendinous constraints and osteolysis and destruction in multiple joints. The progression of the disease leads to secondary displacement and soft tissue attenuation with imbalance at proximal and distal joints. Rheumatoid arthritis and degenerative arthrosis in the PIP joint (Bouchard's arthrosis) are more common in women; however, posttraumatic arthrosis is increasing in women as well as in men as a result of increasing numbers of athletic injuries. Nevertheless, angulation, pain, and limited motion impose severe functional restrictions on the hand.

PREOPERATIVE PLANNING

The decision for performing a PIP joint fusion, a joint arthroplasty, or another treatment option should be made in the office after the examination of the patient. The patient's expectations and needs have to be respected. When choosing a PIP joint fusion the position most appropriate for the particular finger and needs of the patient has to be achieved. Thirty-five to 45 degrees of flexion is optimal for most patients. Radial and ulnar angulation must be avoided.

There are numerous techniques for fusion of the PIP joint or for PIP joint arthroplasties. Those currently considered most reasonable and successful as well as our preferred methods of treatment will be discussed in this article.

TECHNIQUES

PIP Joint Arthrodesis

There are many techniques described for the operative treatment of the arthrotic PIP joint, each with its proponents and

applications. Fixation techniques of the PIP joint described in the literature include a single Kirschner wire, crossed Kirschner wires, intraosseous wiring, mini-plate fixation, compression clamping, tension band wiring, screw fixation, and others (7–10,16). PIP joint arthrodesis has remained an effective and often used option for treating diseased or damaged digital joints of the hand. It provides stability, relieves pain, corrects deformity of the joint, and can restore function provided that motion is present in adjacent joints and the fusion is in a proper position.

Interosseus wiring is recommended for patients with posttraumatic or osteoarthrosis of the PIP joint, but proper alignment of the bone ends is critical (9). The bone ends can be prepared by flat resection of the joint surfaces or with the "cup-and-cone" technique. Holes are drilled 2 to 3 mm proximal and distal from both bone ends with a 0.8-mm Kirschner wire through which a 0.6-mm stainless steel wire cerclage is passed in a single adaptation. One or two 1.0-mm K-wires directed in dorsal palmar directions should be used to achieve additional fixation. The 90-90 loop is also a popular option for fusion.

In patients with rheumatoid arthritis these techniques must be used with caution to avoid the tension in the wires from cutting through the osteopenic bone (6).

Another popular option of treatment is tension band wiring (Fig. 5.1) (7). Its compression is well-known. It can be used for arthrodesis of the PIP joint and the MP and DIP joint as well. It is also a useful option in the treatment of large fragments of mallet fingers.

For this technique the articular surfaces are resected with a power saw at the appropriate 35- and 40-degree angle. Five mm distal to the base of the middle phalanx of the finger a transverse hole is drilled with a 0.8-mm K-wire. A 0.6-mm stainless steel gauge is inserted through the hole. Then 2 par-

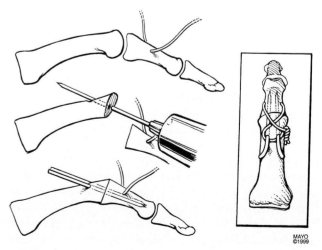

FIGURE 5.1. Schematic drawing of a PIP joint arthrodesis with tension-band wiring.

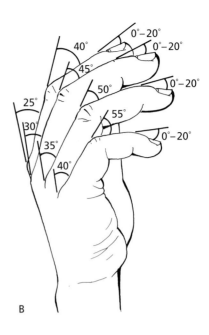

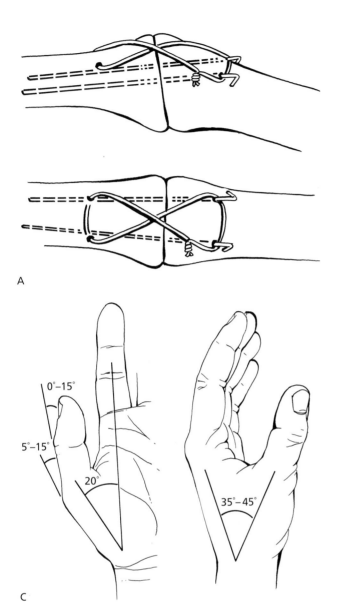

FIGURE 5.2. An illustration detailing the correct placement of the K-wires and tension band wire (**A**). Optimal angles of joint fusion increase as one moves toward the ulnar digits (**B**). Fusion of thumb joints requires a 3-dimensional placement (**C**).

allel K-wires (1.0 mm) are drilled retrograde from the center of the anterior surface through the dorsal cortex of the proximal phalanx and then forwarded into the middle phalanx after reduction of the fusion site. After that, the gauge stainless steel wire is criss-crossed over the joint in a figure-eight fashion and passed around both protruding Kirschner wires. The wire is pulled tight to achieve rigid fixation, compression, lie flat on the bone to avoid irritation of the extensor mechanism, and to achieve the correct amount of flexion in the fused PIP joint (Fig. 5.2). The Kirschner wires should also lie flat on the bone after they are bent (Fig. 5.3). Percutaneous pinning is not recommended in this procedure. Other reliable options can be interfragmentary compression techniques with AO screws or PIP joint arthrodesis with a Herbert screw using a free-hand technique (16). Fusion with a

dorsal mini-plate as described by Büchler and Aiken is a safe technique for procedures immediately after trauma if there is minimal soft tissue damage (10). It also can be used for arthrodesis following arthrosis and has the advantage of immediate postoperative motion because of the highly stable osteosynthesis. An external fixator can also be used immediately after trauma to avoid further soft tissue damage.

Bone grafting is seldom needed for PIP joint arthrodesis unless indicated for a significant loss of bone after trauma, infections, tumor resections, failed fusions, or failed arthroplasties. For small loss of bone, grafting of bone from the distal radius is appropriate. Implantation of a corticocancellous strut can be used to bridge extensive defects. A compound island joint transfer is reserved for significant loss of bone after trauma (17,18).

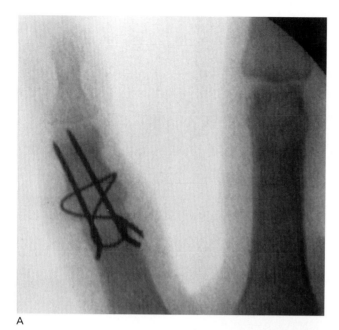

A

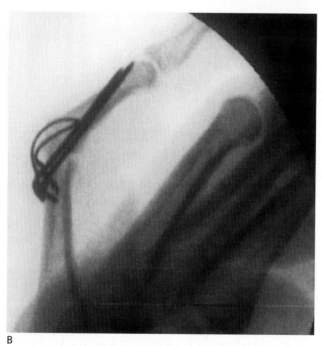

B

FIGURE 5.3. Intraoperative anteroposterior **(A)** and lateral **(B)** x-rays of a PIP joint fusion with tension-band wiring.

Joint Arthroplasties, Total Joint Replacement

Various arthroplastic techniques are available in degenerative and traumatic arthrosis as well as rheumatoid arthritis joint replacement. Resurfacing of destroyed joints with perichondral grafts has been described (19), but the durability of the remodeled joint has been disappointing. Fibrous ingrowth or

fibrous interposition was initially described by Carroll and Taber (11). Palmar plate advancement was first described by Eaton in 1980 (20,21). The Carroll-Taber arthroplasty resects the head proximal to the neck of the proximal phalanx through a lateral approach (11). The indications for this procedure have been largely superseded by insertion of an elastomer spacer.

Silicone replacements (15) are still currently popular, but there is increasing interest in total joint prostheses. The Swanson silicone elastomer arthroplasty has been used for painful, degenerative, or posttraumatic destruction of the PIP joint as well as stiffness that cannot be corrected with soft tissue reconstruction alone. Adequate bone stock, soft tissue coverage, and muscle/tendon balance with an intact extensor tendon apparatus are necessary for the success of this procedure. A newer PIP joint silicone implant, based on the NeuFlex metacarpophalangeal joint design from DePuy (Warsaw, Indiana), has just been released designed with finite element analysis to improve functional range of motion and decrease breakage. These types of advances in joint design may significantly improve silicone joint replacement longevity. Such procedures are preferred for isolated disability of one PIP joint.

A C-shaped incision performed over the dorsum of the PIP joint avoids contact of the skin sutures with the tendon repair. If flexor tendon surgery is also necessary, a mid-lateral or palmar incision is used. The exposure of the joint is made between the lateral band and central tendon on both sides of the joint. The collateral ligaments and the palmar plate are released proximally to allow dislocation of the joint laterally. The head of the proximal phalanx is resected at the metaphyseal flare and hypertrophic spurs are removed from the base of the middle phalanx. After reaming the medullary canals of the proximal and the middle phalanges, the largest feasible size implant is used. To permit reattachment of the collateral ligaments, 4-0 sutures are placed through drill holes in the proximal phalanx. The sutures are placed before implant insertion. The incisions between the lateral bands are sutured to the central tendon of the extensor apparatus. After closure of the skin, a hand dressing is applied and the finger carefully aligned to protect the collateral ligaments and especially to prevent ulnar angulation. Alternatively, a palmar approach to the PIP joint for silicone arthroplasty may be performed (Fig. 5.4).

Despite the improvements in small-joint arthroplasty there is some frustration in not being able to match the success that is obtainable in large-joint implants. Silastic joint spacers have provided a means of treatment for painful degenerative arthrosis and rheumatoid arthritis of the PIP joint, but are criticized because of limited range of motion and instability. These deformable implants depend for their stability solely on the integrity of the surrounding soft tissue. In the long-term, problems associated with component loosening and breakage have tempered enthusiasm for their use (22,23).

The development of an efficacious design for the PIP joint on the principle of total joint design has been difficult largely

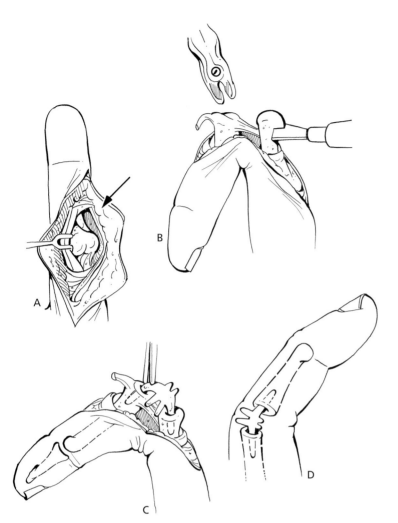

FIGURE 5.4. Following a Bruner incision over the palmar PIP joint, the palmar plate is elevated exposing the PIP joint (**A**). The head of the proximal phalanx is resected by a saw, and any osteophytes at the base of the middle phalanx are removed by a ronguer (**B**). With the PIP joint hyperextended, a PIP silicone joint implant is inserted (**C**). The joint is reduced and the soft tissues closed providing a stable construct (**D**).

because of the problems with stability as mentioned above (24). There have been a number of constrained and semiconstrained designs. These have been used in relatively small series primarily by their originators (12,25). The senior author of this article (R.L.L.) has developed a surface replacement prosthesis based on a series of anatomical, biomechanical, and histologic evaluations of the normal geometry of the articular surfaces of the PIP joint (Fig. 5.5) (5,24,26). The assumption was that an unconstrained surface replacement would simulate a physiologic articulation, and if performed with preservation of the collateral ligaments would provide lateral stability for the PIP joint. It was felt the minimal constraint would divert lateral forces and axial torques from the stem endosteal interface to the capsule and cortex so as to diminish the mechanical contribution to osteolysis and subsidence at the bone prosthesis interface. Also a centered rotational axis should provide balanced tendon moment arms to ensure a functional range of motion. The components of this prosthesis (Avanta™, San Diego, CA, USA) are designed to be either press fit or cemented in place. The proximal component is a cast chromium cobalt alloy composed of a polished articular surface and a shot-blasted stem. The articular surface is semicircular in the sagittal plane and chevron-shaped in the frontal plane. The distal component has a UHMWPE articular surface affixed to a titanium base and stem. The form

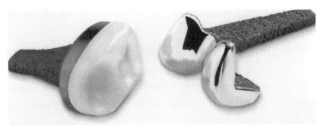

FIGURE 5.5. Surface replacement arthroplasty components for the proximal interphalangeal joint (Figures 5.5–5.8 and 5.10 are courtesy of Avanta Orthopedics, San Diego, CA).

For preoperative planning, transparent templates can be used to measure the implant size on posterior-anterior and lateral x-rays of the involved finger.

As a surgical approach we prefer a dorsal curvilinear incision centered over the PIP joint, but an ulnar mid-lateral or a palmar approach are options. The dorsal approach allows the easiest orientation by providing a wide exposure of the extensor mechanism and PIP joint. The extensor apparatus is incised to either side of the central slip for 1.5 cm. A modified distally based flap originally described by Chamay in 1988 (27) preserves the attachment of the central slip (Fig. 5.6). The articular surfaces of the head of the proximal phalanx and base of the middle phalanx have to be removed with a power saw preserving the capsuloligamentous structures in so far as possible (Fig. 5.7). The intramedullary cavities are opened first with a series of progressively larger awls. Rasps

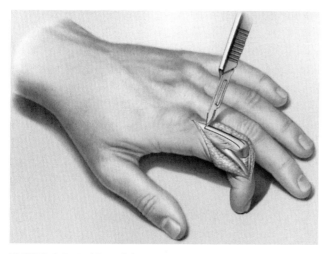

FIGURE 5.6. Incision of the extensor mechanism in a manner of a distally based modified "Chamay-flap" while preserving distal attachment of the central slip.

is highly congruent to the proximal articular surface. The stems in cross-section are flattened palmarly and arched dorsally to simulate the contours of the endosteal surfaces, and are slightly curved longitudinally to match the curvature of the medullary canal. The prosthesis kit comes with paired components in extra small, small, medium, and large sizes.

The indications and the criteria for implantation of this prothesis are similar to those for implantation of a silicone prosthesis. Ideally the surrounding soft tissue of the joint should be intact, the extensor and flexor tendon apparatus functioning, and the collateral ligaments intact. It should be noted that the clinical experience of this implant outside of the author's institution is extremely limited, and the wider acceptance of this device remains to be seen.

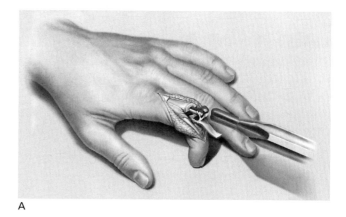

A

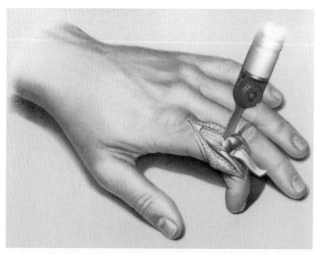

FIGURE 5.7. With a small powered saw a transverse osteotomy is carried out to remove the distal 2 and 3 mm of the proximal phalanx. The collateral ligaments are protected as much as possible.

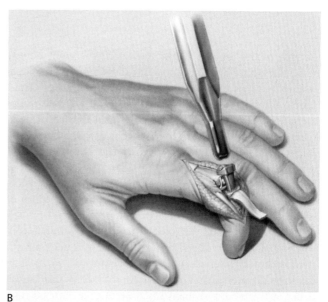

B

FIGURE 5.8. After removing of the trial components, injection of cement (PMMA) into the medullary canals is performed through a shortened # 14 Intracath. The proximal (**A**) and middle phalanx (**B**) components are implanted and seated with an impactor.

sized to the prosthetic stems are then used to prepare the intramedullary cavities. The final adjustments are made with a power bur.

Each trial component is inserted to check for proper alignment and orientation. Adjustments are made as necessary. When both components fit properly, the joint is reduced. Free flexion from 0–90° should be possible. The joint is checked for lateral stability. When satisfied the trials are removed and the permanent components inserted. If a press fit is selected each component is seated by applying the impactor and tapping the joint into place.

If cement fixation is selected, the cement (Polymethyl methacrylate; Simplex, Howmedica, Rutherford, NJ) is injected using a syringe through a size 14 Intracath catheter (BD Vascular Accessories, Sandy, UT).

After injection of cement into the medullary canals the components are implanted and firmly seated with the impactor (Fig. 5.8). Afterwards, reduction of the joint is necessary, and it should be held until the cement has set. When satisfactory fit of the implanted prosthesis is obtained, the finger is moved until a functional passive ROM is achieved. After wound irrigation with cool saline, excess cement must be removed. X-rays are obtained to verify component placement and to identify extruded cement before closing the layers.

If sufficient joint capsule is present dorsally, it may be closed as a separate layer with 3-0 multiple filament suture. The extensor mechanism is repaired with nonabsorbable suture material and the skin closure performed.

RESULTS / OUTCOMES FOR EACH TECHNIQUE

PIP Joint Arthrodesis

PIP joint fusions are not without complications. From the surgeons point of view they should not be approached as easy operations. Complications such as nonunion, rotational malunion, infection, or osteomyelitis can occur frequently. A common problem is postoperative pin tract infection if the K-wires are not buried underneath the skin. Pseudoarthrosis rates after PIP joint fusions by several techniques are reported from 0% to 12% (28).

Proximal Interphalangeal Surface Replacement Arthroplasty

Linscheid has experience over a 20-year period with PIP surface replacements in 60 patients (5,14,26,29). Eighty-two PIP surface replacement proximal interphalangeal (SR-PIP) prostheses were used. The average age of the patients was 60 years, follow-up averaged 6 years. Surgical indications were degenerative arthrosis in 44 (Fig. 5.9), posttraumatic arthrosis in 24, and rheumatoid arthritis in 14 fingers. Average duration of complaint was six years. All patients complained of pain, deformity, or limited motion. Preoperative range of motion was from 15° hypoextension to 95° flexion with an average of 35°. The static deformities included swan neck in

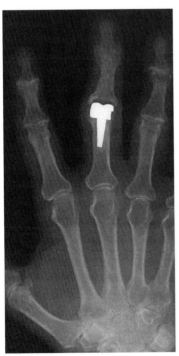
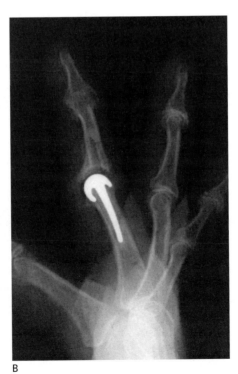

A   B

FIGURE 5.9. Patient anteroposterior (**A**) and lateral (**B**) x-rays with a surface replacement arthroplasty at the PIP joint of the right middle finger at five-year follow-up (forms prosthesis with distal component completely made out of UHMWPE).

eight, boutonniere deformities in five, and lateral deviations from 10° to 35° in 23 fingers. Seventy-eight of the original 82 joints were followed up for a minimum of two years—the average was 60 months. Sixty joints were without pain. In 8 PIP joints mild aching and in another 8 discomfort with activity was seen. Of the 23 fingers with 10° or more deviation preoperatively, only 4 were deviated that far postoperatively. The average range of motion reached 14° of hypoextension to 90° of flexion with an arc of 47°. The late results mirrored the preoperative status in that fingers with a swanneck tendency were more likely to have some residual hyperextension and a flexion deficit while fingers with preoperative extension deficits were likely to have persistent extension deficits postoperatively.

The results were separated in good, fair, and poor. Overall 40 patients had a good result, 22 a fair result, and only 18 patients a poor outcome (29).

Condamine et al. used a prosthesis of similar principle for both the MP and PIP joints (12,25). The implant is a semiconstrained sliding arthroplasty. Their results were satisfactory with an improved range of motion, a complete anteroposterior stability, and a good stem fixation. The best results were achieved in patients with posttraumatic degeneration of the PIP joint. Sixty percent of their patients were pain-free, and 40% presented occasional slight pain. Stem loosening occurred only in rheumatoid arthritis patients. For overall assessments their results were good or very good in 75% of the patients.

PIP Joint Silicone Arthroplasty

Two- and three-year follow-up of early silicone implants revealed a significant incidence of loosening and fracture. In response to this, the implants were strengthened and the technique adjusted to diminish the occurrence of these complications.

In addition, cemented implants have been developed with a fixed-fulcrum prosthesis in an attempt to improve the overall results.

REHABILITATION

Following PIP joint fusion, immobilization for six weeks is recommended by most of the authors. Early active motion of the MP and DIP joint can be started on the second day after surgery with the support of a hand therapist. The fixation material can be left in place or be removed after solid bony union is achieved.

After replacement arthroplasty the PIP joints are held firmly in neutral to 10° flexion. Gentle DIP motions are begun immediately to encourage lateral band excursion. Active PIP motions are allowed with a special splint (Fig. 5.10). Gentle motion at 10°–20° may commence in the first week if optimal extensor repair was obtained and as long as complete

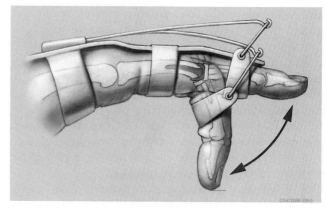

FIGURE 5.10. Exercises and splinting of the joints may begin early. A dynamic splint is often helpful in the early phases of rehabilitation. This should prevent hyperextension at the PIP joint with a static extension block, but provide an elastic sling to help return the finger to neutral after the joint has been flexed.

extension is obtained. The finger is splinted in full extension during rest and is supported by dynamic extension assistance during exercise periods if extension is incomplete.

COMPLICATIONS

The various complications of PIP joint fusions have been addressed in this article previously.

Complications after PIP surface replacement arthroplasty tended to reflect the preoperative status. Instability as shown by subluxation or angulation recurred in seven joints, each of which had a poor result. Implant loosening could be observed after a late postoperative fracture of a proximal phalanx in one patient and in the index and midfinger proximal components after two years in a patient with severe degenerative arthrosis. In two fingers a lag of extension of 50° with unstable boutonniere deformities was observed, and all eight fingers had extension lags of 45° in otherwise stable joints. Seven of the poor results were from fingers with stiffness in extension. An isolated rheumatoid finger with a fair result originally worsened with disintegration of the central slip over a year.

Twelve secondary operative procedures were performed in eleven fingers, including extensor tenolysis, radial collateral ligament reconstruction, and realignment of a proximal component. After five or more years' duration mild hypertrophic bone growth was seen around the head of the proximal component in some X-rays.

At the authors' institution, results of silicone implants were unsatisfactory because of loosening, periosteal bone formation and recurrence of deformity through plastic deformation of the polyethylene component (30). Our experience is quite similar to that reported by Pelligrini and Burton in 1990 (31).

Complications in general after total joint arthroplasty can include reflex sympathetic dystrophy, infection related to skin necrosis, stem loosening, dislocation of the device, joint capsular contractures, and tendon adhesions.

Total joint arthroplasties of the hand have a poorer record than those in the large joints of extremities. This is related to a variety of problems inherent to the hand, including joints situated within a complex kinetic chain, multiple parallel rays, and small size. Simulation of normal kinematics requires restoration of an anatomic joint including its capsuloligamentous supports. The ideal PIP joint replacement is not yet available; however, some progress has been made in this field over the past several years. Although our reported results are varied, it is worth noting that the severity of the problems was sometimes marked and that the indications for arthroplasty in many cases could be considered as salvage procedures. Even in some patients with limited movement, pain relief was satisfactory.

The best results can be expected in traumatic and degenerative arthrosis. Our results have shown little tendency to deteriorate over time, as has been noted in some other arthroplasties. With experience our confidence in the procedure has increased.

SALVAGE PROCEDURES

Splinting

Extended cast immobilization or splinting can be useful if delayed union after PIP joint fusion occurs.

Splinting can also be extended occasionally beyond six weeks if extension lags of 30° or more develop after surface replacement arthroplasty.

Revision

Secondary operations after surface replacement arthroplasty can include extensor plication for extension lag, lateral collateral ligament reconstruction, tenolysis of the extensor apparatus for extension deficit, and joint capsule contracture release.

Silastic Arthroplasty

If sufficient cortical bone is present following excision of a total joint, salvage of some motion may be obtained by converting to a silicone arthroplasty.

Arthrodesis Intercalated Bone Graft

If persistent nonunion after PIP joint fusion occurs, re-arthrodesis is indicated. To have adequate length of the particular finger, an intercalated bone graft from the radius or the iliac crest is a worthwhile option. This technique is also necessary after failed surface replacement or other arthroplasties with multiple prior operative procedures.

Amputation

Amputation can be a salvage procedure if persistent infection occurs. It is considered as an "ultima ratio" or last line of defense for swollen, painful, and useless fingers and can be performed as disarticulation at the PIP joint or, for a more aesthetically pleasing result, as a ray amputation.

REFERENCES

1. Littler JW. On the adaptability of man's hand (with reference to equiangular curve). *Hand* 1973;5:187–191.
2. An KN, Chao EYS, Linscheid RL, Cooney WP III. Functional forces in normal and abnormal fingers. *Orthop Trans* 1978; 168–170.
3. Linscheid RL, Chao YS. Biomechanical assessment of finger function in prosthetic joint design. *Orthop Clin North Am* 1973;4: 317–330.
4. Kiefhaber TR, Stern PJ, Grood ES. Lateral stability of the proximal interphalangeal joint. *J Hand Surg* 1986;11A:661–669.
5. Linscheid RL, Murray PM, Vidal MA, Beckenbaugh RD. Development of a surface replacement arthroplasty for proximal interphalangeal joints. *J Hand Surg* 1997;22A:286–298.
6. Millender LH, Nalebuff EA. Reconstructive surgery in the rheumatoid hand. *Orthop Clin North Am* 1975;6:709–732.
7. Allende BT, Engelem JC. Tension-band arthrodesis in the finger joints. *J Hand Surg* 1980;5A:269–271.
8. Ayres JR, Goldstrom GL, Miller GJ, et al. Proximal interphalangeal joint arthrodesis with the Herbert screw. *J Hand Surg* 1988;13A: 600–603.
9. Zimmerman NB, Weiland AJ. Ninety-nine intraosseous wiring for internal fixation of the digital skeleton. *Orthopedics* 1989;12:99–104.
10. Büchler U, Aiken MA. Arthrodesis of the proximal interphalangeal joint by solid bone grafting and plate fixation in extensive injuries to the dorsal aspect of the finger. *J Hand Surg* 1988;13A:589–594.
11. Carroll RE, Taber TH. Digital arthroplasty of the proximal interphalangeal joint. *J Bone Joint Surg* 1954;36A:912–920.
12. Condamine JL, Benoit JY, Comtet JJ, Aubriot JH. Proposed digital arthroplasty critical study of the preliminary results. *Ann Chir Main* 1988;7:282–297.
13. Iselin F. Arthroplasty of the proximal interphalangeal joint after trauma. *Hand* 1975;7:41–42.
14. Linscheid RL, Dobyns JH. Total joint arthroplasty: the hand. *Mayo Clin Proc* 1979;54:516–526.
15. Swanson AB, Maupin BK, Gajjar NV, Swanson GD. Flexible implant arthroplasty in the proximal interphalangeal joint of the hand. *J Hand Surg* 1985;10A:796–805.
16. Faithful, DK, Herbert TJ. Small joint fusions of the hand using the Herbert bone screw. *J Hand Surg* 1984;9B:167–168.
17. Foucher G. Reconstruction after traumatic destruction of the finger joints. *Chirurgie* 1990;116:176–179.
18. Foucher G, Citron N, Sammut D. Compound vascularized joint transfer in hand surgery. Apropos of a series of 16 cases. *Rev Chir Orthop Reparatrice Appar Mot* 1991:77:34–41.
19. Hasegawa T, Yamano Y. Arthroplasty of the proximal interphalangeal joint using costal cartilage grafts. *J Hand Surg* 1992;17B: 583–585.
20. Eaton RG, Malerich MM. Volar plate arthroplasty of the proximal interphalangeal joint: a review of ten years' experience. *J Hand Surg* 1980;5:260–268.
21. Dionysian E, Eaton RG. The long-term outcome of volar plate arthroplasty of the proximal interphalangeal joint. *J Hand Surg* 2000;25A:429–437.

22. Foliart DE. Swanson silicone finger joint implants: A review of the literature regarding long-term complications. *J Hand Surg* 1995; 20A:445–449.

23. Lin HH, Wyrick JD, Stern PJ. Proximal interphalangeal joint silicone replacement arthroplasty: clinical results using an anterior approach. *J Hand Surg* 1995;20:123–132.

24. Minamikawa Y, Imaeda T, Amadio PC, et al. Lateral stability of proximal interphalangeal joint replacement. *J Hand Surg* 1994; 19A:1050–1054.

25. Condamine JL, Fourquet M, Marcucci L, Pichereau D. Primary metacarpophalangeal and proximal interphalangeal arthrosis of the hand. Indications and results of 27 DJOA arthroplasty. *Ann Chir Main* 1997;16:66–78.

26. Uchiyama S, Cooney WP III, Linscheid RL, et al. Kinematics of the proximal interphalangeal joint of the finger after surface replacement. *J Hand Surg* 2000;25A:305–312.

27. Chamay A. A distally based dorsal and triangular tendinous flap for direct access to the proximal interphalangeal joint. *Ann Chir Main* 1988;7:179–183.

28. Lister G. Intraosseous wiring of the digital skeleton. *J Hand Surg* 1978;13A:595–599.

29. Sauerbier M, Cooney WP, Berger RA, Linscheid RL. Kompletter Oberflächenersatz des Fingermittelgelenks – Langzeitresultate und chirurgische Technik. *Handchir Mikrochir Plast Chir* 2000;32: 411–418

30. Takigawa S, Cooney WP III, Meletiou S, et al. Review of Swanson implant arthroplasty in the proximal interphalangeal joint of the hand. *J Hand Surg* 2001;submitted.

31. Pelligrini VD Jr, Burton RI. Osteoarthritis of the proximal interphalangeal joint of the hand: arthroplasty or fusion? *J Hand Surg* 1990;15A:194–209.

THE METACARPOPHALANGEAL JOINT

STEPHEN D. TRIGG

HISTORICAL PERSPECTIVE

Anatomic Considerations

The metacarpophalangeal (MCP) joint is an anatomically complex condyloid joint that lies centrally within the mobile longitudinal and distal transverse arches of the hand (1). Unlike the more simple ginglymoid interphalangeal (IP) joint, which has but a single, nearly congruent flexion-extension arc of motion, the condyloid MCP joint is diarthrodial, that is, allowing flexion-extension, abduction-adduction, and limited rotation (1–4). While the basic form of the MCP and IP joints are anatomically similar (comprised of the bony articular elements, capsule, and collateral ligaments), the more complex motion of the MCP joint is largely allowable by the shape of the metacarpal head. In the sagittal plane the metacarpal head is eccentrically shaped with the distance between the center axis of motion being greater palmarly than dorsally. In the coronal plane the metacarpal head is nearly wedge-shaped, flaring palmarly, and becomes bicondylar, articulating centrally with the base of the proximal phalanx in neutral, laterally in abduction/adduction, and palmarly in the bicondylar region in flexion (4–6).

Another biomechanical result of the complex wedge-like shape of the metacarpal head is that in extension the major portion of the collateral ligaments is lax, allowing for abduction/adduction of the proximal phalanx. In flexion, however, the ligaments become taut, which stabilizes the base of the proximal phalanx against the condylar portion of the metacarpal head. The proximal phalanx is further stabilized through the arc of motion by the palmar plate, sagittal bands, and dorsal capsule (4–7). In extension, the phalanx is weakly stabilized through the dynamic action of the extrinsic extensor expansion apparatus and by the tension of the intrinsic muscle tendons via their dorsal insertion into the extensor hood (1,2).

The foregoing details of the anatomic complexity of the MCP joint are inherently proportional to the joint's contribution to the composite complexity of hand function, arguably one of the most distinguishing features of the human species. Even the simplest of functional patterns of prehension, that of grip and pinch, requires that the digits both extend and abduct at the MCP joint (along with reciprocal extension of the IP joints) to allow spatial accommodation of diverse objects (1,2,4–7). For precision handling of objects, the palmar pulp tissue of the fingers (particularly of index and long fingers) must be brought into working opposition with the thumb, which requires a composite of MCP joint flexion, rotation, and ulnar deviation. During pinch, the lateral stresses applied by the thumb to the phalanges of the index (and to a lesser extent the long finger) are considerable and must be resisted by the dynamic action of the radial intrinsic muscles (1,4,7). Firm grasp and pinch bring into play even greater perpendicular, parallel, and rotational stresses upon the collateral ligaments, capsule, palmar plate, and require more forceful contraction of the intrinsic and extrinsic muscle tendon groups acting over the joint (1,2,4).

Disease Considerations

The principal example of a progressive inflammatory arthritic condition that commonly affects MCP joints is rheumatoid arthritis (RA). It has been in no small part through the study of RA and its destructive effects upon the digital joints that the body of knowledge of hand anatomy, kinesiology, and pathology has been significantly furthered. It therefore is entirely appropriate that RA joint deformities should serve as the primary model for further discussion of MCP joint pathology and reconstruction. RA is a systemic autoimmune disorder of unknown etiology, which is characterized by symmetrical erosive synovitis, articular cartilage destruction, and periarticular structural degeneration. The structural changes if untreated progress toward fixed deformity and significantly altered hand function.

Sterling Bunnell is credited with originating the term *ulnar drift* to describe the abnormal progressive ulnarward deviation of the proximal phalanges at the MCP joints affected by RA, and this deformity is the most distinguishing visual characteristic of rheumatoid hand deformity (Fig. 6.1) (1). Although ulnar drift is a descriptively useful term, the pathological progression of the deformity is in reality a decidedly more complex sequence of changes than the semantics would suggest. Indeed, ulnar drift is the result of the combination of structural attenuation of the supportive ligamentous and capsular elements and the development of pathologic imbalances of the involved dynamic muscles/tendon forces

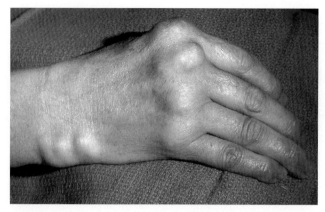

FIGURE 6.1. An example of a hand affected by long-standing rheumatoid arthritis. Note the ulnar drift deformity with subluxation of the fingers. Marked synovial proliferation is seen about the MCP joints and at the distal radioulnar joints. Early swan-neck deformity is noted in the ulnar three digits.

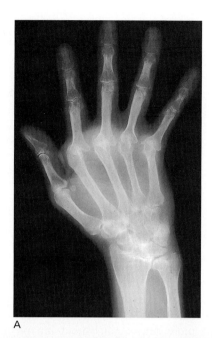

A

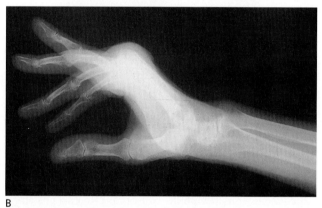

B

FIGURE 6.2. Posteroanterior and lateral X-rays of the hand shown in Figure 6.1. Note the dislocation of the proximal phalanges and the destructive effects of RA about the wrist. The carpus has translated both ulnarly and palmarly allowing for the development of the rheumatoid zig-zag deformity along the phalangeal-carpometacarpal-forearm axis.

acting over the joint, which results in a progression toward ulnar translation, palmar subluxation, and rotatory supination of the proximal phalanges (Fig. 6.2) (1,4–6). The clinical and experimental investigation of the etiology and structural anatomic basis for the onset and progression of ulnar drift deformity is certainly among the most scholarly pursuits in all of reconstructive hand surgery (1,2,4,7–23). From careful review of these investigations, while there are certainly notable differences in the stated importance of the involved pathologic factors, there are several areas of mutual agreement. First is the recognition that in the normal hand at rest there is naturally a degree of ulnar deviation of the proximal phalanges relative to the long axis of the metacarpals, which is greatest in the index finger. Second, the trajectory of dynamic muscle action upon the extrinsic flexor tendons is not linear; rather it is proximally convergent at or near the base of the fourth metacarpal. This eccentric ulnar directed line of pull by extrinsic flexors is most pronounced in the index and long fingers, thus placing considerable lateral (ulnar torque) strain upon the flexor sheath and pulley system during pinch and grip. In addition, the flexor tendons exert a considerable palmar-directed (dislocating) force upon the flexor sheath and thus to the base of the proximal phalanges. Other important ulnar deviating forces present in the normal hand include the observations that (a) the ulnar intrinsic insertions tend to be stronger and so oriented as to produce an increased mechanical advantage compared to their radial intrinsic counterpart, and (b) Zancolli's concept of the palmar and ulnarward traction upon the palmar plate produced via the intermetacarpal ligament that occurs with flexion of the fourth and fifth metacarpals during grip (1,2,7).

The details of these outlined ulnarward directed forces present in the normal hand have considerable importance with respect to the onset of destructive effects of RA upon the MCP joint. It is generally agreed upon that the initial causative insult to the MCP joint in RA is the presence of the inflammatory synovitis, which results in capsular distention and collateral ligament attenuation. This results in periarticular instability and sets up the potential for the normal ulnar/palmar dynamic forces discussed above to become pathologic and unbalance the normal posture and function of the digits (1,2,4,7,11,12). Unrestrained by the weakened static structural elements the flexors pull the proximal phalanx ulnopalmarward into subluxation. With subluxation of the proximal phalanx, the flexor sheath is displaced volarly resulting in ulnar bowstringing of the flexor tendon, which effectively increases the moment arm upon the MCP joints. On the dorsal aspect of the joint, the extensor tendon translates ulnarward (with stretching of the radial sagittal fibers) toward the intermetacarpal valley. In the ulnarly transposed

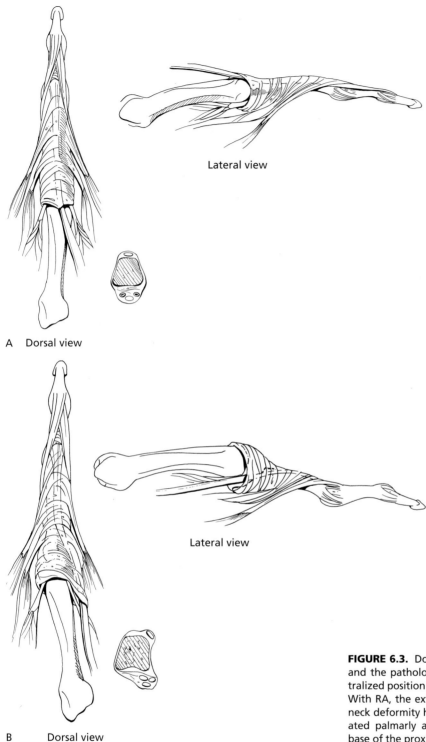

Lateral view

A　Dorsal view

Lateral view

B　Dorsal view

FIGURE 6.3. Dorsal and lateral views of normal finger anatomy and the pathologic changes that result from RA. Note the centralized position of the extensor mechanism in the normal finger. With RA, the extensor tendon is subluxated ulnarly. Early swan-neck deformity has developed. The proximal phalanx has subluxated palmarly and deviated ulnarly. Dorsal erosion about the base of the proximal phalanx is shown.

position, the extrinsic extensors and flexors become powerful ulnar deviating forces while concurrently losing their ability to efficiently extend and flex the proximal phalanx (Fig. 6.3). The pathologic tendon imbalances are not restricted to the MCP joint level alone, for in the transposed position the tension upon the lateral bands and central slip is increased, thus, initiating the tendency toward middle phalanx extension and

development swan-neck deformity (1,2,4,6,18,19,22). In cases of mild ulnar drift where the deformity can be easily corrected, splinting may be considered. Unfortunately, most splints, which truly correct ulnar drift, are bulky and cumbersome, and are only moderately effective over the long term. With progression or persistence of the deformity the radial intrinsics can no longer actively overcome the ulnar deviating forces and over time, the ulnar sagittal bands, collateral ligaments, ulnar intrinsics, and ulnar joint capsule all become contracted resulting in fixed ulnar deviation of the digits (1,4,7,11).

As the disease progresses, destruction is not limited to the soft-tissues. The inflammatory synovium also destroys the articular cartilage, presumably through direct enzymatic degradation. Concurrent with articular cartilage degeneration, the joint contact of the subluxated proximal phalanx with the metacarpal head is no longer congruent and bone erosion may occur about the dorsal rim of the base of the proximal phalanx and about the palmar aspect of the metacarpal head (4,7,12,20,24,25). The intercarpal and radiocarpal articulations of the wrist may be similarly affected by RA resulting in degenerative articular collapse. With progressive ligamentous attenuation the carpus often translates ulnarly causing reciprocal radial deviation of the carpometacarpal segment and yielding the so-called rheumatoid zig-zag deformity along the forearm-carpometacarpal-phalangeal orientation (4,7,15,16,26) (see Fig. 6.2A). Radial deviation of the wrist has been demonstrated to exacerbate ulnar deviation of the fingers through imbalance of the extrinsic muscle dynamic forces (15,16).

NONOPERATIVE TREATMENT

The care of a patient with complex rheumatoid hand and wrist deformities is always an involved and generally a prolonged process. The patient may remain under observation for years prior to proceeding to surgical treatment. Many discussions of the surgical treatment of rheumatoid hand deformities fail to note the importance of effective preoperative and postoperative pharmacologic management of the disease. Recurrences of synovitis and/or progression of disease in adjacent joints can negate previous effective reconstructive surgical efforts. Therefore, it is imperative that the rheumatologist and the surgeon establish a coordinated treatment plan for each patient.

The manifestation and degree of polyarticular involvement of RA is individually variable and every patient's activity level, employment, family assistance, and own psychosocial attributes for dealing with their condition is unique. Most often, the direction of nonoperative treatment falls to the supervision of the hand surgeon who then initiates the course of hand therapy. While it is certainly beyond the scope of this chapter to discuss in detail the professional techniques and disciplines of preventative and preoperative hand therapy and splinting, a comprehensive working knowledge of these should be considered an obligation of the directing surgeon. This necessarily dictates confidence in and the development of a close working relationship with a qualified and interested hand therapist. An experienced hand therapist will likely spend considerably more direct, individual time with the patient and often is a principal educator in the rehabilitation process. Joint protection protocols, splinting, appropriate therapeutic modalities, and selection of adaptive/assistive devices should be considered only with the patient allowed to directly participate in the process, otherwise compliance may be compromised. Through this type of comprehensive team approach, the patient will come to clearly understand the goals of treatment and the expectations for their degree of involvement and commitment. This reduces the potential for misunderstanding, disillusionment, and false expectations from the patient.

PREOPERATIVE PLANNING AND SURGICAL STAGING

The defined goals of reconstructive surgery about the arthritic MCP joint are to relieve pain, correct and prevent recurrence of deformity, and to improve function (1,25,27,28). In the patient with osteoarthritis or posttraumatic degenerative arthritis, the goals are usually more readily defined and stated by the patient with relief of pain almost always foremost. However, in the patient with RA where polyarthritic involvement is more common, clinical judgment must be exercised in order to sort out and prioritize the degree of joint involvement, pain, deformity, and functional deficits. Patients with long-standing RA are often quite stoic, having lived with the experience of prolonged pain and diminishing function. As a result, it may be difficult for them to articulate or objectively define what may be the most painful or dysfunctional part, particularly when there is significant bilateral limb or polyarticular involvement. Therefore, it is incumbent upon the surgeon to facilitate the process and guide the patient toward formulation of a reasonable, systematic treatment approach. To this end, it is also imperative to fully inform the patient what outcomes are most predictable and probable from any proposed surgical procedure(s); specifically, alleviation of pain is usually more predictable than is the restoration of near normal function or the prevention of late recurrences of deformity (27). It further follows that a patient may present with significant, established deformities but report minimal if any pain, and thus it would be imprudent to initially recommend surgery in the short term. Moreover, the degree of hand deformity is not necessarily proportional to the degree of function or to the ability to perform work or activities of daily living (8,27,29,30).

While there are no absolutes regarding the order of surgical procedures in a patient with polyarticular involvement, I agree in principal with Ferlic's recommendations that the spine and lower extremities should be considered first if they are significantly symptomatic. The use of crutches and walkers may compromise the outcome of previously performed reconstructive surgeries about the upper limb articulations and hand (1,29). However, that stated, a painful wrist or thumb may disallow effective use of these ambulatory aides, and this should be carefully evaluated prior to any proposal for lower extremity surgery should ambulatory aides be necessary for the successful outcome of those procedures.

While RA hand deformities may be the most visually striking, the proximal joints of the upper extremities must be assessed carefully as part of the staging process. It would be pointless to proceed with major reconstruction of digital deformities in a patient with a stiff and painful shoulder or elbow, which would limit the placement of the reconstructed hand for purposeful use. As previously stated, degenerative collapse and ulnar deviation of the wrist (zig-zag deformity) affect the dynamic soft-tissue balance about the MCP joint, and thus the wrist must be treated first. Flexor tendon rupture repair and tendon transfers should precede reconstruction of the MCP joint, as active flexor power is requisite for rehabilitation following MCP joint surgery (1,27). Extensor tendon ruptures can be delayed, or less commonly be repaired/reconstructed at the time of MCP joint surgery as extension of the joint can be accomplished by postoperative dynamic splinting (14,27,30).

The interdependence of PIP joint deformity upon primary MCP joint pathology has been previously noted and therefore, MCP joint deformities are usually corrected first. Oftentimes, following the restoration of MCP joint alignment and function the reciprocal PIP joint deformity will be significantly improved or at least later correction of the deformity will be simplified (4,22,25,28).

OPERATIVE TREATMENT OF THE MCP JOINT

Indications

The range of operative procedures about the MCP joints are broadly classified as correction of early imbalances and mild deformity or reconstruction of established deformity. Synovectomy of the MCP joint has been considered by some to be a useful prophylactic or preventative measure against progression of further deformity when performed early (1,9,31). Flatt recommends that one should proceed with synovectomy as a singular procedure only with caution, as it is often difficult to accurately define the degree of synovial involvement by clinical examination and/or X-rays. Furthermore, RA is a disease characterized by periods of remission and recurrences, and as such it is difficult to assess the effectiveness of synovectomy over the long term. Most have advocated proceeding with synovectomy alone only in MCP joints with persistent synovitis but without degenerative articular changes or established soft-tissue imbalances that have failed to resolve following pharmacologic treatment (inclusive of joint injections) over a six-month period (1,27). Beyond this fairly narrow indication, synovectomy is most often performed in conjunction with other procedures about the MCP joint.

Contraindications to MCP joint surgery are few. The presence of deformity but without pain and with reasonable hand function should in general be considered a relative contraindication for surgery (1,27). Nonetheless, should deformity progress and function decline coexistent with a continued absence of pain, the patient should be informed

that more favorable outcomes from reconstructive surgery about the MCP joints are more predictable when there are less severe soft-tissue contractures and articular destruction (1,4,7,14,22,25,27–29,32).

SURGICAL TREATMENTS

Soft-tissue Procedures

Implant replacement arthroplasty is the most commonly performed reconstructive procedure on MCP joints affected by RA. However, the restoration of joint alignment and balance of the dynamic tendon forces about MCP joint without implant arthroplasty should be considered in those patients who have demonstrated progression of ulnar drift but have minimal proximal phalangeal subluxation and without significant articular destruction. The most commonly performed soft-tissue procedures are synovectomy, intrinsic release, crossed intrinsic transfer, and extensor tendon realignment. Current PA, lateral, and Brewerton tangential projection radiographs should be obtained to note any evidence for early cortical erosions at the capsular reflections and ligament insertions, which would suggest more advanced articular destruction. Clinically, the intrinsic tightness and differential intrinsic tightness tests are necessarily performed preoperatively to evaluate the degree of intrinsic contracture contributing to the deformity (1).

Operative Technique

The operative exposure to the MCP joint(s) can be performed either through a single dorsal transverse incision or through curvilinear longitudinal incisions (1,4,25,28,33). Historically, a single transverse incision centered over the MCP joints is recommended when multiple joints are involved. Weiss and Strickland prefer longitudinal incisions between the index/long and ring/small MCP joints for nearly all arthroplasties at this joint level (34). The exposure of the index and long finger MCP joints and the ring and small finger MCP joints can be accomplished through longitudinal incisions placed between the joints in the respective intermetacarpal space extending from proximal to the junctura to the mid-web space distally. The argument for the longitudinal incision(s) is that the approach is extensile and reportedly reduces the disruption to the dorsal veins, thereby lessening postoperative swelling. Proponents of the transverse incision argue that the exposure of the articular and periarticular structures is significantly greater and that postoperative swelling can be minimized through careful dissection and retraction of the neurovascular structures, which are reliably found in the loose intermetacarpal adipose tissue. Exposure of a single joint is easily accomplished through a longitudinal incision.

No matter which skin incision is chosen, the skin flaps should be developed as thickly as possible and made sufficiently wide so that retraction tension upon the skin is minimized.

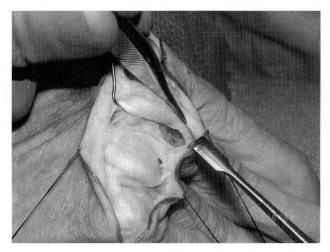

FIGURE 6.4. Exposure of the finger MCP joints and extensor mechanisms through a single transverse incision. The extensor tendons are subluxated ulnarly with associated stretching and attenuation of the radial sagittal band fibers. (See Color Fig. 6.4.)

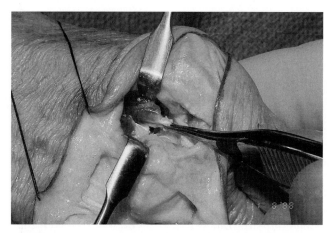

FIGURE 6.6. Exposure of the ulnar intrinsic tendon, which has been incised at the muscular tendonous junction (distal end of the tendon held in the forceps) accomplishing the ulnar intrinsic release. (See Color Fig. 6.6.)

The extensor tendon and hood fibers, sagittal bands, and intrinsic tendon mechanisms (oblique and transverse portion) are exposed, usually most extensively about the ulnar aspect (Fig. 6.4). Direct exposure of the joint capsule requires retraction of the extensor tendon mechanism, which is accomplished by division of a single, sagittal band directly adjacent to the tendon itself. The more contracted ulnar sagittal band is divided when there is significant ulnar translation of the extensor tendon (Fig. 6.5) (1,4,25,28). In cases where there is minimal extensor tendon displacement, some prefer a radial approach to the joint by division of the radial sagittal band (4). Swanson advocates that for exposure of the index and small finger MCP joints the approach should be made directly through the interval between the extensor digitorum communis and proprius tendons (25).

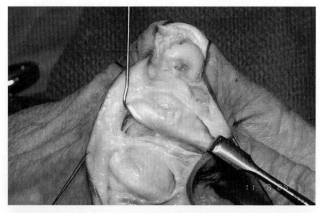

FIGURE 6.5. The ulnar sagittal band fibers are markedly contracted. Note that with traction applied through the hook cannot centralize the tendon without release of the contracted ulnar sagittal band, as has been performed in the index digit shown at the top of the photograph. (See Color Fig. 6.5.)

Further exposure of the joint for synovectomy requires that extensor tendon and hood be dissected from the underlying joint capsule. In cases where the synovitis is florid or long involved, oftentimes the capsule is indistinct from the underlying synovial tissue or is adherent, making separation difficult. Once the extensor mechanism is dissected and retracted, the joint capsule is incised and a comprehensive synovectomy is performed, including the recesses at the capsular reflections and between the metacarpal head and collateral ligaments. I have found that a small dental rougeur is the most effective single instrument to accomplish digital joint synovectomy.

The need for intrinsic release is further assessed directly at this stage, prior to proceeding with extensor tendon realignment. When judged necessary, the ulnar aspect of the extensor mechanism is more extensively exposed by blunt spreading dissection. Through the previously created dorsal incision through the sagittal band fibers, a blunt curved probe or small curved hemostat is passed volarly so as to hook around and deliver into full view the transverse and volar thickened oblique fibers of the intrinsic tendon. Several methods of intrinsic release have been proposed. Flatt recommends that if crossed intrinsic transfer is not planned, then a triangle portion of the intrinsic mechanism may be excised, which includes the thickened volar fibers and a portion of the transverse (vertical) fibers. This leaves a proximal portion of the transverse fibers intact, so as to provide assistance with MCP joint flexion (1,2,18,19,36,37). Alternatively, simple division at the musculotendinous junction may accomplish the intrinsic release (Fig. 6.6). The deep insertion of the intrinsic into the proximal phalanx may also require release if further efforts at realignment prove difficult (2,18,19,25,28). In the small finger, owing to the differences of the intrinsic anatomy about the ulnar aspect of this digit, one must be careful to be certain to dissect the abductor digiti minimi from the flexor digiti mini and release only the abductor (1).

Crossed Intrinsic Transfer

Crossed intrinsic transfer (CIT) should be considered a modification of ulnar intrinsic release. In this procedure, the ulnar intrinsic tendon of the index, long, and ring finger is distally released but preserved proximally mobilizing it to its musculotendinous junction. The preserved tendon is then transferred to the radial aspect of the adjacent digit to act as a dynamic stabilizer against recurrence of ulnar deviation (1,2,9,21,38,39). CIT is most often performed in addition to synovectomy and extensor tendon realignment. With Straub's method of CIT, the distally released ulnar intrinsic tendon is sutured to the adjacent radial intrinsic wing tendon or lateral band (1,21). Flatt modified Straub's original CIT method after reporting the frequent disturbing postoperative development of swan-neck deformity (1,9). Flatt's modification of CIT sutures the ulnar intrinsic tendon to the distal portion of the adjacent radial collateral ligament negating any contribution to PIP joint extension (1,9). The tendon is sutured with nonabsorbable sutures under sufficient tension so that ulnar deviation of the digit is corrected with hand placed in a position at rest (1).

Extensor Mechanism Realignment

The pathologic ulnar deviating forces of the subluxated extrinsic extensor and flexor tendons have been previously discussed. Unfortunately, there is to date no satisfactory direct method for anatomically repositioning the flexor tendon and sheath. Therefore, it is imperative that the extensor mechanism be correctly realigned and stabilized, so as to reduce its potential for contributing to the reoccurrence of ulnar drift deformity (4,33). Extensor mechanism realignment follows MCP joint synovectomy and ulnar intrinsic release and/or CIT, and the details of the operative exposure and release of the contracted ulnar sagittal band fibers are as previously noted. Following careful dissection of the extensor mechanism from the underlying capsule and ulnar intrinsic release, the extensor tendon should centrally realign after repositioning of the proximal phalanx. If there is significant insufficiency of the radial sagittal fibers, one may encounter the tendency for the extensor tendon to redisplace ulnarly. Swanson proposes that reefing (imbrication) of the stretched radial sagittal band fibers is usually sufficient in most cases to prevent redisplacement of the tendon (25). However, if following imbrication of the radial sagittal band there is any doubt that the repair is not competent enough to resist ulnar translation of the centralized tendon, several techniques have been proposed to further augment the centralization. Harrison's extensor loop method, in effect, creates a dorsal extensor tenodesis (1,40). A radial slip of the extensor tendon is raised proximally and left intact distally whereupon the free end

passed through a bone channel created by a drilling through the dorsal rim of the proximal phalanx. The slip of extensor tendon is the looped back to the main portion of the intact tendon where it is sutured creating an extensor loop tenodesis (40). Swanson simplifies Harrison's loop tenodesis by suturing the extensor tendon directly to the dorsal rim of the base of the proximal phalanx with stout nonabsorbable suture passed through small drill holes (25). Nalebuff and associates have also modified Harrison's extensor loop method by raising a similar distally based extensor tendon strip, but which is harvested from the ulnar side of the tendon. The free end is then passed under the main portion of the tendon by passing it through the dorsal joint capsule where it is then sutured to the radial side of the main portion of extensor tendon (24,27). Following extensor tendon realignment hemostasis is obtained, following release of the tourniquet. The skin incision is closed over small drains.

Soft-tissue Reconstruction

Postoperative Care

Following completion of the procedure, the hand is placed in a bulky, soft compression dressing incorporating a palmar plaster splint. The dressing should be constructed so as to immobilize the wrist in neutral to slight extension and to maintain the corrected finger alignment of neutral MCP joint flexion and normal longitudinal alignment. The interphalangeal (IP) joints are placed in slight flexion. The subcutaneous drains are removed on the first or second postoperative day and a similar bulky, soft-tissue dressing is reapplied. As soon as favorable wound conditions allow (usually four to five days), the hand is placed in a dynamic MCP joint extension wrist-hand arthrosis with alignment outriggers and rubber bands similar to that which would be used following MCP joint replacement arthroplasty. A static night splint is also fabricated to maintain the optimum corrected finger alignment (1,9,38,39,41,42).

Closely supervised hand therapy in the early postoperative period is important to ensure optimum results from intrinsic release, CIT, and extensor tendon realignment. The patient is instructed to perform active MCP flexion exercises, in the dynamic splint, at least three to four times a day for the initial three to five weeks following surgery, depending on the combination of procedures, number of digits involved, and individual wound healing. Brief daily periods of active range of motion, out of the splint, are encouraged to minimize MCP joint stiffness. During the early postoperative phase, both splints are used. The dynamic splint may be discontinued thereafter, but the static night splint is retained for ten to twelve weeks. Following cessation of the dynamic splint, the therapy should be advanced along an individualized gradual resumption of simple activities of daily living at six to eight weeks, then progressing towards normal activity beyond three months (38). If correction was performed only to a single digit, a static splint alone is fabricated foregoing the dynamic splint. Therapeutic range-of-motion exercises are performed out of the splint often that may incorporate adjacent finger buddy strapping to facilitate the ROM program.

Outcomes

The difficulty in accurately assessing the success of synovectomy when performed as a singular procedure has been previously discussed, and in a majority of cases, some combination of synovectomy, intrinsic release with or without CIT and extensor mechanism realignment will be performed together. The criteria for evaluation of these soft-tissue reconstructive procedures has been based upon the success of correction of ulnar drift, ROM about the MCP joint (and IP joints), and prevention of further digital deformity (e.g., swan-neck) over the long term.

Intrinsic release with CIT and extensor mechanism realignment have been shown to be effective in correcting ulnar drift. Wood et al. maintained an average of 6° ulnar drift at 81 months postoperatively; Oster et al. reported maintenance of an average correction of ulnar drift of 5° at 12 years postoperatively (1,9,38,39,41,42). Owing to the magnitude of surgical dissection and soft-tissue realignment involved, one would expect a potential for diminishment in postoperative joint ROM. Wood reported an average postoperative active MCP joint motion of 56° at 81 months, and Oster et al. observed an average of 47° at 12.7 years. El-Gammel and Blair reported an average loss of 18° MCP joint ROM at 5 years postoperatively but observed an increase in PIP joint motion. Oster et al. found no statistically significant differences in outcome between transfer of the intrinsic tendon into the adjacent lateral band or to the collateral ligament despite Flatt's earlier findings. Nonetheless, these authors recommended that should there be any observed preoperative tendency toward swan-neck deformity, the transfer is made into the collateral ligament (1,9,38,39,41,42).

The findings of these larger series of soft-tissue reconstruction of the MCP joint deformity, without implant arthroplasty, performed in those patients without significant articular destruction would strongly suggest that this form of arthroplasty be considered when there is an established progression of deformity and loss of function. Wood states that soft-tissue arthroplasty does not preclude later implant replacement arthroplasty should subsequent articular destruction ensue (39). Patient acceptance, long-term range of motion, and function compare favorably to silicone implant arthroplasty (39,41). Soft-tissue reconstruction should also be considered in patients with systemic lupus erythematosus where articular cartilage destruction is generally less severe than observed in RA. With recent improvement in the pharmacologic management of RA, especially in controlling recurrences of synovitis, soft-tissue arthroplasty may deserve further consideration as an alternative to implant replacement arthroplasty.

Resection Interposition Arthroplasty

Resection arthroplasty for severe joint degeneration of the hip and knee following sepsis or trauma was performed as early as the late 1800s. In 1958, Fowler and Riordan reported their early results of a dorsopalmar wedge-shaped resection arthroplasty of the metacarpal head inpatients with RA (1,43). The rationale for this procedure (performed in the pre-implant arthroplasty era) was to resect a sufficient amount of the metacarpal head so that the proximal phalanx could be realigned colinear with the metacarpal. Dorsal tenodesis of the extensor mechanism to the base of the phalanx was performed to prevent recurrence of palmar subluxation and ulnar displacement of the extensor mechanism (43). Lateral stability was conferred by preserving the width of the metacarpal bone. Fowler considered that any remaining articular cartilage about the base of the proximal phalanx would act as an articular interface to the raw wedge-shaped cancellous surface of the resected metacarpal head (43,44). Kestler, Kuhns, and Harrison also devised modifications of resection-type joint arthroplasties that have been reported in limited series (1,40,45,46).

In 1972, Tupper introduced an important modified resection arthroplasty technique whereby the palmar plate was utilized as an articular interposition material. The palmar plate was proximally released from the metacarpal following transverse resection of the metacarpal head at the neck level. The proximal edge of the palmar plate was then sutured to the dorsal aspect of the remaining metacarpal neck through drill holes. This, in effect, created an interposition membrane between the two bone ends and additionally acted as a checkrein against recurrent palmar subluxation of the proximal phalanx. The radial collateral ligament, which was incised from the resected metacarpal head, was reattached dorsoradially to the metacarpal neck in an attempt to restore radial stability. Capsulorrhaphy and centralization of the extensor tendon was then performed (1,47,48).

Vainio described another method of resection interpositional arthroplasty whereby a portion of the extensor tendon is used as the interposition material (1,33,49). Similar to the Tupper method, the metacarpal head is excised at the neck level and the collateral ligaments are proximally released. The extensor tendon is then incised at such a position so that there is a sufficient length for the free end of the remaining distal portion of the tendon to be sutured directly to the palmar plate near the base of the proximal phalanx. The collateral ligaments are then reattached to the metacarpal neck by suture passed through drill holes. The proximal incised end of the extensor incised tendon is then sutured to its distal portion at the point that is courses palmarly. In the index finger the indicis proprius tendon is transferred radially to the tendon of the first dorsal interosseous muscle to improve abduction power (49,50).

Following either the Tupper or Vainio resection arthroplasty, the hand is initially splinted for three weeks before initiating controlled mobilization. Tupper recommends the use of a dynamic alignment outrigger splint be a part of a progressive ROM program (1,47,49,50).

The clinical outcomes following resection interposition arthroplasty are limited as these procedures have neither become universally accepted nor are they as frequently performed as implant arthroplasty. Flatt correctly points out that the results of the originating surgeons are always better than those who later attempt the procedure (1). Nonetheless, from the available limited study data on resection interposition arthroplasty methods, the outcomes are sufficiently favorable (average long-term MCP joint ROM 40° to 60°) that these procedures warrant consideration in certain circumstances including severe bone loss, previous sepsis, or as a salvage procedure for failed implant arthroplasty (47,49).

Perichondrial Graft Arthroplasty

Various transplanted autologous tissues have been used on a limited basis as interposition material in degenerative joints including fat, dermis, fascia, tendon, and joint capsule (27,51). In the 1970s, several Swedish investigators experimented with the use of perichondrial tissue to resurface damaged articular surfaces after it was shown that perichondrial tissue harvested from rabbit ear and distally implanted would produce chondroid tissue (52–54). Subsequent animal studies showed that implantation of perichondrial grafts had the potential to regenerate articular cartilage defects (54,55). In 1976, Skoog and Johansson reported a human case report where autogenous rib perichondrium graft tissue was utilized to resurface an MCP joint damaged by trauma and sepsis (55). The rib perichondrium was obtained from inferior costal margin with the tissue elevated as a strip by sharp dissection. Laboratory studies had shown that the deeper layer (cambium layer) held the largest concentration of cartilage cells with the potential for regeneration. The joint surface(s) were prepared by removal of any remaining damaged articular cartilage. The harvested perichondrial tissue was then draped over the bone ends and sutured in place with the deep layer facing the joint surface. Should both joint surfaces require resurfacing a thin sheet of silicone film was placed between the joint surfaces and the digits immobilized for approximately two weeks, whereupon a controlled program of ROM was begun, usually with the aid of dynamic splinting. The silicone sheet was removed at three months.

Following initial reports of short-term clinical success, the Swedish technique of perichondrial grafting was subsequently broadened to other joints about the hand and included joints affected by RA and osteoarthritis (33,56,57). In contrast to the Swedish experience, others have reported poor or unpredictable outcomes in patients older than 40 years of age and in nearly all joints with a preoperative diagnosis of septic arthritis (33). The most promising results were in younger patients (less than 20 years) with posttraumatic arthritis. Perichondrial graft resurfacing is a conceptually promising technique; however, more controlled studies with longer-term follow-up are required to determine both the applicability and durability of this type of arthroplasty before it can be further recommended.

Arthrodesis

The finger MCP joints are the keystone articulation of the mobile longitudinal arch of the hand. As such, arthrodesis of any MCP joint is rarely indicated as significant alteration of hand function ensues. Historically, MCP joint arthrodesis was recommended primarily in the border digits (index and small fingers) in manual laborers or in those patients with persistent pain from previous sepsis, post-burn arthrosis, failed implant arthroplasty, or in cases of severe instability secondary to bone loss or neuromuscular dysfunction (1,58). Beyond these conditions, other forms of arthroplasty, which preserve motion, are preferable.

The selection of position (flexion angle) of MCP joint arthrodesis should be individualized to the specific functional needs of the patient. In general the angle of fusion should approximate the normal postural flexion cascade of the proximal phalanges of the hand at rest; that is, adding 5° of flexion to each finger ulnar to an index angle of 25° to 30° (58). In addition to the flexion angle, careful consideration should be directed toward making certain that no malrotation or lateral malangulation is allowed, otherwise overlapping or abutment with adjacent digits will occur with attempted grasp (58).

The details of the operative exposure for arthrodesis of a single joint (usually through a longitudinal incision) have been discussed in detail in a previous section. Preparation of the bone surfaces for arthrodesis should preserve as much length as possible yet produce a maximum area of cancellous bone-to-bone apposition. Two methods for bone shaping and surface preparation have been most advocated: the so-called cup-and-cone method of Carroll and matching angular osteotomy (59,60). Both methods have proven equally successful (58–61). The cup-and-cone method allows for a greater freedom for incremental adjustments in position without requiring further bone resection (58,59).

Many techniques for internal fixation for digital joint arthrodesis have been proposed and biomechanical analysis of various methods have been widely reported (58). Because of ease of insertion, familiarity, and lower costs, those methods, which utilize K-wire fixation and/or stainless steel wire have wide appeal. Tension band wiring over K-wires, 90-90 intraosseous wiring, and dorsal plating have superior biomechanical strength to that of crossed or parallel K-wires and are sufficiently strong so as to allow an early protected postoperative ROM of the IP joints (58). Bioabsorbable pins and rods, external fixators, and intrafragmentary compression screw fixation techniques have been advocated as alternative methods to achieve arthrodesis of the IP joints. Their application for MCP joint is too limited to recommend any of these methods over tension band wiring, intraosseous wiring, or plate fixation. Bone grafts should be strongly considered in instances where there is bone loss, or in cases of previously failed arthroplasty or arthrodesis (58).

Joint Replacement Arthroplasty

Ever since Burman in 1940 introduced a vitallium replacement cap for the metacarpal head, numerous MCP joint implant arthroplasty designs have been proposed (1,4,12, 33,62). However, in distinct contrast to the continued improvements in durability of implant arthroplasty devices for lower and upper extremity articulations other than in the hand, virtually all finger prosthetic implants have developed problems over the long term (4,33,36,63–77). Such problems include material failure, fixation failure, bone erosion, stress shielding, recurrence of deformity, and microparticulate inflammatory response.

In terms of both numbers and complexity, the majority of MCP joint replacement arthroplasty has been performed in patients with RA (4,12). The complex sequence of pathologic changes that occur about the MCP joint affected by RA and that subsequently result in ulnar drift deformity has been previously discussed in detail and clearly elucidates the many challenges to successful implant design. From a historical perspective, following Burman's MCP joint arthroplasty, Flatt developed a metallic-coupled hinge MCP joint implant with double prong intramedullary fixation stems. The implant hinge allowed only flexion and extension without any tolerances for lateral motion. The implants provided excellent pain relief and correction of ulnar drift deformity. Over the long term, however, the author reported a significant incidence of stress shielding, bone erosion, loosening, and implant fracture, and the design were subsequently abandoned (1,66).

In the 1960s, Swanson and Niebauer nearly simultaneously developed viscoelastic silicone elastomer MCP joint implants (22,25,28,32,78,79). Both designs require resection of the metacarpal head and preparation of intramedullary canals of the metacarpal and proximal phalanx for placement of the implant. The concept behind Swanson's design was that the implant would act as a spacer allowing for subsequent fibrous capsular development about the implant (4,28). The Niebauer viscoelastic silicone implant was designed more as a true hinge and incorporated a Dacron mesh about the intramedullary stems to allow for fibrous ingrowth fixation (1,78,79). By contrast the Swanson implant allows for a sliding of the intramedullary stems within the canals (pistoning). The central hub of the Swanson implant is crescent-shaped palmarly which allows for bending yet acts as a true spacer separating the resected bone surfaces.

The early clinical success of their silicone implant designs was favorable and essentially revolutionized the surgical management of digital RA hand deformities. In particular, the Swanson design has achieved wide acceptance from the 1970s onward. However, upon the scrutiny of longer-term follow-up, particularly as noted in several larger retrospective studies, was the observance of a consistent percentage of material failures and gradual recurrence of deformity. As well, functional improvements in grip and pinch strengths as compared to preoperative measurements were inconsistent and motion often deteriorated over time (29,64,67,68,70,71,73).

With the emerging reality for the potential for long-term problems with silicone as an implant material and with recognition of the rapidly evolving success of the cemented hip endoprosthesis during the early 1970s, several investigators developed cemented metal and polyethylene implants. The majority of these implants were either modified hinges or balls and socket designs coupled by a snap fit linkage (1,4, 65). The cemented implants never achieved wide acceptance as compared to the silicone implants. Longer-term follow-up of these devices exposed problems of cement fixation failure and with implant loosening and implant material deterioration (1,4,74).

In 1974 the Swanson design silicone elastomer was reformulated and was reported to increase the resistance for tear propagation (26,76). Later, Swanson introduced the use of circumferential titanium grommets to protect the implant spacer and proximal stems from the bone interface in order to reduce the potential for implant wear and fracture and for proximal bone erosion (80). The use of these grommets adds an additional step to an already technically detailed procedure and requires sufficient bone stock to allow proper fit of the grommets into the intramedullary canal. Furthermore, it has not been established that the grommets significantly reduce osteolysis about the implants, although a slightly decreased incidence of implant fracture has been reported (33,80,81). Despite the material and technique alterations to the Swanson design, silicone elastomer remains a highly deformable material, which provides little resistance to either rotation or lateral compression and therefore the stability of the arthroplasty construct depends largely upon the integrity of the soft-tissue reconstruction.

Linscheid et al. have comprehensively studied the biomechanics of digital implant arthroplasty, and their work has furthered our understanding of how difficult it is to design an MCP joint replacement implant that replicates the complex anatomy of this articulation (4,5,12,82). Several important findings from their investigations are particularly noteworthy. First they have shown how critical is the need to preserve the near normal bone length relationship in order to minimize the development of internal stresses upon any MCP joint implant (4,12). Second, with resection of the metacarpal head (and any portion of the proximal phalanx), it is exceedingly difficult to replicate the normal center of joint motion, particularly with any internally constrained or coupled implant design. Furthermore, with any technique that resects the metacarpal head, the collateral ligaments are often released, allowing the flexor sheath and palmar plate to bowstring palmarly increasing the movement arm that the flexors can exert upon the joint (12). From their research, it was proposed that an uncoupled surface replacement prosthesis,

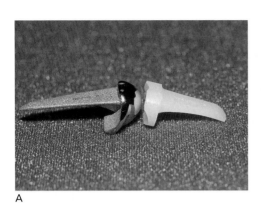
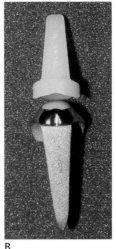
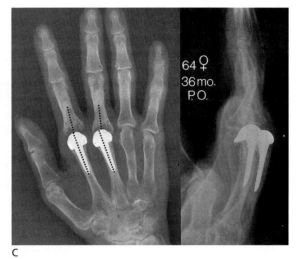

A B C

FIGURE 6.7. The SRA metacarpophalangeal joint implant (courtesy of Avanta Orthopaedics, San Diego, California, USA, 2000).

which would require less bone resection and allow for preservation of the collateral ligament, would more accurately replicate the complex anatomy of the MCP joint and thus potentially lessen the stresses upon the implant. In 1983, Beckenbaugh reported the preliminary experience of a custom noncemented uncoupled pyrolytic carbon MCP joint implant (83). The companion follow-up study from 1999 reported slight improvements in range of motion, implant stability, recurrence of ulnar drift, and implant failure when compared to data from reports of silicone implant arthroplasty. Significant improvements in reducing periprosthetic osteolysis were noted (67).

Recent advances in computer-aided design (CAD), coupled with improvements in the manufacturing of biocompatible materials to exact tolerances, has furthered interest in surface replacement arthroplasty. Linscheid and Avanta Orthopaedics have recently introduced an MCP joint surface replacement arthroplasty implant (SRA) that currently remains under clinical trial (Avanta Orthopaedics, San Diego, CA, USA) (33,82). The SRA implant utilizes a cobalt-chromium metacarpal component and an ultra-high molecular weight polyethylene proximal phalangeal component. Linscheid reports that the metacarpal head portion incorporates CAD geometry, which attempts to replicate the normal eccentric convexity of metacarpal head, thus incorporating palmar flanges, which both increases the contact surface area with the proximal phalangeal component and provides improved stability about the joint in flexion (Linscheid, RL personal communication, 2000) (Fig. 6.7). The surgical technique for implanting this prosthesis requires a minimum of bone resection and allows for preservation or careful reconstruction of the collateral ligaments. The current design requires cement fixation of the components.

In 1987 the Sutter Corporation (recently produced by Avanta Orthopaedics) introduced a modified silicone MCP hinge joint implant with a rectangular shape. The axis of the

hinge joint was placed more palmarly in order to facilitate joint extension and to reduce material impingement at the limits of flexion and extension. The rectangular shape of the implant and broader surfaces of the hub were designed to increase rotational stability (Fig. 6.8). Despite these reported improvements, the durability of the implant and clinical outcomes as compared to the Swanson design have not been proven (33,63).

More recently, DePuy Orthopaedics has introduced a hinge-type silicone MCP joint implant co-designed with

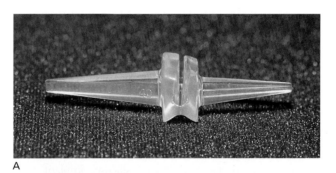

A

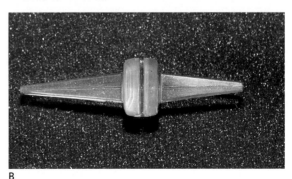

B

FIGURE 6.8. The Avanta silicone MCP joint replacement implant (courtesy of Avanta Orthopaedics, San Diego, CA, USA).

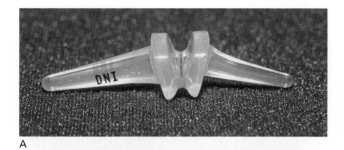

A

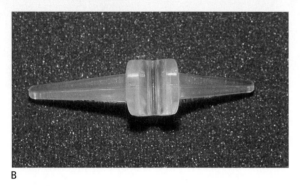

B

FIGURE 6.9. The Neuflex silicone MCP joint implant. Note the 30° neutral flexion incorporated in the prosthesis joint hinge (courtesy of DePuy, Inc., Warsaw, IN, USA).

Weiss. The goal of this design was to reduce the internal stresses upon the implant hinge throughout the arc of motion and to improve flexion. This clever design incorporates a 30° neutral palmar flexion angle at the hinge, which stimulates the observed natural posture of MCP joint flexion of the hand at rest (Fig. 6.9). By incorporating this neutral angle, it was shown that to fully extend the MCP joint would thus require minimal extensor power but throughout flexion from 30° to 90° would require only 60° of further flexion through the implant hinge to accomplish anticipated full motion thus overall reducing internal stresses upon the implant (34). Similar to the Niebauer and Sutter (Avanta) design, the hinge-spacer portion of the implant and stems is largely rectangular to improve rotational stability. The intramedullary canals are machined by sequential rectangular-shaped rasps to provide more precise seating of the stems. In a study by Weiss and Strickland, 50 patients had 168 implants with an average follow-up examination of 14 months. All were satisfied with their hand appearance and had no pain. Furthermore, no radiographic evidence of implant fracture was noted, and an average overall arc of motion of 12° to flexion of 73° was obtained (34).

Silicone Implant Arthroplasty: Surgical Technique

The surgical procedure may be performed under an axillary block regional anesthesia or general anesthesia. In patients with longstanding or severe RA, it is prudent to obtain preoperative lateral cervical spin flexion and extension X-rays to determine whether there is any evidence for vertebral instability, particularly in the upper segments.

The surgical exposure may be accomplished either by a single transverse incision or through several longitudinal incisions as has been previously discussed in the soft-tissue reconstruction section. The transverse incision is more commonly recommended. It is centered just proximal to the MCP joint over the metacarpal necks. The dissection is carried deep by a gentle blunt longitudinal spreading technique developing the skin flaps so as to provide adequate exposure of the extensor mechanism. Considerable care should be directed toward the retraction of the skin, which is often quite thin. Proximal and distal retraction of the skin flaps may be accomplished by placing a braided suture into the dermis at the skin edges, and gentle traction applied by small hemostats (see Fig. 6.4). Considerable care should be directed toward preserving the neurovascular structures, which are reliably found in the intermetacarpal spaces.

In cases of severe ulnar drift, one should expect to find the extensor tendon fully subluxated ulnarly into the intermetacarpal space with resultant stretching and attenuation of the radial sagittal fibers (see Fig. 6.5). Exposure of the joint requires careful dissection of the extensor mechanism from the joint capsule. This necessitates incision of the extensor hood at its ulnar margin directly adjacent to the central tendon. In the index and small fingers, exposure of the joint may be accomplished by a splitting dissection between the extensor digitorum communis and the indicis proprius in the index and extensor digiti minimi tendon in the small finger. Some surgeons advocate that the extensor hood be incised along the radial border, which then allows for imbrication of the radial fibers to the ulnar border of the central tendon upon closure. By this method it is argued that the sling of the extensor mechanism is effectively tightened (33). In cases where the extensor tendon cannot be centralized because of significant ulnar contraction of the ulnar hood fibers, both the radial and ulnar fibers are incised and then later sutured to one another. The freely mobile extensor tendon may then be sutured to the reconstructed hood fibers in a central position, or alternatively may be sutured through drill holes placed through the dorsal rim of the base of the proximal phalanx (4,33).

By whichever method chosen to expose the capsule, the extensor mechanism must be retracted from the dorsal capsule. This often necessitates a release of the junctura between the index and long fingers and longitudinal separation of the conjoined tendon of the ring and small fingers. Radial retraction of the extensor mechanism may also require division of the contracted ulnar intrinsic, thus accomplishing an ulnar intrinsic release. In those patients where CIT is to be performed, the intrinsic tendon is dissected so as to allow sufficient tendon length for transfer as discussed in a previous section. Otherwise, the ulnar intrinsic tendon is exposed and divided at its musculotendinous junction. Swanson recommends that the index finger ulnar intrinsic be preserved, as it assists supination of the index finger (25,28,33).

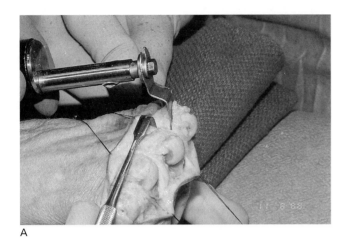

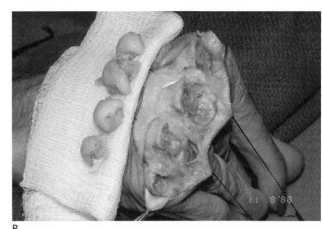

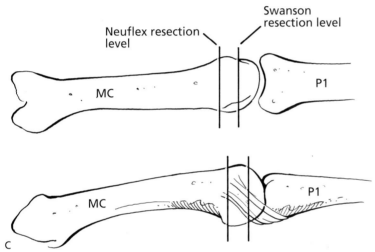

FIGURE 6.10. A. Osteotomy of the metacarpal head through the neck level perpendicular to the long axis of the metacarpal diaphysis. **B.** Completed transection of the metacarpal heads. **C.** Resection level should be precise based on the type of implant chosen for replacement. For the Swanson implant, the narrow design allows minimal joint resection although less stability. For the NeuFlex design, the resection level is at the distal end of the metacarpal flair allowing full seating of the stable block hinge. In both cases, no resection of the base of the proximal phalanx is required. (See Color Fig. 6.10.)

Following the intrinsic release, the hood fibers are dissected from the underlying capsule; often there will be protrusion of rheumatoid synovium through the dorsal capsule and direct exposure of the joint may proceed through this interval. Otherwise, the capsule may be incised longitudinally whereupon a comprehensive synovectomy is then performed. The neck of the metacarpal and base of the proximal phalanx are exposed subperiosteally. Following synovectomy, the metacarpal head is transected perpendicular to the long axis of the diaphysis at the metacarpal flare using an oscillating saw (Fig. 6.10). Most surgeons recommend releasing the collateral ligaments from the metacarpal before head excision (28). Oftentimes, the dorsal base of the subluxated proximal phalanx will be worn (sloped) from abnormal wear contact with the volar aspect of the metacarpal head (see Fig. 6.3B). If such erosion is encountered, the base of the proximal phalanx must then be transected perpendicular to the shaft yet preserving as much length as possible. Even when no sloping is encountered, all of the remaining articular cartilage must be removed from the base of the proximal phalanx. Any osteophytes about the periphery must also be moved, thus preparing a flush surface for the seating of the implant. Following

removal of the bone, the joint is again inspected for any remaining synovium. Swanson and others recommend that the flexor tendons be inspected for evidence of RA synovitis. The flexor sheath is incised longitudinally and the profundus tendon then delivered into the joint space by a smooth, blunt nerve hook whereupon a focal tenosynovectomy of the tendons is performed (4,28,33).

The medullary canals of the metacarpal and proximal phalanx are then prepared for trial implant sizing. A sharp pointed awl is used initially to gain access to the medullary canal and center the pilot hole for subsequent broaching and reaming. For the Swanson implant it is helpful to use blunt-tipped burrs to prepare the canal. The Sutter (Avanta) and NeuFlex implant technique use graduated matched rectangular rasps and broaches to facilitate the reaming process, which also simplifies the sizing process. With the Swanson implant, it is important that the opening of the intramedullary canal of the proximal phalanges be rectangular in shape and so positioned in the index and small fingers that the rectangular opening is angled slightly (from directly parallel to the palmar surface of the proximal phalanx.) In the index finger, the opening is slanted high on the dorsoulnar side, sloping palmar and radialward. This slant allows the stem of the Swanson prosthesis to create a slight supination moment, which is desirable in the index finger. In the small finger, the medullary canal rectangular opening is angled in the opposite direction to impart slight pronation to the digit.

Following the preparation of the medullary canals, prostheses trials are used in order to select the largest possible prosthesis, whereupon no buckling or impingement of the implant is encountered. Oftentimes, the medullary canal of the ring fingers is the narrowest. With the Swanson implant the intramedullary stems must be allowed to slide within the canals so that the tapered ends of the prosthesis do not bottom out, which would cause buckling, rotation, or unwanted compression of the implant. At this point, if circumferential titanium grommets are to be used they are fitted into the medullary canals and must correspond to the size of the selected implant (80).

Should one encounter buckling or impingement of the implant, additional measures must be undertaken to allow proper seating. The palmar plate may be incised or resected if severely contracted, allowing for further extension and of the proximal phalanx. Alternatively, additional bone may be resected in an incremental fashion. Once the proper sized implant has been determined from insertion of trials, the intramedullary canals are copiously irrigated with antibiotic impregnated saline removing any bone fragments from the reaming process. If the collateral ligaments have been released from the metacarpal, the radial ligaments will need to be reattached either to the preserved periosteum or to the metacarpal neck through drill holes. Radial collateral ligament reattachment reconstruction is most critical in the index digit in order to restore lateral stability required during pinch (Fig. 6.11) (1,4,25,28,33). The sutures are placed prior to implant placement. I prefer to use a 3-0 nonabsorbable braided suture, which is placed through the collateral ligament in a Bunnell fashion with the free end of the sutures exiting the prepared drill holes. Similar reattachment or imbrication of the radial collateral ligaments of the long and ring will improve radial stability and may decrease the potential for recurrence of ulnar deviation. The selected implants are gently inserted with smooth instruments to prevent tearing of the silicone material. If the capsule is adequate, it may be closed over the implant using a fine absorbable suture. The reattachment of the radial collateral ligament or imbrication thereof from the previously placed suture then follows often incorporating a portion of the capsule in the repair. Many surgeons do not find it necessary to close the capsule over the implant as often the capsule is quite attenuated or could not be adequately separated from the underlying synovium (4,33,84).

The radial sagittal band fibers are then imbricated by suture and the extensor tendon centralized by any of the means described previously. All suture knots should be buried to prevent dermal initiation. The incised junctura tendinum are repaired using a nonabsorbable 4-0 braided suture. If the

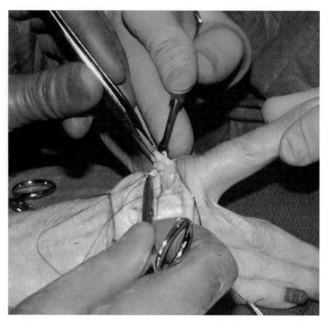

FIGURE 6.11 Reattachment of the radial collateral ligament of the index finger by nonabsorbable suture, which has been previously placed through drill holes in the metacarpal neck. (See Color Fig. 6.11.)

implants are properly selected, the soft tissues properly reconstructed, and the extensor mechanism realigned, the posture of the digits should appear essentially normal. The soft tissues are then infiltrated with 0.5% bupivacaine and the skin is closed over small drains. I prefer small strips of silicone sheeting or the equivalent.

The postoperative dressing is an important part of the operation and should not be applied haphazardly. A bulky conforming soft-tissue dressing using multiple fluffs placed strategically both dorsally and palmarly should be added to provide gentle, even compression to reduce swelling, and also to support the digits in the corrected position. A palmar plaster splint is incorporated to immobilize the wrist in neutral. The MCP joints are held in extension with slight IP joint flexion. Care should be taken not to wrap the dressings so as to create any rotation or ulnar deviation of the digits.

Postoperative Care

The drains are removed on the first or second postoperative day and a similar conforming bulky soft-tissue dressing is reapplied. Beginning 3 to 5 days postoperatively or when local wound conditions allow, the patient is fitted with a dynamic outrigger extension splint using rubber bands with alignment slings to maintain the corrected digit positioning (Fig. 6.12). Supervised instruction of active and active-assisted flexion exercises are then begun, making certain that flexion of the digit occurs at the MCP joint level and not entirely through the PIP joints. The therapist may sequentially remove rubber

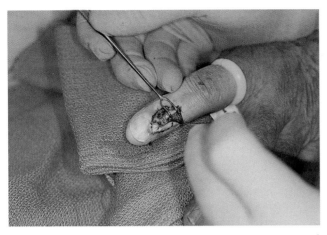

COLOR FIG. 4.10. Elevation of skin flap over mucous cyst and retraction of extensor tendon. (See Fig. 4.10 on page 47.)

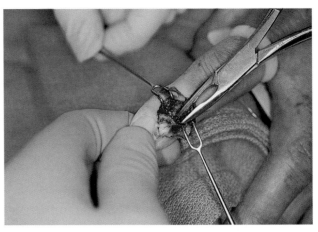

COLOR FIG. 4.11. Debridement of marginal osteophytes along the joint line with a rongeur. (See Fig. 4.11 on page 47.)

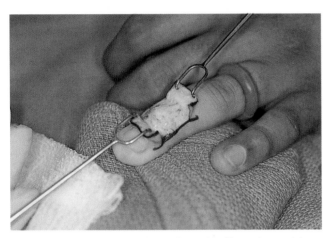

COLOR FIG. 4.15. Full thickness flaps skin flaps elevated from the extensor tendon epitenon during DIP joint exposure. (See Fig. 4.15 on page 48.)

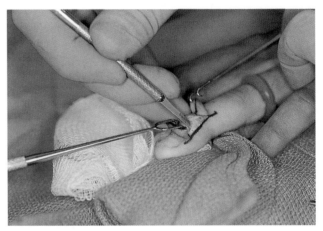

COLOR FIG. 4.16. Technique for "back-cutting" origin of the collateral ligament. Beaver blade is placed between the collateral ligament and head of the middle phalanx. Rotation of the blade releases the collateral ligament from its origin. (See Fig. 4.16 on page 48.)

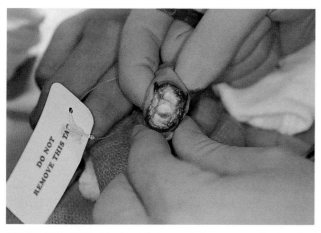

COLOR FIG. 4.17. Flexion of the DIP joint exposes the head of the middle phalanx and the base of the distal phalanx. (See Fig. 4.17 on page 48.)

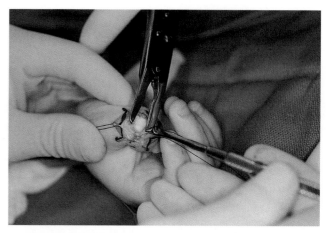

COLOR FIG. 4.21. Following joint exposure, a rongeur is used to fashion the convex curvature of the middle phalanx. (See Fig. 4.21 on page 50.)

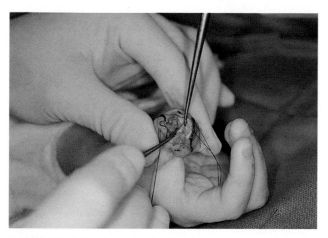

COLOR FIG. 4.22. A curette is utilized to remove any remaining cartilage from the distal phalanx base and create a reciprocal convex surface. (See Fig. 4.22 on page 50.)

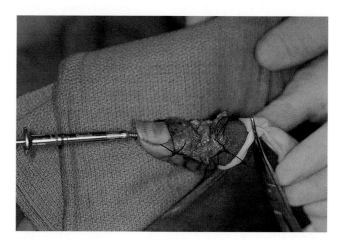

COLOR FIG. 4.32. A self-tapping screw inserted retrograde through the finger pulp and across the reduced DIP joint. (See Fig. 4.32 on page 53.)

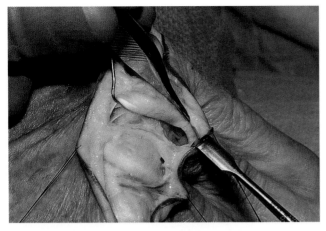

COLOR FIG. 6.4. Exposure of the finger MCP joints and extensor mechanisms through a single transverse incision. The extensor tendons are subluxated ulnarly with associated stretching and attenuation of the radial sagittal band fibers. (See Fig. 6.4 on page 80.)

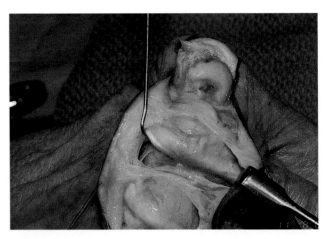

COLOR FIG. 6.5. The ulnar sagittal band fibers are markedly contracted. Note that with traction applied through by the hook cannot centralize the tendon without release of the contracted ulnar sagittal band, as has been performed in the index digit shown at the top of the photograph. (See Fig. 6.5 on page 80.)

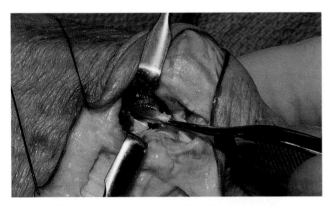

COLOR FIG. 6.6. Exposure of the ulnar intrinsic tendon, which has been incised at the muscular tendonous junction (distal end of the tendon held in the forceps) accomplishing the ulnar intrinsic release. (See Fig. 6.6 on page 80.)

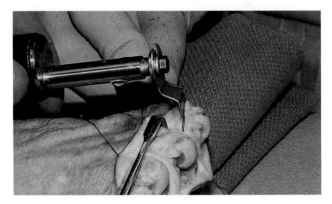

COLOR FIG. 6.10. (A). Osteotomy of the metacarpal head through the neck level perpendicular to the long axis of the metacarpal diaphysis. (See Fig. 6.10 on page 87.)

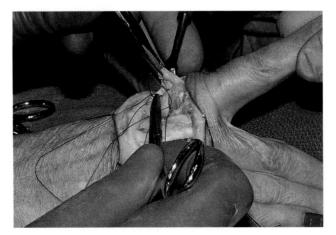

COLOR FIG. 6.11. Reattachment of the radial collateral ligament of the index finger by nonabsorbable suture, which has been previously placed through drill holes in the metacarpal neck. (See Fig. 6.11 on page 88.)

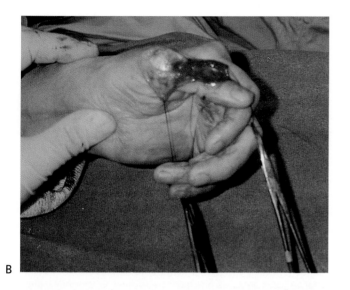

B

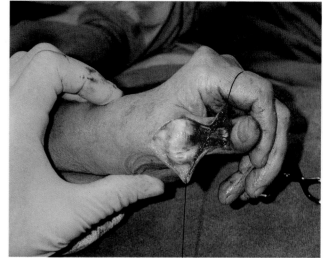

C

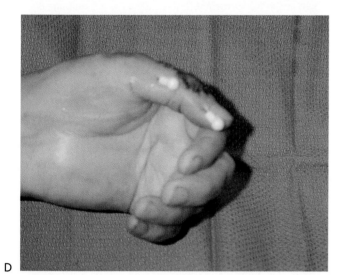

D

COLOR FIG. 7.4. Surgical procedure of the left RA thumb using inter-op photos (B, C) and post-op (D) of Boutonnière reconstruction using Nalebuff modified technique. (See Fig. 7.4 on page 99.)

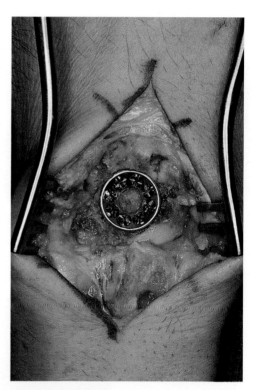

COLOR FIG. 10.17. An intra-operative view of the Spider Plate placed in the dorsal wrist with bone graft augmenting the central hole (A). (See Fig. 10.17 on page 131.)

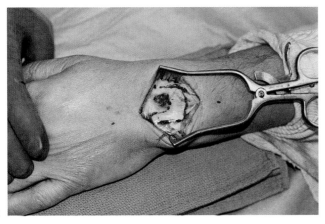
A

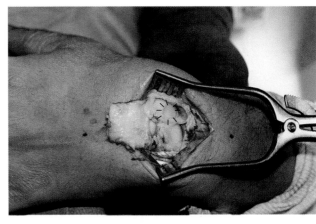
B

COLOR FIG. 11.6. (A). The dorsal capsule is exposed. A distally based capsular flap is marked (solid outer line). The head of the capitate is centered in the flap (dotted inner line). (B) The capsular flap is retracted distally to reveal the carpus. Note the area of exposed subchondral bone on the proximal pole of the scaphoid (small lines). (See Fig. 11.6 on page 146.)

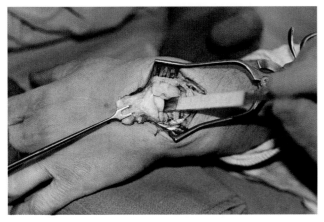

COLOR FIG. 11.7. The wrist is palmar-flexed and the head of the capitate is inspected for arthrosis. The majority of the joint surface is preserved, so excision of the proximal row can proceed. (See Fig. 11.7 on page 146.)

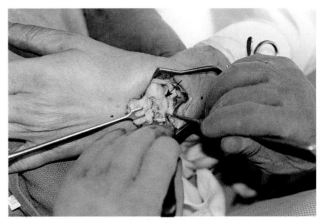

COLOR FIG. 11.8. The wrist is palmar-flexed and the lunotriquetral ligament is sectioned. In this patient the scapholunate ligament (arrow) was incompetent. (See Fig. 11.8 on page 146.)

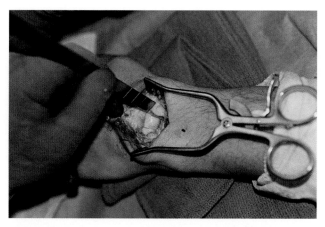

COLOR FIG. 11.9. A small osteotome is placed across the waist of the scaphoid, and it is split. This facilitates removal of the proximal pole and provides access to the distal pole for excision in a piecemeal fashion. (See Fig. 11.9 on page 147.)

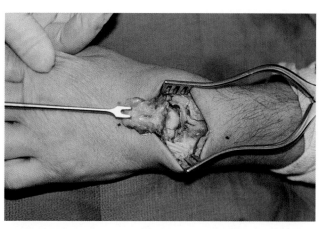

COLOR FIG. 11.10. Following excision of the proximal row, the capitate should rest in the lunate fossa of the radius. Impingement of the trapezium on the radial styloid is assessed at this time by placing the wrist through a range of wrist motion. Impingement is an indication for radial styloidectomy (see text), but the trapezium is usually noted to be volar to the styloid. (See Fig. 11.10 on page 147.)

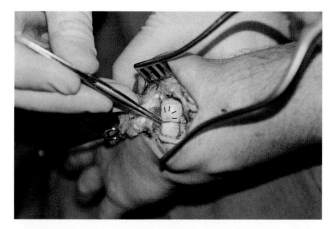

COLOR FIG. 11.12 Following proximal row carpectomy (PRC) (See Figs. 11.5–11.9) the capitate is shown to have early arthritic changes (small lines), primarily in the capitate-triquetral region. These changes do not preclude PRC in our experience, but they are an indication for a capsular interposition. (See Fig. 11.12 on page 150.)

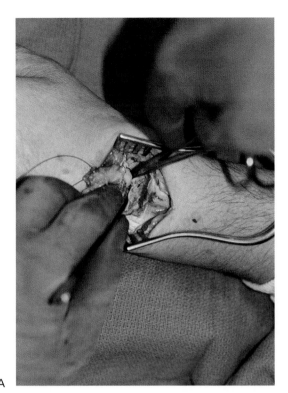

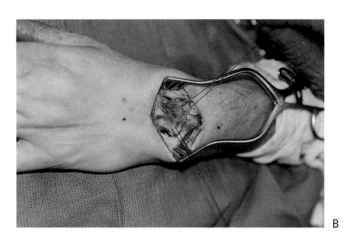

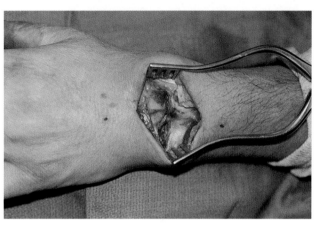

COLOR FIG. 11.13. Dorsal capsular interposition arthroplasty. (A). Sutures are placed in the volar wrist ligaments. (B). These sutures are brought dorsally through the proximal edge of the capsular flap. (C). The capsular flap is then tied down to the volar wrist ligaments, providing an interface between the capitate and radius articular surfaces. (See Fig. 11.13 on page 150.)

A

B

C

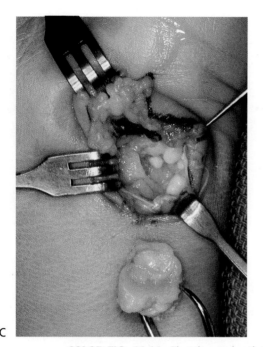

C

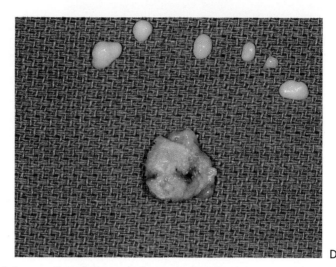

D

COLOR FIG. 11.14. Pisotriquetral arthritis. (C). Intraoperative photograph demonstrating the multiple loose bodies found in the joint, as well as the worn undersurface of the pisiform. (D). The loose bodies excised from the joint as well as the resected pisiform. The patient was diagnosed with synovial chondromatosis. (See Fig. 11.14 on page 152.)

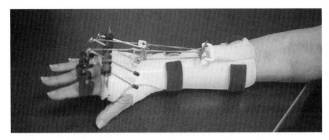

FIGURE 6.12 Postoperative dynamic extension outrigger splint with alignment rods and slings. This is a standard design used following MCP joint replacement arthroplasty and soft tissue realignment.

bands during therapy sessions to direct gentle active-assisted motion of each digit with the goal of obtaining 60–70° of flexion. A static resting night splint, which maintains corrected digit alignment, is also fabricated. Supervised therapy sessions are continued for 10 to 12 weeks with the frequency of visits determined by the individual progress of each patient and with the demonstration of the ability to accomplish the goals of self-directed therapy. Frequent adjustments to the outriggers and slings are common in the early postoperative period. The dynamic alignment splint is generally worn during the day for the first 4 to 6 weeks and thereafter for ROM sessions performed 3 to 4 times a day until approximately 3 months postoperatively. The static splint is worn at night for 3 months following surgery. The patient will often develop stiffness at the MCP joint level several weeks after surgery and may require fitting with a dynamic flexion splint and/or the addition of gentle passive flexion stretching exercises (33,85, 86). The operative technique and postoperative therapy regimen for the Sutter and NeuFlex implants are fundamentally the same as for the Swanson implant described above.

Outcomes

The long-term results of silicone implant arthroplasty of the MCP joint have been widely reported. Swanson's major indication for silicone implant arthroplasty was for the relief of pain and to improve the functional impairments associated with severe ulnar drift (22,25,28). By all accounts, the outcomes from the majority of reports of silicone MCP joint arthroplasty have observed consistent excellent relief of pain. The objective data of the outcomes for functional improvement and ROM of the digits are less consistent and variable. Average ROM of the MCP joint following silicone implant arthroplasty range from 34° to 57°, with an extension lag of 15°. This range of motion represents a modest gain over preoperative measurements, but certainly falls short of a desirable ROM (33,36,64,68,73). Clearly, the magnitude of the soft-tissue reconstruction and realignment is a major factor in the limitation of postoperative ROM. Most long-term studies report both a gradual diminishment in average ROM over

time and a recurrence of ulnar drift (5° average recurrence). Despite the improved finger alignment, postoperative grip and pinch strength measurements are only minimally improved or unchanged from preoperative values. CIT has been shown to lessen the tendency for late recurrence of ulnar drift while not diminishing ROM (4,33,38,39,41).

Fracture of MCP joint silicone implants has been reported as high as 26% (4,63). Despite radiographic evidence of implant fracture, these material failures have not been associated with an increase in pain and usually go unnoticed by the patient. Reactive microparticulate silicone synovitis following placement of silicone carpal implants has been widely reported (87,88). This complication has been infrequently observed in rheumatoid patients undergoing digital implant arthroplasty. Infections are rare (24).

METACARPAL PHALANGEAL JOINT IMPLANT ARTHROPLASTY
Future Considerations

The future of design improvements and research in biocompatible materials for MCP joint implant arthroplasty remains uncertain. At present, the Swanson MCP joint implant should be considered the standard—a design that is fundamentally unchanged since it was first used in the late 1960s. The most recently introduced silicone implants and the surface replacement implants, both of which incorporate intriguing design modifications, remain in clinical trial. Therefore, it is unknown whether these designs will prove to be more durable or result in improved ROM as compared to the Swanson implant. Osteointegration of biocompatible metals shows considerable promise in overcoming the problems of bone cement as an acceptable means of implant fixation, but further applied research for the applicability for digital joint implants is needed (89).

One of the major impediments to fostering any meaningful research in any MCP joint implant development is the current regulatory policies of our own Food and Drug Administration and the cumbersome and expensive process of implementation of proven technology into human trial. Moreover, and perhaps as importantly, the monetary reimbursement to the manufacturers continues to decline in the present medical care cost containment era, which undoubtedly stifles any incentive on their part to incur the cost of research and development. Without a fundamental change to these encumbrances, it is unlikely that there will be any major innovations in MCP joint implant arthroplasty in the near future. Fortunately, there have been significant recent improvements in the pharmacologic management of RA. Methotrexate and other slow-acting antirheumatic drugs (SAARDs) show promise in controlling the manifestations of the disease and may modify the natural course of RA, thus decreasing or delaying the progression of RA hand deformities.

REFERENCES

1. Flatt AE. *Care of the arthritic hand*, 4th ed. St. Louis: Mosby, 1983.
2. Zancolli E. *Structural and dynamic bases of hand surgery*, 2d ed. Philadelphia: Lippincott, 1983.
3. Krishnan J, Chipchase L. Passive axial rotation of the metacarpophalangeal joint. *J Hand Surg [Br]* 1997;22:270–273.
4. Linscheid RL, Beckenbaugh RD. Arthroplasty of the metacarpophalangeal joint. In: Morrey BF, An K-N, eds. *Reconstructive surgery of the joints*, 2nd ed. New York: Churchill Livingstone, 1996:287.
5. An KN, Chao EY, Cooney WP, Linscheid RL. Forces in the normal and abnormal hand. *J Orthop Res* 1985;3:202–211.
6. An KN, Cooney WP. Biomechanics. In: Moffey BF, ed. *Joint replacement arthroplasty*. New York: Churchill Livingstone, 1991: 137–146.
7. Flatt AE. The pathomechanics of ulnar drift. Final Report Social and Rehab Services. Grant No. RD2226M.
8. Clawson DK, Souter WA, Carthum CJ, Hymen Ml. Functional assessment of the rheumatoid hand. *Clin Orthop* 1971;77:203–210.
9. Ellison MR, Flatt AE, Kelly KJ. Ulnar drift of the fingers in rheumatoid disease. Treatment by crossed intrinsic tendon transfer. *J Bone Joint Surg [Am]* 1971;53:1061–1082.
10. Hakstian RW, Tubiana R. Ulnar deviation of the fingers. The role of joint structure and function. *J Bone Joint Surg [Am]* 1967;49: 299–316.
11. James DF, Clark IP, Cotwill JC, Halsall AP. Forces in the metacarpophalangeal joint due to elevated fluid pressure—analysis, measurements and relevance to ulnar drift. *J Biomech* 1982;15:73–84.
12. Linscheid RL, Dobyns JH. Total joint arthroplasty. The hand. *Mayo Clin Proc* 1979;54:516–526.
13. McMaster M. The natural history of the rheumatoid metacarpophalangeal joint. *J Bone Joint Surg [Br]* 1972;54:687–697.
14. Miller-Breslow A, Millender LH, Feldon PG. Treatment considerations in the complicated rheumatoid hand. *Hand Clin* 1989;5: 279–289.
15. Shapiro JS. A new factor in the etiology of ulnar drift. *Clin Orthop* 1970;68:32–43.
16. Shapiro JS, Heij na W, Nasatir S, Ray RD. The relationship of wrist motion to ulnar phalangeal drift in the rheumatoid patient. *Hand* 1971;3:68–75.
17. Smith EM, Juvinall RC, Bender LF, Pearson JR. Flexor forces and rheumatoid metacarpophalangeal deformity. Clinical implications. *JAMA* 1966;198:130–134.
18. Smith RJ. Intrinsic contracture. In: Green DP, Hotchkiss RN, Pederson WC, eds. *Green's operative hand surgery*, 4th ed. New York: Churchill Livingstone, 1999:604.
19. Smith RJ, Kaplan EB. Rheumatoid deformities at the metacarpophalangeal joints of the fingers. *J Bone Joint Surg [Am]* 1967;49: 31–47.
20. Stirrat CR. Metacarpophalangeal joints in rheumatoid arthritis of the hand. *Hand Clin* 1996;12:515–529.
21. Straub L. The rheumatoid hand. *Clin Orthop* 1959;15:127–139.
22. Swanson AB, de Groot GA, Hehl RW, et al. Pathogenesis of rheumatoid deformities of the hand. In: Cruess RL, Mitchell NS, eds. *Surgery of rheumatoid arthritis*. Philadelphia: Lippincott, 1971:143.
23. Taleisnik J. Rheumatoid synovitis of the volar compartment of the wrist joint: its radiological signs and its contribution to wrist and hand deformity. *J Hand Surg [Am]* 1979;4:526–535.
24. Nalebuff EA, Millender LH. Surgical treatment of the swan-neck deformity in rheumatoid arthritis. *Orthop Clin North Am* 1975;6: 733–752.
25. Swanson AB. Flexible implant arthroplasty for arthritic finger joints: rationale, technique, and results of treatment. *J Bone Joint Surg [Am]* 1972;54:435–455.
26. Swanson AB, Swanson G. Flexible implant arthroplasty of the radiocarpal joint. *Semin Arthroplasty* 1991;2:78–84.
27. Feldon PG, Terrono AL, Nalebuff EA, et al. Rheumatoid arthritis and other connective tissue diseases. In: Green DP, Hotchkiss RN, Pederson WC, eds. *Green's operative hand surgery*, 4th ed. New York: Churchill Livingstone, 1999:1651–1739.
28. Swanson AB. Silicone rubber implants for replacement of arthritis or destroyed joints in the hand. *Surg Clin North Am* 1968;48:1113–1127.
29. Ferlic DC, Smyth CJ, Clayton ML. Medical considerations and management of rheumatoid arthritis. *J Hand Surg [Am]* 1983;8: 662–666.
30. Souter WA. Planning treatment of the rheumatoid hand. *Hand* 1979;11:3–16.
31. Ellison MR, Kelly KJ, Flatt AE. The results of surgical synovectomy of the digital joints in rheumatoid disease. *J Bone Joint Surg [Am]* 1971;53:1041–1060.
32. Nalebuff EA. Rheumatoid hand surgery—update. *J Hand Surg [Am]* 1983;8:678–682.
33. Berger RA, Beckenbaugh RD, Linscheid RL. Arthroplasty in the hand and wrist. In: Green DP, Hotchkiss RN, Pederson WC, eds. *Green's operative hand surgery*, 4th ed, Vol 1. New York: Churchill Livingstone, 1999:147–192.
34. Weiss APC. NeuFlex prostheses. In: Simmen BR, Allieu Y, Lluch A, et al, eds. *Hand arthroplasties*. London: Martin Dunitz, 2000:315–322.
35. Sully L, Jackson IT, Sommerlad BC. Perichondrial grafting in rheumatoid metacarpophalangeal joints. *Hand* 1980;12:137–148.
36. Blair WF, Shurr DG, Buckwalter JA. Metacarpophalangeal joint implant arthroplasty with a Silastic spacer. *J Bone Joint Surg [Am]* 1984;66:365–370.
37. Harris CJ, Riordan DC. Intrinsic contracture in the hand and its surgical treatment. *J Bone Joint Surg [Am]* 1954;36A:10–20.
38. Blair WF. Crossed intrinsic transfers. In: Blair WF, Steyers CM, eds. *Techniques in hand surgery*. Baltimore: Williams & Wilkins, 1996: 660–666.
39. Wood VE, Ichtertz DR, Yahiku H. Soft-tissue metacarpophalangeal reconstruction for treatment of rheumatoid hand deformity. *J Hand Surg [Am]* 1989;14:163–174.
40. Harrison SH. Excision arthroplasty of the metacarpophalangeal joints. In: Tubiana R, Achach PC. Groupe d'*tude de la main, eds. *La Main rhumato*de (The Rheumatoid hand)*. Paris: L'Expansion, 1969:269.
41. el-Gammal TA, Blair WF. Motion after metacarpophalangeal joint reconstruction in rheumatoid disease. *J Hand Surg [Am]* 1993;18: 504–511.
42. Oster LH, Blair WF, Steyers CM, Flatt AE. Crossed intrinsic transfer. *J Hand Surg [Am]* 1989;14:963–971.
43. Riordan DC, Fowler SB. Surgical treatment of rheumatoid deformities of the hand (abstract). *J Bone Joint Surg [Am]* 1958;4OA: 1431–1432.
44. Riordan DC, Fowler SB. Arthroplasty of the metacarpophalangeal joints: review of resection-type arthroplasty. *J Hand Surg [Am]* 1989;14:368–371.
45. Kestler OC. Surgical procedure for the painful arthritic hand. *Bull Hosp Jt Dis* 1946;7:114.
46. Kuhns JG. Rehabilitation of the hand in rheumatoid arthritis. *J Bone Joint Surg [Am]* 1958;4OA:1432.
47. Tupper JW. The metacarpophalangeal volar plate arthroplasty. *J Hand Surg [Am]* 1989;14:371–375.
48. Weilby A. Resection arthroplasty of the metacarpophalangeal joint a.m. Tupper using interposition of the volar plate. *Scand J Plast Reconstr Surg* 1977;11:239–242.
49. Vainio K. Vainio arthroplasty of the metacarpophalangeal joints in rheumatoid arthritis. *J Hand Surg [Am]* 1989;14:367–368.
50. Hellum C, Vainio K. Arthroplasty of the metacarpophalangeal joints in rheumatoid arthritis with transposition of the interosseus muscles. *Scand J Plast Reconstr Surg* 1968;2:139–143.

51. Carroll R, Taber T. Digital arthroplasty of the proximal interphalangeal joint. *J Bone Joint Surg Am* 1954;36A:912–920.
52. Ohlsen L. Cartilage formation from free perichondral grafts: an experimental study in rabbits. *Br J Plast Surg* 1976;29:262–267.
53. Ohlsen L. Cartilage regeneration from perichondrium. Experimental studies and clinical applications. *Plast Reconstr Surg* 1978;62: 507–513.
54. Skoog T, Ohlsen L, Sohn SA. Perichondral potential for cartilaginous regeneration. *Scand J Plast Reconstr Surg* 1972;6:123–125.
55. Skoog T, Johansson SH. The formation of articular cartilage from free perichondral grafts. *Plast Reconstr Surg* 1976;57:1–6.
56. Engkvist O, Johansson SH. Perichondral arthroplasty. A clinical study in twenty-six patients. *Scand J Plast Reconstr Surg* 1980;14: 71–87.
57. Engkvist O, Ohlsen L. Reconstruction of articular cartilage with free autologous perichondral grafts. An experimental study in rabbits. *Scand J Plast Reconstr Surg* 1979;13:269–274.
58. Weiland AJ. Small joint arthrodesis. In: Green DP, Hotchkiss RN, Pederson WC, eds. *Green's operative hand surgery*, 4th ed. New York: Churchill Livingstone, 1999:95–107.
59. Carroll RE, Hill NA. Small joint arthrodesis in hand reconstruction. *J Bone Joint Surg [Am]* 1969;51:1219–1221.
60. Wright CS, McMurtry RY. AO arthrodesis in the hand. *J Hand Surg [Am]* 1983;8:932–935.
61. Moberg E. Arthrodesis of the finger joint. *Surg Cling North Am* 1969;40:465–470.
62. Burman MS. Vitallium cap arthroplasty of the metacarpophalangeal and interphalangeal joints of the fingers. *Bull Hosp Jt Dis* 1940;1:79–80.
63. Bass RL, Stern PJ, Nairus JG. High implant fracture incidence with Sutter silicone metacarpophalangeal joint arthroplasty. *J Hand Surg [Am]* 1996;21:813–818.
64. Beckenbaugh RD, Dobyns JH, Linscheid RL, Bryan RS. Review and analysis of silicone-rubber metacarpophalangeal implants. *J Bone Joint Surg [Am]* 1976;58:483–487.
65. Beckenbaugh RD, Steffee AD. Total joint arthroplasty for the metacarpophalangeal joint of the thumb. A preliminary report. *Orthopedics* 1981;4:298.
66. Blair WF, Shurr DG, Buckwalter JA. Metacarpophalangeal joint arthroplasty with a metallic hinged prosthesis. *Clin Orthop* 1984; 156–163.
67. Cook SD, Beckenbaugh RD, Redondo J, et al. Long-term follow-up of pyrolytic carbon metacarpophalangeal implants. *J Bone Joint Surg [Am]* 1999;81:635–648.
68. Derkash RS, Niebauer JJ, Jr., Lane CS. Long-term follow-up of metacarpal phalangeal arthroplasty with silicone Dacron prostheses. *J Hand Surg [Am]* 1986;11:553–558.
69. Ferlic DC, Clayton ML, Holloway M. Complications of silicone implant surgery in the metacarpophalangeal joint. *J Bone Joint Surg [Am]* 1975;57:991–994.
70. Goldner JL, Gould JS, Urbaniak JR, McCollum DE. Metacarpophalangeal joint arthroplasty with silicone-Dacron prostheses (Niebauer type): six and a half years' experience. *J Hand Surg [Am]* 1977;2:200–211.
71. Kirschenbaum D, Schneider LH, Adams DC, Cody RP. Arthroplasty of the metacarpophalangeal joints with use of silicone-rubber implants in patients who have rheumatoid arthritis. Long-term results. *J Bone Joint Surg [Am]* 1993;75:3–12.
72. Levack B, Stewart HD, Flierenga H, Helal B. Metacarpophalangeal joint replacement with a new prosthesis: description and preliminary results of treatment with the Helal flap joint. *J Hand Surg [Br]* 1987;12:377–381.
73. Mannerfelt L, Andersson K. Silastic arthroplasty of the metacarpophalangeal joints in rheumatoid arthritis. *J Bone Joint Surg [Am]* 1975;57:484–489.
74. Steffee AD, Beckenbaugh RD, Linscheid RL, Dobyns JH. The development, technique and early results of total joint replacement of the metacarpophalangeal joints of the fingers. *Orthopedics* 1981; 4:175–180.
75. Stothard J, Thompson AE, Sherris D. Correction of ulnar drift during silastic metacarpo-phalangeal joint arthroplasty. *J Hand Surg [Br]* 1991;16:61–65.
76. Swanson AB, Poitevin LA, de Groot Swanson G, Kearney J. Bone remodeling phenomena in flexible implant arthroplasty in the metacarpophalangeal joints. Long-term study. *Clin Orthop* April 1986;(205):254–267.
77. Wilson YG, Sykes PJ, Niranjan NS. Long-term follow-up of Swanson's silastic arthroplasty of the metacarpophalangeal joints in rheumatoid arthritis. *J Hand Surg [Br]* 1993;18:81–91.
78. Niebauer JJ, Landry RM. Dacron-silicone prosthesis for the metacarpophalangeal and interphalangeal joints. *Hand* 1971;3: 55–61.
79. Niebauer JJ, Shaw JL, Doren WW. Silicone-dacron hinge prosthesis. Design, evaluation, and application. *Ann Rheum Dis* 1969;28: Suppl:56–58.
80. Swanson AB, de Groot Swanson G, Ishikawa H. Use of grommets for flexible implant resection arthroplasty of the metacarpophalangeal joint. *Clin Orthop* Sept 1997;(342):22–33.
81. Schmidt K, Willburger R, Ossowski A, Miehlke RK. The effect of the additional use of grommets in silicone implant arthroplasty of the metacarpophalangeal joints. *J Hand Surg [Br]* 1999;24:561–564.
82. Linscheid RL, Murray PM, Vidal MA, Beckenbaugh RD. Development of a surface replacement arthroplasty for proximal interphalangeal joints. *J Hand Surg [Am]* 1997;22:286–298.
83. Beckenbaugh RD. Preliminary experience with a noncemented nonconstrained total joint arthroplasty for the metacarpophalangeal joint. *Orthopedics* 1983;6:962–965.
84. Millender LH, Nalebuff EA. Metacarpophalangeal joint arthroplasty utilizing the silicone rubber prosthesis. *Orthop Clin North Am* 1973;4:349–371.
85. Madden JW, De Vore G, Arem AJ. A rational postoperative management program for metacarpophalangeal joint implant arthroplasty. *J Hand Surg [Am]* 1977;2:358–366.
86. Swanson AB, Swanson GD, Leonard J, Boozer J. Postoperative rehabilitation programs in flexible implant arthroplasty of the digits. In: Hunter JM, Schneider LH, Mackin PT, Callahan AD, eds. *Rehabilitation of the hand: surgery and therapy*, 3rd ed. St. Louis: Mosby, 1990:912–928.
87. Carter PR, Benton LJ, Dysert PA. Silicone rubber carpal implants: a study of the incidence of late osseous complications. *J Hand Surg [Am]* 1986;11:639–644.
88. Peimer CA, Medige J, Eckert BS, et al. Reactive synovitis after silicone arthroplasty. *J Hand Surg [Am]* 1986;11:624–638.
89. Hagert CG, Branemark PI, Albrektsson T, et al. Metacarpophalangeal joint replacement with osseointegrated endoprostheses. *Scand J Plast Reconstr Surg* 1986;20:207–218.

7

THUMB INTERPHALANGEAL AND METACARPOPHALANGEAL JOINTS

EDWARD DIAO

HISTORICAL PERSPECTIVE

The first significant report of rheumatoid arthritis and its treatment in the thumb was presented by Clayton at the 1962 American Society for Surgery of the Hand meeting in Chicago (1). Most notably this study looked at contracture of the thumb, subsequent deformities, and methods of release. Subsequent works by Flatt (2), Vainio (3), Inglis (4), and Marmor (5) each offer important expansions upon Clayton's original article.

Nalebuff presents the most influential work on the subject in the 1968 Bulletin for the Hospital of Joint Diseases (6). Here Nalebuff devises the first classification of rheumatoid thumb deformities as well as outlining treatments. The previous authors had all addressed aspects of rheumatoid thumb deformities such as the adduction deformity, boutonnière deformity, and ulnar drift in their work, but it is Nalebuff who first proposes a comprehensive classification scheme to include both the most common deformities (i.e., the boutonnière deformity) as well as some of the less common patterns. Throughout the 1970s, papers by Inglis, Harrison, and further writings by Nalebuff consolidate the surgical approaches to joint deformity and muscle imbalances about the thumb and IP joint.

INDICATIONS/CONTRAINDICATIONS

In previous chapters, the pathophysiology of joint deformities was discussed. In this section, the patterns of disease and deformity in rheumatoid arthritis and osteoarthritis will be reviewed more specifically with indications and contraindications for various surgical treatments in the thumb interphalangeal and metacarpophalangeal joints.

In the thumb ray itself, the joint most commonly affected by osteoarthritis is the carpometacarpal, or trapezial metacarpal joint. Given this general pattern, the incidence of isolated treatment for thumb metacarpalphalangeal, or interphalangeal arthritis that would necessitate surgery is relatively limited. Thus the focus of this chapter will be on connective

tissue diseases, namely rheumatoid arthritis as an etiology for thumb interphalangeal, and metacarpalphalangeal joint surgery.

In 1968, Nalebuff proposed a classification of thumb deformities. In this classification scheme, the type I was the boutonnière deformity. It was the most common type, comprising 50% to 74% of all thumb deformities (7,8). Since Nalebuff's original description and classification system, he and others have modified the system and provided additional clinical categories (9).

Boutonnière deformity is characterized by metacarpophalangeal (MP) joint flexion and distal interphalangeal (DIP) joint hyperextension. It is caused by a proliferative MP joint synovitis, which results in stretching and attenuation of the extensor mechanism at the level of the MCP joint, including the dorsal capsule, extensor pollicis brevis (EPB) tendon, and extensor pollicis longus (EPL) tendon within the extensor hood. The pathomechanics of this synovitis result in the attenuation of the EPB tendon insertion as the structure stretches.

Simultaneously, attenuation and stretching of the extensor hood occurs. This allows for displacement of the EPL, which normally sits just ulnar to the dorsal midline of the digit at the MP joint, to a more ulnar and ultimately a volar position. Concomitant collateral ligament attenuation, volar plate attenuation, and/or intra-articular joint destruction occurs. The result of these events is volar subluxation of the metacarpal proximal phalanx and MCP flexion deformity. As this occurs, the ability to actively extend the MCP joint diminishes.

Secondary effects of this joint flexion deformity occur both distally at the IP joint and proximally at the carpometacarpal (CMC) joint. IP joint hypertension results from the altered pull vector of the intrinsic muscles in the displaced EPL tendon. Simultaneously, synovitis or attenuation of the volar plate of the IP joint will result in further hyperextension. Additionally, metacarpal radial abduction occurs as compensation to allow abduction of the entire thumb ray with the flexed MP joint. All of these unbalanced forces are accentuated when pinch forces occur. Initially in the early stages both the MP and the IP joint deformities are passively correctable, but over time fixed deformities may develop in the MP joint, the IP joint, and ultimately, even the carpometacarpal (CMC) joint.

Indications for operative treatment are based on the three clinical stages of type I deformity. Each stage requires a different surgical approach. These are outlined in Table 7.1.

In the early stage, both the MP joint deformities (MP joint subluxation) and the IPJ deformity (IP joint hypertension) are passively correctable. At this stage, the surgical treatments include (a) synovectomy of the MP joint and (b) reconstruction of the extensor mechanism, to rebalance the forces about the MP joint.

In the second stage, the MP joint deformity is fixed. However the IP joint remains passively correctable. At this stage, there is more alteration of hand function in comparison to the first stage, and thus more patients are candidates for surgical reconstruction.

If the MP joint has a fixed deformity without much joint destruction, soft-tissue release of the joint at the volar plate and collateral ligaments may be appropriate, followed by a stage one type approach utilizing synovectomy and capsular tightening. However the majority of patients with second stage type I deformity will have some element of joint destruction. If the two adjacent joints, i.e., the IP joint distally and the CMC proximally, are minimally involved, then arthrodesis is the treatment of choice at the MP joint. If, however, degenerative changes are already developing or are likely to develop at either the IP joint or the CMC joint, then MP joint arthroplasty or arthroplasty combined with EPL rerouting should be considered. Feldon and others believe that correction of boutonnière deformity at the second stage helps prevent the third stage from occurring (10).

The third and most severe stage of type I deformity is the situation in which both fixed MP joint flexion deformity and fixed IP joint hyperextension deformity occur. Treatment is

dependent on the status of these two joints, as well as the condition of the more proximal carpal metacarpal joint. If the IP joint deformity is mild, a dorsal capsulotomy can be considered with some preservation of IP joint motion. However with moderate arthritic changes at the IP joint, recurrence is likely (11). With more severe IP joint destruction, IP joint arthrodesis is indicated.

Additionally, the status of the MP joint must be considered. Common factors affecting the procedure to be performed at the MP joint include severity of deformity, the status of articular cartilage and subchondral bone, and the procedure required for the distal IP joint. Ideally, if IP joint fusion is performed, preservation of MP joint motion is desirable. This can be achieved through with synovectomy and EPL rerouting, or with silicone implant arthroplasty (12).

Nalebuff type II deformity is a rare phenomena. It is most easily characterized as a combination of Nalebuff type I (boutonnière) deformity and Nalebuff type III (swan-neck) deformity. Distal to the thumb metacarpal, the deformity is similar to that of type I, with MP joint flexion and IP joint hypertension. Proximal to the metacarpal, however, the deformity is similar to that of type III, with CMC joint subluxation or dislocation. Treatment for type II deformity is similar to that of type I for the thumb IP and MCP joints, and to that of type III for the CMC joint.

The type III or swan-neck deformity is the second most common rheumatoid thumb deformity. Type III thumb deformity, like type II, originates at the carpometacarpal joint level with metacarpal subluxation of the trapezium and resultant adduction of the thumb metacarpal.

In type III deformity, primary CMC joint subluxation and disease is accompanied by MP joint hyperextension and IP joint flexion. The imbalance of extensor forces and CMC joint subluxation combine with volar plate laxity at the MP joint, thus leading to MP joint hyperextension. With the resultant change in muscle forces about the joint, distal IP joint flexion occurs. As type III patients attempt to open the first web space to accommodate grasp, the fixed CMC joint deformity prevents metacarpal abduction and extension. Therefore extension forces are transmitted externally to the MP joint resulting in MP joint hyperextension.

Indications for operative treatment of patients with type III deformity are also based on three general stages of disease. In the first stage, patients exhibit a symptomatic painful CMC joint with varying degrees of radiographic CMC joint destruction. Consequently, there is weak pinch and moderate degree of dysfunction. In the event of such mild to moderate joint changes, surgical treatment is indicated only after failure of conservative management of the arthritis with systemic medications, thumb opposition splinting, and at least a trial of steroid injections. In the event these treatments fail, and given minimal involvement of MP joint pathology, the recommended treatments are either hemi- or full resection arthroplasty at the carpal metacarpal joint with or without ligament reconstruction. Distal to the CMC joint procedure,

TABLE 7.1. TREATMENT OPTIONS FOR TYPE I THUMB DEFORMITY (BOUTONNIÈRE DEFORMITY)

Stage	MP Joint Treatment	IP Joint Treatment
Early	Supple-Flexion Synovectomy Extensor Mechanism Reconstruction EPL rerouting	Supple-Hyperextension Synovectomy

Moderate	Fixed ± Joint Destruction
	Capsular Tightening
	Arthrodesis (If CMC & IP
	  are supple)
	Arthroplasty (If CMC & IP
	  are involved)
		Passively Correctable
		Synovectomy

Advanced	Fixed-Flexion
	Arthrodesis
	Arthroplasty (EPL
	  Rerouting/Synovectomy
	  or Silicone Implant)
	Arthrodesis
		Fixed-Hyperextension
		IPJ Capsular Release
		Rebalance Forces
		Arthrodesis
		Arthrodesis

0.035-inch K-wires and 25 or 26 gauge stainless steel wires through threaded holes. They reported a 3% nonunion rate and a 9% incidence requiring hardware removal. Four patients had a painless pseudoarthrosis at the operation site. The authors concluded that tension bands provided reliable, stable fixation with some compression, and, in compliant patients, they were able to dispense with external splinting.

The Indiana Hand Center experience with small joint arthrodesis was reviewed by Leibovic and Strickland (24). In this series, K-wires were associated with the highest nonunion rate, tension bands had an intermediate nonunion rate, and Herbert screws had the lowest nonunion rate. They found a 50% failure rate in the plates compared to a 21% failure rate of K-wires, a 5% failure rate of tension bands, and a 0.5% failure rate of Herbert screws. Traditionally, the most common type of fixation for arthrodesis has been crossed K-wires. In a review by Burton, Margles, and Lunseth (25) 171 consecutive arthrodeses of small joints of the hand were performed on 134 patients using the technique described by Littler (26). Excellent alignment of bone surfaces with flat bone cuts, accurate placement of crossed K-wires, and use of supplemental cancellous bone graft were the hallmarks of this technique. These authors achieved union in 170 out of 171 arthrodesis, for nonunion rate of 0.6%. There were no infections and only four delayed unions. Uhl and Schneider (27) reviewed 76 consecutive cases of tension band arthrodesis with a fusion rate of 99%. Ijsselstein and coauthors (28) did a retrospective review of 203 arthrodesis to compare tension bands and various conventional K-wire techniques, including single K-wire, crossed K-wires, and crossed K-wires with interosseous wires. There was an 18% incidence of pin-site infection and a 15% reoperation rate in the K-wire groups. There was a 2% rate of infection in the tension band group and a 5% reoperation rate. In their hands, tension bands offered the best results. McGlynn and coauthors (29) used K-wires for fixation of bones prepared by a high-speed burr and achieved bone union in ten weeks or less in 86% of digits. This modification of the Carroll and Hill technique using a power burr proved effective in these authors' hands, and when combined with three K-wires, they found external mobilization may be unnecessary. Evolving from Kirschner and interosseous wires, various types of screws, plates, external fixators, and bone plugs have been used to effect arthrodesis. Faithfull and Herbert (30) reviewed use of the Herbert bone screw and achieved a 100% union rate in the small joints of the finger and thumb in 25 patients. Using lag screws, Wright and McMurtry (31) reported a 96% fusion rate in 110 joints in 83 patients. There was a 100% fusion rate at the PIP joint and 96% at the MP joint. Of their four failures, two had surgical infections. A more recent study by Katzman et al. (32) of 51 Herbert screw arthrodesis in IP joints in patients with both degenerative or posttraumatic arthritis as well as rheumatoid arthritis or mallet finger deformities, solid osseous union occurred in all patients, with an average interval of fusion at eight weeks. Nine of 33 rheumatoid joints required

supplemental K-wires to prevent rotation. There were 6 complications, mostly in rheumatoid patients.

The first large tension band arthrodesis series in the finger joints was reported by Allende and Engelem (33). They had a total of 26 digits, with only 5 complications, 2 infections, 2 with malunion or delayed union, and only 1 case of carpal-metacarpal joint arthrodesis.

An alternative method of AO screw fixation using an oblique lag screw was described by Teoh, Yeo, and Singh (34) with a 96% union rate in 23 joints. More recently, biodegradable pins have been introduced in hand surgery. Jensen and Jensen (35) compared biodegradable pins to K-wires. They found no difference in time to union or complication rates. They felt that biodegradable pins offered certain advantages as no additional procedures were needed in the 11 patients with pins compared to the 12 patients in the K-wire group. A historically interesting variation on this procedure is the bone peg as a method of bone grafting in those patients with severe bone loss. The original technique described in 1960 by Moberg and Henrikson (36) used bone grafts cut in straight square sections. Baruch and Kahanovich (37) described an angulated bone peg taken from the ulna or iliac crest for patients with bone loss and instability after trauma to the finger and failed arthroplasty.

Stern and Fulton (38) performed a study that looked specifically at complications of small joint arthrodesis. They looked at 181 arthrodesis of DIP and/or thumb IP joints. They compared various techniques including crossed K-pins (111 joints), interfragmentary wires and longitudinal K-pin (43 joints), and Herbert screws (27 joints). The nonunion rate was similar in each technique. There were 21 nonunions, of which 13 were pain free and 6 required subsequent arthrodesis (with one amputation and one patient who refused further surgery). Twenty percent of the arthrodesed joints had major complications: nonunion, malunion, deep infection, and osteomyelitis. Sixteen percent developed minor complications such as superficial wound infections, dorsal skin necrosis, cold intolerance, PIP stiffness, paresthesias, and prominent hardware. This study highlights the potential complications associated with small-joint arthrodesis. Nonetheless, arthrodesis in the thumb IP or MP joint is, on the whole, a very useful and predictable treatment and certainly the best treatment for some of the rheumatoid thumb deformities.

I feel that the Herbert screw provides excellent bone fixation when bone stock is adequate and the cross-sectional dimensions of the bone are large enough to accommodate the screw. Alternatively, a mini Herbert screw can be used for smaller fingers. Preparation for hand drilling with a standard retrograde technique is performed by first establishing the core hole, with the drill, then tapping for the screw threads, and finally placing the appropriately sized screw in a retrograde position.

Proper placement of the Herbert screw is crucial. It is difficult to reposition an improperly placed screw, and intraoperative fluoroscopy is essential for accurate placement of implants. An appropriate depth screw is selected and then placed to provide compression at the arthrodesis site. Splinting is advocated for the first four weeks.

The quality and quantity of bone available at the thumb IP joint determines the techniques of fixation. The surgeon may need to select K-wire instead of screw fixation. I feel that interosseous wires, although they provide good compression, require more significant surgical exposure than the Herbert screw or K-wire fixation, and thus have more limited applications.

For osteoarthritis patients, and many patients suffering from rheumatoid arthritis where bone quality is an issue, K-wire fixation may be the most expedient solution. Generally, 0.045 inch is the minimum viable size for K-wires. The IP joint position should be established in terms of mild flexion position, 15–25° of flexion. The K-wire can be drilled longitudinally retrograde from the distal pulp across the IP joint into the middle phalanx, or crossed with two oblique pins. If bone quality is sufficient to accept more sophisticated fixation, Herbert screw, Herbert Whipple screw, tension band wiring, or other compression screw fixation techniques can be used. These systems have advantages for better internal fixation. However, the critical factor in success with these implants is bone quality.

The terminal retrograde insertion of the Herbert screw is my favorite technique in patients with adequate bone stock. In this technique as well as others for interphalangeal joint arthrodesis, an operative/interoperative imaging system, ideally a mini C-arm type fluoroscopic imaging device is helpful. AP and lateral X-rays should be evaluated to assess the size of the distal phalanx intramedullary canal. It must be wide enough to accept the screw. The advantage of the Herbert screw is that the midsection of its shaft is unthreaded. The IP arthrodesis site should be prepared with curettes and rongeurs after exposure. We then favor two techniques that are possible for screw insertion. The retrograde preparation of both distal phalanx and proximal phalanx guide holes can be done by first drilling a 0.035-inch K-wire retrograde, then using this hole to pass the smaller Herbert drill to prepare the canal from distal phalanx to proximal phalanx, followed by the passage of the tap across the interphalangeal joint from distal to proximal phalanx. Measurement is made for the appropriate screw length, then the larger drill is inserted into the terminal phalanx to prepare for the seating of the screw's trailing threads. The screw is advanced with the screwdriver while control of the rotation is carefully maintained. If a properly sized screw has been selected then compression should occur as the leading screw threads traverse the interphalangeal joint and engage the middle phalanx. Rotary stability can be augmented with a secondary K-wire of 0.028 inch or 0.035 inch. If the screw is too short, it won't sufficiently traverse the interphalangeal joint and engage the middle phalanx. If the screw is too long however, the screw will either cut out of the trapezial portion of the middle phalanx or enter the softer intramedullary bone with poor fixation.

An alternative technique for screw placement is a two-step preparation technique. First, the IP joint is hyper-flexed.

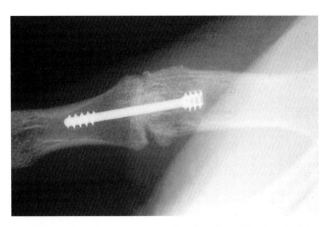

FIGURE 7.1. Herbert screw fixation for the MCP thumb joint arthrodesis.

Then, a guide wire is drilled antegrade from the IP joint through the distal phalanx and out the tip. Then the proximal phalanx is prepared by retrograde wire passage through the IP joint to the proximal phalanx. This is followed by the drill from the tip, then the tap, then the proximal screw thread drill and finally, the screw placement (Fig. 7.1).

METACARPALPHALANGEAL JOINT

Operative procedures for the rheumatoid metacarpalphalangeal joint include synovectomy alone, synovectomy with extensor mechanism reconstruction, capsular release, arthrodesis, and arthroplasty. For synovectomy, an S-shaped curved incision is best for exposure. The extensor mechanism is exposed, which will contain elements of the extensor pollicis brevis, extensor pollicis longus, and the dorsal capsule of the hood mechanism (39). Synovium can bulge around these extensor mechanisms and often between the extensor pollicis longus, which is ulnar in position, and the extensor pollicis brevis, which is radial in position. Synovectomy is performed with rongeurs and curettes, with limited capsulotomies performed. As this space is relatively tight, small curettes such as a dental curette are helpful, as is careful retraction of the synovium with forceps and scissor dissection. Occasionally, small defects in the cartilage are seen, which may also require curetage.

In simple cases concerning mildly affected joints without much soft-tissue deformity, the dorsal extensor mechanism can simply be reapproximated with absorbable sutures if that was the mode of entry into the joint. However, for more severe cases with significant extensor mechanism disruption, varying degrees of operative intervention can be performed at the extensor mechanism level. In the mildest cases where the extensor pollicis brevis and extensor pollicis longus have a diastasis, a simple reapproximation with a pants-over-vest suturing of the capsular tissue surrounding EPL and EPB tendon can be performed. There are several ways to do these reconstructions (4,40,41). In Nalebuff's technique, the

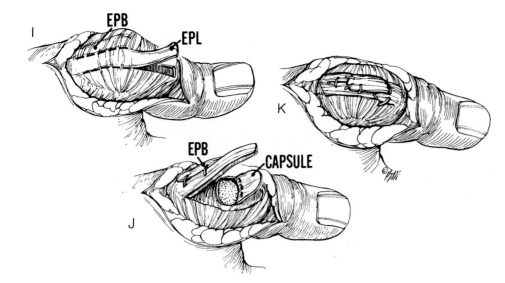

FIGURE 7.2. (I) In the standard method of extensor pollicis longus (EPL) rerouting, the extensor pollicis longus tendon is transected between the MP and IP joints and elevated proximally. In Nalebuff's modified technique, the extensor pollicis longus is transected more proximally, and the distal stump is sutured to the extensor pollicis brevis (EPB) tendon. The proximal stump is passed through the MP joint capsule and sutured back onto itself in both methods (J& K).

extensor pollicis longus is transected at the proximal first third of the proximal phalanx, between the interphalangeal joint and the metacarpalphalangeal joint. This is then freed up proximally by dividing the tendon proper from the extensor mechanism. Next the attenuated extensor pollicis brevis tendon is dissected from its insertion, dissected from the base of the proximal phalanx, and detached from the extensor hood mechanism. Next the key is to expose the dorsum of the MP joint, taking care to preserve the thickest portion of the dorsal joint capsule, whose attachment to the base of the proximal phalanx should be maintained.

Now the extensor pollicis longus will be passed through a small buttonhole made in this distally based capsular flap through which the extensor pollicis longus tendon will be passed and pulled back over itself (Fig. 7.2).

With the joint in full extension, the tendon is sutured with good tension. The thumb should now be unsupported and the resting position noted to be in less deformity than preoperatively. Next the extensor pollicis brevis is pulled distally and sutured into the side of the extensor pollicis longus (Nalebuff original technique). The extensor pollicis brevis tendon can also be sutured to the extensor pollicis longus thumb to improve interphalangeal joint extension (Nalebuff modified technique).

Nalebuff has subsequently modified his technique (19). In the modified technique, the extensor pollicis brevis and extensor pollicis longus are both divided and then transferred to each other. In other words, the proximal extensor pollicis brevis is sutured to the distal portion of the extensor pollicis longus near its insertion. Conversely, the proximal extensor pollicis longus is sutured to the insertion of the extensor pollicis brevis. In the transfer of the EPL proximally to EPB distally, the capsular reefing is still performed to enhance the insertion of the original extensor pollicis brevis. Nalebuff feels that more reliable terminal joint (IPJ) extension is achieved this way, and I concur (Figs. 7.3 and 7.4).

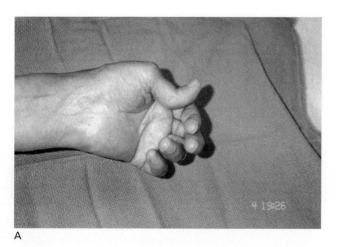

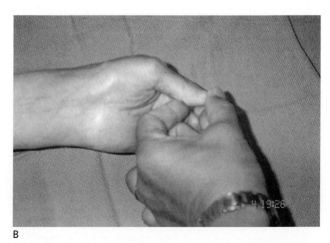

FIGURE 7.3. Pre-operation photo (**A, B**) of the left RA hand test before surgery.

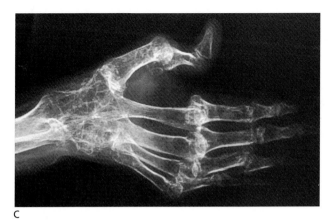 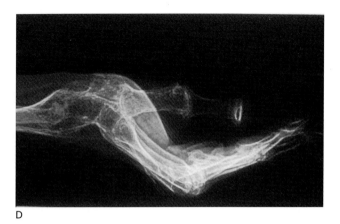

C D

FIGURE 7.3. (*continued*) Pre-operation x-ray (**C, D**) of the left RA hand test before surgery.

Ingles described a procedure in which the extensor mechanism was split between extensor pollicis longus and brevis, and a tenosynovectomy was performed. The abductor pollicis brevis and adductor pollicis are then detached from the extensor hood and retracted proximally and laterally. After synovectomy, the extensor pollicis brevis is advanced to the base of the proximal phalanx through a drill hole (Fig. 7.5). The abductor pollicis brevis and adductor pollicis tendons are then advanced distally and attached to either side of the extensor pollicis longus tendon (1). The importance of Ingles' contribution lies not only in recognizing the necessity of rebalancing EPL and EPB forces when reconstructing the

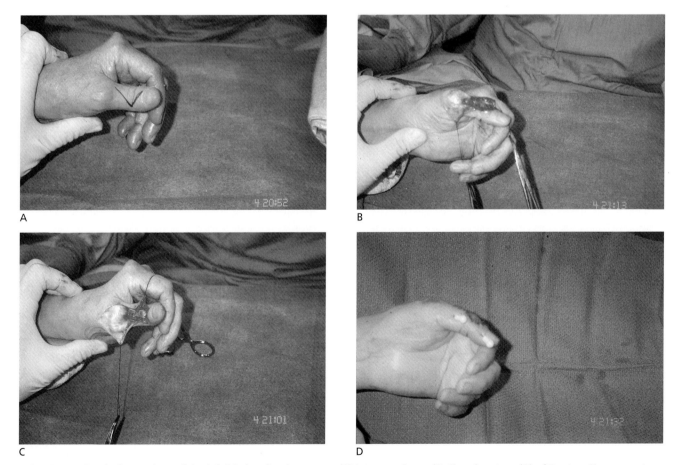

A B

C D

FIGURE 7.4. Surgical procedure of the left RA thumb using pre-op (**A**) inter-op photos (**B, C**) and post-op (**D**) of Boutonnière reconstruction using Nalebuff modified technique. (See Color Fig. 7.4.)

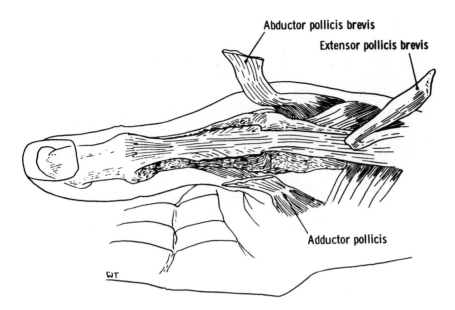

Abductor pollicis brevis

Extensor pollicis brevis

Adductor pollicis

FIGURE 7.5. The abductor pollicis brevis and adductor pollicis are dissected free from the remaining, attenuated extensor hood.

dorsal hood mechanism's MCP joint, but also in noting the contribution of the abductor pollicis and the adductor pollicis to the deformity (Fig. 7.6).

Harrison's procedure is similar to the original Nalebuff description. After splitting the EPL tendon, it is passed through a hole in the base of the proximal phalanx and then sutured back to itself. This is a modification or variation of the Nalebuff technique in that the passage of the extensor pollicis longus passes through a bone tunnel rather than a capsular flap with a buttonhole.

I favor the modified Nalebuff technique as the simplest, most reliable and most reproducible technique. I find that in severe deformities the EPL/EPB/dorsal hood procedure alone does not correct the entire deformity. In these cases, releasing the abductor/adductor pollicis and reattaching these muscles in a more proximal position reduces the intrinsic pull on the IP joint and helps to reduce the extension deformity.

In type IV deformities, the extensor mechanism of the thumb must be reconstructed, along with the attenuated ulnar collateral ligament. Therefore, the operative technique is to perform an extensor reconstruction as previously described, while additionally exposing the ulnar collateral ligament complex. Generally, there will be a firmer bony attachment that is preserved and a more attenuated one that is divided. The ulnar collateral ligament can be divided in midsubstance, and soft-tissue sutures of 2×0 ethibond or ticron applied. If there is severe deficiency of the ligament to bone attachment, pullout suture or suture anchors can be employed. Generally, along with reconstruction of the ulnar collateral ligament, an adductor tendon advancement can be added to the procedure to provide additional tissue for the deficient ulnar collateral complex.

In patients who have fixed metacarpalphalangeal joint contractures, capsular releases to alleviate the flexion deformity

may need to be combined with extensor reconstructions. In cases of mild intra-articular joint involvement and when severe MP contractures with severe intra-articular pathology and extensive cartilage loss exist, further addition of either arthrodesis or arthroplasty techniques may be warranted.

In cases of fixed MP flexion, Flatt describes a soft-tissue release (1). This procedure is performed with a dorsal approach. Abductor and adductor pollicis are detached from the extensor pollicis longus just distal to the MP joint on either side. This may improve some of the IP joint extension and contracture distally. A dorsal capsulotomy of the IP joint can be done to allow further IP joint flexion. The extensor mechanism is mobilized proximally by releasing bony attachments of the extensor mechanism to the base of the proximal phalanx on the radial and ulnar sides, combined with manipulation of the metacarpalphalangeal joint into extension. If MP extension cannot be performed, then division of the accessory collateral ligament, the collateral ligament proper, and/or volar plate release may be necessary. After synovectomy, the extensor pollicis brevis is attached to the proximal phalanx through either the capsule or the bone. The previously divided muscle tendons can now be attached to the soft-tissues at the neck of the metacarpal. Improved MP joint extension is maintained with a temporary K-wire fixation.

Arthrodesis is an excellent and effective treatment for metacarpalphalangeal joint pathology in the rheumatoid or arthritic thumb. An important function of the metacarpalphalangeal joint is stability; motion can easily be sacrificed in order to reduce pain, deformity, and to achieve a stable thumb skeleton. In fixed deformities of the rheumatoid thumb with significant bone destruction, the MP joint is ideally treated with arthrodesis, provided mobility at other joints along the thumb ray can be maintained at either the interphalangeal or trapezial metacarpal joints.

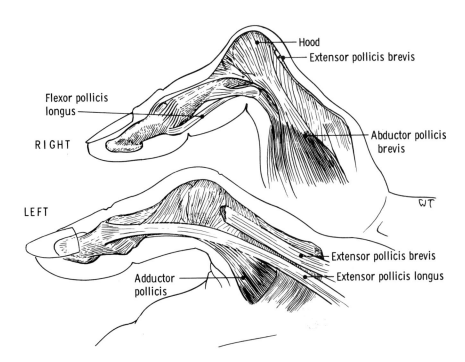

FIGURE 7.6. The metacarpophalangeal joint of the thumb showing extensive tendon damage. The insertion of the extensor pollicis longus into the base of the proximal phalanx is ruptured and has retracted proximally. The extensor hood becomes attenuated, allowing the abductor pollicis brevis and the extensor pollicis longus to migrate volarward, below the center of rotation of the metacarpophalangeal joint.

The many techniques used for arthrodesis of the small joints of the fingers are applicable to the thumb as well. These include Kirshner wire, or K-wire fixation, cross K-wire techniques, tension band wiring techniques, bone screws, AO screws using the lag screw technique, the Herbert screw, bone pegs, or plate fixation. In cases of severe deformity of the MCP, IP, and CMC joints, there may be indications to perform arthrodesis of both the MCP and the IP joint.

The MP joint has larger bones and bone surfaces than the IP joint, and therefore acceptance of screw fixation is not an issue. However, in order to have good bone purchase at both the head of the screw proximally and the screw threads distally, relatively larger screws must be employed in an oblique or intramedullary fashion. Therefore, the bone resection and bone removal that may be required can be significant. Moreover, to use an AO lag screw, the surgeon may be forced to remove a significant amount of cortical bone in order to allow adequate "seating" of the head of the screw in an antegrade placement with proximal phalangeal bone removal. Therefore, K-wires supplemented by tension bands provide an excellent surgical alternative (5). There is usually sufficient bone stock to allow for this technique, and minimal bone removal is required. Several clinical studies also support the use of this as a treatment method. The technique is illustrated in Figure 7.7.

Bone can be fashioned either through flat cuts or the cup-and-cone technique of Carroll and Hill (23). Two longitudinal K-wires, either 0.035 inch or 0.045 inch, are passed antegrade from the distal metaphyseal portion of the metacarpal down the intramedullary space of the proximal phalanx, to engage the palmar cortex at the midportion of the proximal phalanx.

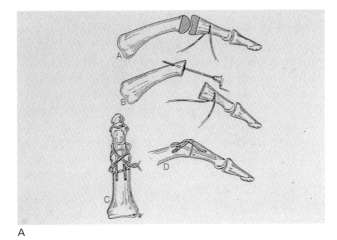

A

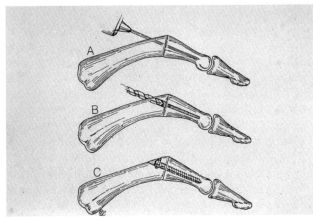

B

FIGURE 7.7. A. Tension band technique. **B.** AO lag screw technique.

Joint angles are determined using the guidelines mentioned previously. A transverse bone tunnel is made with a K-wire in the junction of the proximal first third to the proximal first half of the middle phalanx. A 25-gauge wire is passed through the bone tunnel, looped in a figure-eight fashion over the longitudinal pins, and tightened. The extensor mechanism is repaired with 5-0 nylon suture, and the skin is closed. Temporary splinting is provided, and depending on the patient, early mobilization is possible with good bone stock and adequate surgical technique in the compliant patient.

In general the MP joint of the thumb should be fixed in a position of mild flexion, approximately 15°, as recommended by Inglis (4). Additionally, there should be mild (in general) abduction of the proximal phalanx. Internal rotation or supination is helpful to allow the thumb to pinch against the digits. However, the most important consideration is the position of the thumb relative to the opposing digits. In the rheumatoid arthritis patient with rheumatoid disease and deformity, obviously the thumb may have to be adjusted from the "ideal" angles and positions in order to affect the most useful relationship between the thumb and fingers. Also, depending on the degree of carpalmetacarpal joint pathology and instability, MP joint position may be adjusted accordingly.

The previous discussion centered around the most common deformities of the interphalangeal joint and metacarpalphalangeal joint of the thumb, namely IP joint hyperextension and MP joint flexion, as exhibited in the type I boutonnière deformity. Some additional procedures are important to discuss regarding the swan-neck or Nalebuff type III deformity. For the IP joint diagnosed with type III deformities, wherein the flexion deformity is passively correctable or is fixed but with good preservation of bone stock, the soft-tissue procedure would initially consist of proximally freeing up the extensor pollicis longus mechanism to allow satisfactory pull-through of tension via the proximal muscles to effect IP joint extension. If, after freeing up the insertion of the intrinsic muscles from the extensor mechanism, as in the Flatt technique, and separating the extensor pollicis brevis and extensor pollicis longus, there remains residual IP joint flexion, rebalancing can then be performed by resecting of a portion of the extensor pollicis longus, then repairing proximal and distal segments. This procedure, in effect, shortens the extensor pollicis longus tendon to improve terminal joint extension and resting position. Alternatively, this can be done if there is significant attrition of the tendon, without formal resection of the intervening portion, with use of a Kessler or mattress suture to shorten the length of the attenuated tendon.

If the attrition of the extensor pollicis longus is so severe as to essentially resemble a mallet deformity, then the mal-let repair, suturing of the tendon to its insertion, can be performed. If the bony attachment is deficient, a repair of the extensor mechanism using pull-through sutures through the terminal phalanx to be sewn over a button is appropriate.

In cases of IP joint flexion deformity surgery, temporary K-wire fixation may be useful.

In the metacarpophalangeal joint with type III swan-neck deformities, MP hyperextension may be supple or fixed. Surgical treatment for fixed deformities would start out with a dorsal extensor mechanism release. Separation of the extensor pollicis longus and extensor pollicis brevis portions of the hood mechanisms with or without the attachment of the intrinsic muscle contributions is the first step. Both of these tendons can be mobilized with a scissor dissection, if this is appropriate. Alternatively, a partial or full longitudinal release of the dorsal hood mechanism between the extensor pollicis brevis and extensor pollicis longus may be required. For passive correction of the MP joint hyperextension, further dorsal capsular release and release of the dorsal portions of the collateral ligament may be necessary. Once passive MP joint flexion is obtained, a decision should be made on maintaining this position. Volar capsulodesis is one of the operative choices ideally in the manner described by Floyd and Eaton. The radial volar margin of the abductor aponeurosis is split in line with its oblique fibers and retracted dorsally. The radial collateral ligament and the volar plate are incised, and the retrocondylar portion of the joint is visualized. The palmar metacarpal cortex 5 mm proximal to the condyle is decorticated to bleeding bone. A 3-0 Ethibond suture is put in place to imbricate the volar plate. The volar plate is attached to the proximal phalanx and can then be rerouted toward the metacarpal and sutured subperiosteally to the radial border of the metacarpal (4,13). Another choice for maintaining MCP flexion position is a sesmoidesis, performed in the manner described by Tonkin et al. (42).

Either volar capsulodesis or sesmoidesis is appropriate if there is reasonable MP joint preservation. However, in cases of severe destruction or severe deformity, metacarpalphalangeal joint fusion in mild flexion is the most reliable technique, as described previously. In general, the type III deformities require surgical treatment of the carpalmetacarpal joint, usually with excision using ligament reconstruction, or excision in temporary pin fixation (see Chapter 8).

The indications for metacarpalphalangeal arthroplasty by silicone replacement are quite rare (43). In general, stability without motion is preferable over preservation of motion with the prospect of chronic instability.

There are special considerations for both IP joint, and MP joint treatment in cases of severe bone loss, as is seen with *arthritis mutilans*. In these cases, joint destruction is combined with severe bone loss. In general, it may be appropriate to consider supplementation of lost bone stock with bone grafting techniques. Sources may include resected metacarpal hands or iliac crest bone. In general, these are the most difficult cases given the significant skeletal deformity. Generally, longitudinal oblique or crossed K-wire techniques are most appropriate for skeletal fixation, followed by extended immobilization until bony healing occurs.

RESULTS

When assessing the efficacy of soft-tissue procedures for the thumb IP and MP joints, one must take into account both the durability and functional limitations of a given procedure, as well as the likelihood that future procedures will be necessary. In some respects, the key question becomes whether or not the soft-tissue procedures affect the overall natural history of the disease. Obviously, in a condition as complicated as rheumatoid arthritis, isolating specific factors when performing comparison studies can prove quite difficult.

In Inglis' study, (44) metacarpalphalangeal joint of the thumb reconstructions were assessed by reviewing overall surgical strategies including both soft-tissue reconstructions and arthrodesis. Arthrodesis procedures proved successful in all instances, offering a desirable degree of pain relief. Soft-tissue reconstructions were equally successful, particularly in terms of functional reliability. Arthrodesis patients previously suffering significant pain during rest or mild activity experienced dramatic improvements in their condition, to the point that they experienced either no pain or only minimal pain during strenuous activities. In the soft-tissue reconstruction group there was a somewhat lesser degree of pain relief.

Inglis' long-term results found lateral instability developing in 9 of the 21 hands after undergoing dorsal hood reconstructions. Of these 9, 5 patients developed subluxations and 2 of these 5 required arthrodesis during a second operation. Two-thirds of the patients undergoing metacarpophalangeal arthrodesis developed carpal/metacarpal joint pain (10 of 16 hands), whereas only one-third of patients undergoing synovectomies or knee dorsal hood reconstruction suffered similar effects (7 of 21 hands). Two of the patients who underwent arthrodesis of the metacarpal phalangeal joint also underwent late trapezial excision for pain. Two-thirds or 10 of 16 hands with arthrodesis of the MP joint developed severe hyperextension deformity of the interphalangeal joint, whereas only one-third of the hands undergoing dorsal hood reconstruction developed the same condition (7 of 21 hands).

In Flatt's *Care of the Arthritic Hand*, the author observes an 11% recurrence of synovitis in the metacarpophalangeal joint and a 50% recurrence of synovitis in the interphalangeal joint after synovectomy in soft-tissue reconstructions. Flatt's observed recurrence rates are significantly higher than other reported rates of recurrent synovitis after synovectomy of the MP joint, which generally range between 6% and 13% (45).

The review by Sälgeback, Eiken, and Haga (46) describes 142 thumb operations on 84 patients in a 7-year period from 1960–1970. These patients were given four clinical grades from fully functional to chair or bedridden. The operations performed were synovectomies, tendon extensor pollicis longus advancement, or rerouting of EPB or EPL and arthrodesis of the MP joint. Sixty-seven of the 88 patients undergoing synovectomies reported decreases in the amount of pain they experienced, 19 reported no change, and 2 patients

reported failure of the synovectomy to correct their condition. Five patients experienced a recurrence of deformity. Eighteen patients underwent tendon advancement procedures of which 15 were improved and 3 were unchanged.

Thirty-five of 36 patients undergoing arthrodesis achieved bone union. In Harrison's original study, (47) 216 operations on rheumatoid thumbs were reviewed, which included synovectomy, extensor tendon repair, flexor tendon repair, MCP joint arthrodesis, and terminal joint arthrodesis among others.

In Millender's review (48) 74 procedures were reviewed over a 7-year period. The average length of involvement with the patients in this study was 4.4 years, with a minimum of 2 years. Of these 74, 14 were diagnosed with early type I rheumatoid thumb deformities, 36 with moderate deformities, and 16 with advanced deformities. The MP synovectomy and extensor pollicis longus rerouting had a 64% recurrence rate, necessitating a more definitive postoperative procedure at an average of 6 years after the original surgery. The authors therefore recommend these soft-tissue procedures for patients suffering early joint involvement with full passive correction and normal radiographs, with the understanding that these procedures will likely require further revision in the future. After a 9-year follow-up, MP joint fusions remained durable on average. For MP joint arthroplasties, there was a higher instance of IP joint collapse at 23% (47).

In Harrison and Ansell's review, 16.6% of MP joint arthrodesis procedures failed to achieve bone union (47). These procedures were conducted using a bone graft and interosis wire type technique, but without longitudinal K-wires. Gregor, reviewed by Maneuddu, Bogoch, and Hastings (49), evaluated 11 cases of early stage I or early boutonnière thumb deformity with an average lag of the MP joint ranging from 10° to 60° and a 38-month follow-up. Upon re-examination, nine had equal active and passive MP joint extension, with two thumbs displaying moderate extensor lag. Interestingly, the long extensor was completely sacrificed in these reconstructions.

Rehabilitation

In general, soft-tissue reconstructions should be supported with several weeks of immobilization, after which time fixation can be considered for significant deformities. The challenge in rheumatoid soft-tissue reconstructive surgery is to improve the soft-tissue balance through a combination of surgery and therapy. The main obstacle to this is, of course, the patient's rheumatoid disease itself. Within these guidelines, there is not a strict method of rehabilitation.

Soft-tissue rehabilitation is based on immobilization of the affected area to provide enough support for soft-tissue reconstructions, while at the same time allowing eventual restoration of some motion. To this end, removable thumb opponens splinting is generally recommended.

Rehabilitation for arthrodesis procedures depends very much on the quality of the bone immobilization. If removable implants such as K-wires are used, splinting should be incorporated as long as these implants remain in position. If, however, screws, tension band wires, or bone pegs are used, the joints should be supported until there is evidence of stability with loss of joint pain suggestive of clinical healing. This generally occurs within four to eight weeks.

There are several studies that review the results of silicone metacarpophalangeal joint arthroplasties or Swanson implants for rheumatoid disease. Figgie monitored 59 implants in 50 patients from the Hospital for Special Surgery (43). The majority of patients suffered from type I boutonnière deformity with flexible inner phalangeal joints. The average range of motion was 25° with a flexion arch between 15° and 40°, with an average key pinch strength of 4 pounds. After surgery, 40 of 50 patients reported improvements in the performance of daily tasks. One patient required a second operation for instability of the MCP joint and received arthrodesis. Throughout the follow-up period (a minimum of 3 years and average of 6 1/2), only one patient suffered significant progression of the disease in the inner-phalangeal joint and two in the carpal metacarpal joint.

Swanson and Herndon (1977) and Bechanbaugh and Steffy (1981) conducted two of the original studies of the Swanson implant for the MP joint (43). Both works propose that patients with early disease of the MP joint and joint dislocations and patients with severe disease and bone loss in the collateral ligaments make ideal candidates for arthrodesis. Furthermore, the authors propose that patients suffering erosion of the MP joint with satisfactory collateral ligaments make suitable candidates for implant or supplasty, depending on the specific assessment of the patients' hand and functional requirements. If the deformities of the MP and IP joint necessitate IP joint fusion, then implant osteoplasty of the MP joint is recommended.

Salvage Procedures

Salvage of one failed procedure necessitates another, more definitive procedure. This applies to synovectomy, soft-tissue, arthroplasty, and arthrodesis procedures. In general, the salvage procedure will be an arthrodesis. The decision to use arthrodesis to salvage a single joint is fairly straightforward. However, in instances involving several joints, such as the interphalangeal joint, metacarpal phalangeal joint and carpal metacarpal joint, arthrodesis, while offering stability, will leave the patient with little or no motion. Thus, the physician must make a decision as to which joints will be salvaged through arthrodesis, and which ones will be maintained with some mobility. This is the trade-off that the patient and the surgeon face when planning thumb reconstructions.

REFERENCES

1. Clayton M. Surgery of the thumb in rheumatoid arthritis. *JBJS* 1962;44A:1376–1386.
2. Ferlic DC, Serot DI, Clayton ML. The use of the Flatt Hinge Prosthesis in the rheumatoid thumb. *Hand* 1978;10(1):94.
3. Vainio K. Hand. In: Milch RA, ed. *Surgery of arthritis*. Baltimore: Williams & Wilkins, 1964:130–157.
4. Inglis AE, Hamlin C, Sengelmann R, Straub LR. Reconstruction of the metacarpophalangeal joint of the thumb in rheumatoid arthritis. *J Bone Joint Surg* 1965;704.
5. Marmor L. *Surgery of rheumatoid arthritis*. Philadelphia: Lea & Febiger, 1967.
6. Nalebuff, EA. Diagnosis, classification and management of rheumatoid thumb deformities. *Bulletin of the Hospital for Joint Diseases* 1968;Oct. 29(2):119–137.
7. Brumfield RH, Conaty IP. Reconstructive surgery of the thumb in rheumatoid arthritis. *Ortho* 1980;3:529–533.
8. Nalebuff EA. The recognition and treatment of tendon ruptures in the rheumatoid hand. American Academy of Orthopaedic Surgeons: Symposium on Tendon Surgery in the Hand. St. Louis, MO: CV Mosby, 1975.
9. Swanson AB. Flexible implant Arthroplasty for arthritic finger joints. *J Bone Joint Surg* 1972;54A:435–455.
10. Dray GJ, Millender LH, Nalebuff EA, Philips C. The surgical treatment of hand deformities in systematic lupus erythematosus. *J Hand Surg* 1981;6(4):339–345.
11. Swanson AB, Herndon JH. Flexible (silicone) implant Arthroplasty of the metacarpophalangeal joint of the thumb. *J Bone Joint Surg* 1977;59A:362–368.
12. Ferlic DL, Turner BD, Clayton ML. Compression arthrodesis of the thumb. *J Hand Surg* 1983;8:207–210.
13. Eaton RG, Floyd WE III. Thumb metacarpophalangeal capsulodesis: an adjunct procedure to basal joint arthroplasty for collapse of deformity of the first ray. *J Hand Surg [Am]* 1988;May, 13(3): 449–453.
14. Nalebuff EA, Millender LH. Reconstructive surgery and rehabilitation of the hand. In: Kelley WN, ed. *Textbook of rheumatology*. Philadelphia: WB Saunders, 1985:1818–1833.
15. Smith RJ. Tendon Transfers of the hand and forearm, 1st ed. Boston: Little, Brown and Company, 1987.
16. Flatt AE. The care of the rheumatoid hand, 3rd ed. St. Louis: Mosby, 1974.
17. Diao E, Eaton RG. Total collateral ligament incision for contractures of the proximal interphalangeal joint. *J Hand Surg [Am]* 1993;18(3):395–402.
18. Lipscomb PR. Synovectomy of the thumb and fingers in rheumatoid arthritis. *J Bone Joint Surg* 1967;49A(6):1135.
19. Feldon P, Terrono AL, Nalebuff EA, Millender LH. Rheumatoid arthritis and other connective tissue diseases. In: Green, Hotchkiss, Pederson, eds. *Green's operative hand surgery*, 4th ed. Philadelphia: Churchill Livingstone, 1999:1651–1740.
20. Wyrsch B, Dawson J, Aufranc S, et al. Distal interphalangeal joint arthrodesis comparing tension-band wire and Herbert screw: a biomechanical and dimensional analysis. *J Hand Surg [Am]* 1996;21: 438–443.
21. Vanik RK, Weber RC, Matloub HS, et al. The comparative strengths of internal fixation techniques. *J Hand Surg [Am]* 1984;9:216–221.
22. Kovach JC, Werner FW, Palmer AK, et al. Biomechanical analysis of internal fixation techniques for proximal interphalangeal joint arthrodesis. *J Hand Surg [Am]* 1986;11:562–566.
23. Stern PJ, Gates NT, Jones TB. Tension band arthrodesis of small joints in the hand. *J Hand Surg [Am]* 1993;18:194–197.

24. Leibovic SJ, Strickland JW. Arthrodesis of the proximal interphalangeal joint of the finger: comparison of the use of the Herbert screw with other fixation methods. *J Hand Surg [Am]* 1994;19:181–188.
25. Burton RI, Margles SW, Lunseth PA. Small-joint arthrodesis in the hand. *J Hand Surg* 1986;11A:678–682.
26. Littler JW. Tendon transfers and arthrodesis in combined median and ulnar nerve paralysis. *J Bone Joint Surg* 1949;31A:225–234.
27. Uhl RL, Schneider LH. Tension band arthrodesis of finger joints: a retrospective review of 76 consecutive cases. *J Hand Surg [Am]* 1992;17:518–522.
28. Isselstein CB, Hovius SE, ten Have BL, et al. Is the pectoralis myocutaneous flap in intraoral and oropharyngeal reconstruction outdated? *Am J Surg* 1996;Sep, 172(3):259–262.
29. McGlynn JT, Smith RA, Bogumill GP. Arthrodesis of small joint of the hand: a rapid and effective technique. *J Hand Surg [Am]* 1988;13:595–599.
30. Faithfull DK, Herbert TJ. Small joint fusions of the hand using the Herbert Bone Screw. *J Hand Surg [Br]* 1984;9:167–168.
31. Wright CS, McMurtry RY. AO arthrodesis in the hand. *J Hand Surg [Am]* 1983;8:932–935.
32. Katzman SS, Gibeault JD, Dickson K, Thompson JD. Use of a Herbert screw for interphalangeal joint arthrodesis. Clinical orthopaedics and related research. 1993;Nov.,296:127–132.
33. Allende BT, Engelem JC. Tension-band arthrodesis in the finger joints. *J Hand Surg [Am]*1980;5:269–271.
34. Teoh LC, Yeo SJ, Singh I. Interphalangeal joint arthrodesis with oblique placement of an AO lag screw. *J Hand Surg [Br]* 1994;19:208–211.
35. Jensen CH, Jensen CM. Biodegradable pins versus Kirschner wires in hand surgery. *J Hand Surg [Br]* 1996;21:507–510.
36. Moberg E, Henrikson B. Technique for digital arthrodesis. A study of 150 cases. *Acta Chirurgica Scandinavia* 1959–1960;118:331.
37. Baruch A, Kahanovich S. Angulated bone peg. *Plastic and Reconstructive Surgery* 1980;66:471–473.
38. Stern PJ, Fulton DB. Distal interphalangeal joint arthrodesis: an analysis of complications. *J Hand Surg [Am]* 1992;17:1139–1145.
39. Hatano I, Suga T, Diao E, et al. Adhesions from flexor-tendon surgery: An animal study comparing surgical techniques. *J Hand Surg* 2000;25(2):252–259.
40. Nalebuff EA. Surgical treatment of finger deformities in the rheumatoid hand. *Surg Clin North Am* 1969;49:833–846.
41. Harrison SH. Reconstruction arthroplasty of the metacarpophalangeal joint using the extensor loop operation. *Br J Plast Surg* 1971;24:307–309.
42. Tonkin MA, Beard AJ, Kemp SJ, Eakins DF. Sesamoid arthrodesis for hyperextension of the thumb metacarpal joint. *J Hand Surg* 1995;20A:334–338.
43. Figgie MP, Inglis AE, Sobel M, et al. Metacarpalphalangeal joint arthroplasty of the rheumatoid thumb.*J Hand Surg [Am]* 1990;Mar,15(2):210–216.
44. Inglis AE, Hamlin C, Sengelmann RP, Straub LR. Reconstruction of the metacarpophalangeal joint of the thumb in rheumatoid arthritis. *J Bone Joint Surg [Am]* 1972;June,54(4):704–712.
45. Stein, Terrono. Rheumatorial thumb. *Hand Clinics* 1996;Aug., 12(3):153–156.
46. Sälgeback S, Eiken O, Haga T. Surgical treatment of the rheumatoid thumb. Special reference to the metacarpophalangeal joint. *Scandinavian Journal of Plastic and Reconstructive Surgery* 1976;10(2):153–156.
47. Harrison, Ansell. Surgery of the rheumatoid thumb. *Br J Bone Joint Surg* 1974;27:242–247.
48. Millender. Surgical treatment of the boutonnière rheumatoid thumb deformity. *Hand Clinics* 1989;5 number 2, may 9.
49. Manueddu CA, Bogoch ER, Hastings DE. Restoration of metacarpophalangeal extension of the thumb in inflammatory arthritis. *J Hand Surg [Br]* 1996;Oct., 21(5)633–639.

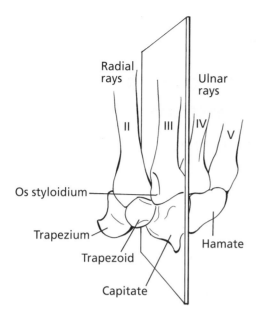

FIGURE 9.1. The lesser carpometacarpal joints can be categorized into the radial (second and third) and the ulnar (fourth and fifth) rays.

develop sometime well after the initial injury. This is true whether the arthrosis occurs despite meticulous surgical restoration or as the sequelae of a missed diagnosis.

A carpal boss, or *carpe bossu* as it was originally described by Foille in 1931, is a bony prominence on the dorsum of the proximal hand at the base of the third metacarpal (13). Other authors have described the boss as originating from either the second or the third CMC joints (5,13). In a study by Cuono and Watson, two-thirds of their symptomatic carpal boss patients had a co-existent os styloideum or accessory ossicle. They hypothesized that a symptomatic carpal boss represented the maldevelopment of the quadrangular joint (capitate-trapezoid-metacarpal articulation) secondary to the accessory ossicle (14). Some authors have postulated that carpal bossing is a form of periostitis, possibly secondary to repetitive microtrauma to the dorsal capsule (5). The lack of subchondral sclerosis, cystic change, and preservation of both joint space and articular cartilage would disfavor an osteoarthritic origin to this condition.

Despite the relative protection of the mid-axis of the hand, injuries to the radial rays have been described. In 1986 Mueller reviewed the literature on CMC dislocations (15). He found 143 reported CMC dislocations with 9 isolated third metacarpal dislocations and 12 combined second and third dislocations. Multiple carpometacarpal dislocations have been reported (16,17). Imbriglia has even reported a chronic dislocation of the index, long, ring, and small digits, which was treated successfully with an open reduction 3 months after the initial injury (17).

While the lesser CMC joints can be involved in rheumatoid arthritis, there is limited discussion of this in the litera-

ture. The joints appear to be somewhat spared in comparison to both the intercarpal and the metacarpal phalangeal joints (MCP). Gunther believes that this is due to two factors. First, thick, strong capsular ligaments support these joints. Second, the extrinsic wrist tendons insert distal to the joints and act as a compressive force (5).

INDICATIONS

The patient with arthritis of the lesser carpometacarpal joint typically presents with pain localized to the joint or joints involved. At times a more nondescript dull ache may be the primary complaint. The pain is frequently exacerbated by activity, though it occasionally is present at rest. The patient may suffer significant functional impairment. There may be marked difficulty in carrying out work tasks or even activities of daily living. This is especially true if work involves repetitive gripping activities when the disease is present in the fourth or fifth CMC joints. Activity-related pain might be less problematic when arthritis involves the index or middle ray CMC joints. This may be due to the inherently more constrained motion at the radial-sided lesser carpometacarpal joints. If radial ray involvement is associated with a metacarpal boss, the appearance of a prominent mass over the dorsal of the hand may be cosmetically unacceptable to the patient. Treatment is typically not indicated if this prominence is painless. Surgical intervention is indicated when symptoms remain refractory to conservative care and reasonable activity restriction.

CONTRAINDICATIONS

An inadequate or incomplete trial of conservative nonoperative care is a contraindication to surgical treatment of lesser CMC joint arthritis. A patient incapable or unwilling to participate in postoperative restrictions and rehabilitation should not be offered surgical treatment for CMC arthritis. Surgery should not be performed in the presence of active systemic or local infections, inadequate local soft-tissue coverage, or in the face of untreated systemic illness.

PREOPERATIVE PLANNING

A detailed history of the patient's occupation should be elicited as well as specific tasks and job activities that exacerbate the pain. Recent changes in a patient's job should be recorded and their relative role in the patient's presentation evaluated. A detailed history of the patient's work activity underscores the treatment principle that it is easier to modify the job activity than to modify the patient. Ergonomic consultation and workstation analysis may be a fruitful adjunct to treatment.

In the case of inflammatory arthritides, potential cervical spine pathology and/or instability should be determined. Appropriate radiographic screening should be performed prior to general anesthesia.

On physical examination, the involved CMC joints should be palpated directly, and provocative maneuvers to elicit joint tenderness are performed. Cuono and Watson describe longitudinal traction coupled with passive pronation and supination of the index finger while the MCP joint is in a fully flexed position (14). This test can easily be done to any of the lesser digits. Gurland describes a test where the MCP joint is flexed, thus locking the collateral ligaments. The proximal phalanx is then grasped and used to flex and extend the ray. He states that this tests the stability of the CMC joint (18). This provocative test should elicit symptoms in patients with CMC joint disease. Range of motion of the digits as well as the ulnar CMC joints should be documented and compared to the uninjured side. Distance of digital tips to the digital palmar crease can be measured and recorded, but goniometric measurements are preferred and may be more reproducible. Grip and pinch strength testing should be measured. An average of three readings should be made for both the affected and unaffected side. Neurovascular examination of the hand should be performed.

If a boss of the index or middle CMC joint is suspected, a dorsal carpal ganglion or an accessory extensor digitorum manus brevis muscle belly must be included in the differential diagnosis. Typically, dorsal carpal ganglions arise from the scapholunate interval and are proximal to the radial CMC joints. In some instances, however, a ganglion cyst may arise from the arthritic spur at the CMC joint. There have even been reported cases of intratendinous ganglions overlying carpal bosses (19).

Tendinopathies and enthesitis should be ruled out, as nonoperative treatment for the control of tendon insertion pain rather than arthritis pain may be indicated. In the event that ring or small CMC joint arthrodesis is being considered, the presence of triquetral-hamate tenderness should be elicited. If other ulnar-sided carpal or metacarpal pathology (such as triangular fibrocartilage tears, ulnar carpal abutment, or lunotriquetral ligament tears) is suspected, precise localization of the painful site is imperative.

The dorsum of the hand should be inspected for any previous scars that would suggest prior trauma and that might interfere with the surgical exposure of the CMC joints. Obvious prominence may suggest a boss, joint luxation, or an unreduced dislocation.

After thorough physical examination, radiographic examination can then proceed. A postcroanterior (PA) zero rotation and oblique and lateral view of the hand should be obtained initially. Gurland has highlighted the importance of the hand being placed flat on the radiograph cassette (18). This allows the parallel relationship of the metacarpal bases to the distal trapezoid, capitate, and hamate to form an elongated letter M. In addition, should targeted views of the

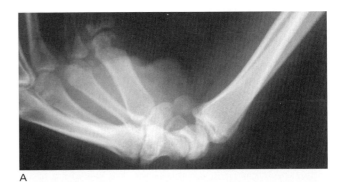

A

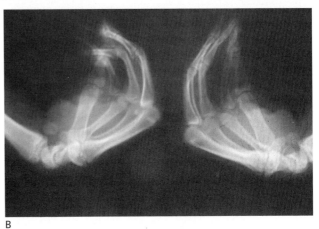

B

FIGURE 9.2. Carpal boss view of right hand/wrist. The forearm is supinated and the wrist is ulnarly deviated. While the patient has carpal bossing bilaterally, she is symptomatic only on the right. Note also the accessory ossicle of the lunate.

index and middle CMC joints be desired a lateral view in 30° of forearm supination and 30° ulnar deviation of the wrist can be obtained. This has been referred to as the carpal boss view (Fig. 9.2) (14). Visualization of the ulnar-sided CMC joints in a lateral plane can be accomplished by pronating the hand by 10° to 30° to place the hamatometacarpal joints into unencumbered view. Bora and Didizian recommended obtaining an anteroposterior (AP) radiograph with the wrist pronated 30° (20). They believed this eliminated the bony overlap of the ulnar rays and better defined the intra-articular congruency of those joints. Kaye and Lister believed the Brewerton view was especially useful in diagnosing acute periarticular injuries to the ring and small metacarpal bases (21). Comparison views to the uninvolved contralateral side can be useful at times. If plain radiographs are inconclusive, secondary radiographic evaluation can be undertaken. Planar tomography or, at most institutions, computed tomography (CT) can be utilized. If the diagnosis remains elusive, an even more sensitive evaluation of the involved joints can be performed. Radionuclide studies, such as a Technetium-99m bone scans can be helpful in the face of normal radiographic studies when posttraumatic synovitis is suspected.

Localization of the painful nidus is facilitated through the use of local anesthetic injections. Local anesthetic coupled with corticosteroids may prove equally therapeutic and diagnostic. Fluoroscopic guidance, when available, allows for precise localization of the articulation and direct instillation of the medication.

Nonoperative modalities are tried initially. Nonsteroidal anti-inflammatory drugs (NSAID) are prescribed. Warm or cold compresses, depending on patient preference and response, are utilized. Splinting or casting of the wrist and hand is performed. As previously discussed, an injection of corticosteroids into the affected joint may be performed. The author's preference is to anesthetize the skin first with a small amount (1–2 cc) of 1% to 2% lidocaine without epinephrine. Then, a mixture of 2 cc of Celestone (40 mg/ml), 1 cc of 0.5% Marcaine without epinephrine, and 1 cc of 1% to 2% lidocaine without epinephrine is introduced directly into the joint with a 21–25 g needle. This is followed by a 4-week period of immobilization with either a forearm-based splint or a short arm cast.

If job modifications and an adequate trial of conservative management do not lead to resolution of disability and pain, surgical treatment of the CMC arthritis may be considered.

TECHNIQUES

For arthrosis of the lesser CMC joints, arthrodesis is our surgical treatment of choice. The option of biological or prosthetic interpositional arthroplasty may be considered for the treatment of arthritis in the more mobile fourth or fifth CMC joints. For the symptomatic boss without arthrosis, a simple dorsal ostectomy may be performed. In select cases of malunited fractures of the base of the fifth metacarpal, intra-articular osteotomy or resection arthroplasty may be performed. Once secondary joint changes have arisen, however, osteotomy is unlikely to yield satisfactory relief of symptoms.

Arthrodesis Technique

While a variety of surgical techniques exist for the treatment of CMC joint arthrosis refractory to conservative care, arthrodesis may provide the most predictable outcome. Therefore, we prefer arthrodesis to soft-tissue or implant arthroplasty or osteotomy.

Arthrodesis can be performed under regional anesthesia if a local sliding corticocancellous block or the distal radius is selected as the bone graft donor site. General anesthesia is utilized if the iliac crest is to be used as the bone graft site. A pneumatic tourniquet is essential in creating a bloodless operative field. Both longitudinal and transverse incisions have been described for the exposure of the lesser CMC joints. For a single CMC joint, a single longitudinal incision (4 cm) is centered directly over the affected site. If one or more joints are involved the incisions may be centered longitudinally between the affected articulations. Care must be taken not to injure the dorsal sensory branches of the radial or ulnar nerves during the superficial dissection. The joints can be exposed through a longitudinal or transverse incision. A longitudinal incision may allow for a capsular/periosteal sleeve to be created and closed over the arthrodesis site. Once identified, the CMC joint is prepared by removing the

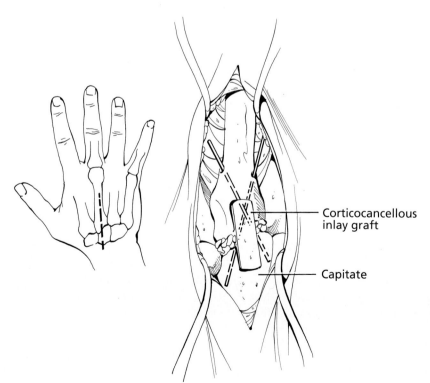

Corticocancellous inlay graft

Capitate

FIGURE 9.3. A corticocancellous inlay graft spans the third CMC joint. Additional cancellous bone graft has been packed into the remaining joint space. Fixation is with obliquely placed K-wires. Care has been taken to insure that the wires do not cross at the joint line.

osteophytes, damaged cartilage and hard subchondral bone. Curettes, rongeurs, and osteotomes are preferred over high-speed burs so as to lessen the risk of thermal injury. The fusion site is then packed with either cancellous or cortico-cancellous autograft (Fig. 9.3). Several authors have recommended corticocancellous grafts, utilizing either a tricortical iliac crest graft or a local sliding corticocancellous graft (22, 23). Fixation may be achieved by a variety of means. Kirschner (K) wires are a relatively simple method that allows for easy removal of hardware in the future. They do, however, lack the ability to compress the arthrodesis site. The border rays are amenable to obliquely placed compression screws (Fig. 9.4). To our knowledge, no series have reported the use of plate fixation. Theoretically, dorsal plating may provide the most rigid fixation, but the involved osseous architecture must be of sufficient size to allow for adequate cortical purchase proximally and distally. The relatively limited distal to proximal dimensions of the carpal bones would seem to make such fixation difficult. The potential for symptomatic hardware or extensor tendon adhesions necessitating tenolysis may also arise at a later date.

The recommended fusion posture is 0° for the index, long, and ring rays while 30° of flexion is described for the fifth CMC joint (6,18). Gurland points out that with fusion in this flexed position the patient may lose the ability to rest his hand flat on a planar surface. He believed that this causes no significant disability, and the ability to maintain the normal curvature of the distal metacarpal arch during grasp is functionally more important. Clendenin and Smith stated that even with arthrodesis of the fourth and fifth CMC joints, the ulnar rays are capable of some flexion through compensatory motion at the midcarpal joint (24,25). Additional bone graft is packed around the fusion site. Hemostasis is secured, then the wound is closed with interrupted sutures in a layered fashion. A bulky dressing and short arm splint is applied.

Of interest, only Green and Kilgore describe incorporation of the MCP joints in the postoperative dressing/splint. It would seem, based on the orthopaedic principle of stabilizing both the joints proximal and distal to an injury, that a splint or cast that immobilizes the wrist and the MCP joints may better shield the CMC joints from inadvertent flexion and extension. Theoretically, the use of such an orthosis in the early convalescence, especially when fixation is stable but not truly rigid, may prove more effective. This concept has been advocated previously by Watson for triscaphe arthrodesis (26).

If the distal radius is chosen as a bone graft donor site, we prefer a separate short longitudinal incision (2 cm) just proximal to Lister's tubercle. This site is easy to palpate, typically free from any directly overlying tendons, and provides easy access to the rich cancellous bone of the radial metaphysis and styloid. When possible, the periosteum is preserved so that it may be closed over the cortical defect. For cancellous graft, trepanning a small ellipse (1 cm) with a drill or K-wire creates a cortical window. A series of straight and curved curettes aid in bone harvesting. A thrombin-soaked piece of Gelfoam is useful for hemostasis and in supporting the cortical window. For corticocancellous grafts a longer incision may be necessary. The cortical dimensions can then be established by a combination of trephination with K-wires and cleavage with small, slender osteotomes.

If a general anesthetic is utilized, local infiltration with Marcaine at the arthrodesis and bone graft donor sites is helpful with postoperative pain control. When the iliac crest is chosen as a bone graft donor site, care must be taken to insure that the incision is sufficiently proximal and lateral from the anterior superior iliac spine (ASIS) so that the lateral femoral cutaneous nerve is safe from injury.

Arthrodesis Results

The largest arthrodesis study is that of Joseph et al. from 1981. Lesser joint arthrodeses were performed on a total of 37 joints in 28 patients. Follow-up was an average 27 months and ranged from 3 to 27 months. Two patients required revision surgery for nonunion, ultimately yielding solid arthrodeses in all 28 patients. Eighteen patients rated their outcome as good and 10 rated their result as good (22).

ALTERNATIVES

Alternatives to arthrodesis include soft-tissue and prosthetic arthroplasties as well as partial resection arthroplasties and intra-articular osteotomies. Typically, these are used for the

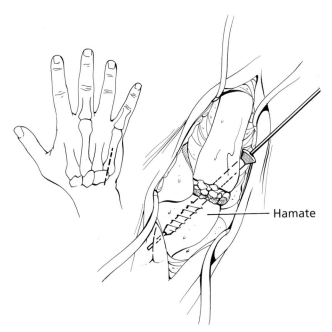

— Hamate

FIGURE 9.4. After excision of the irregular joint surfaces and dense subchondral bone, the joint has been filled with cancellous bone graft. A cannulated screw has been used to compress the arthrodesis site.

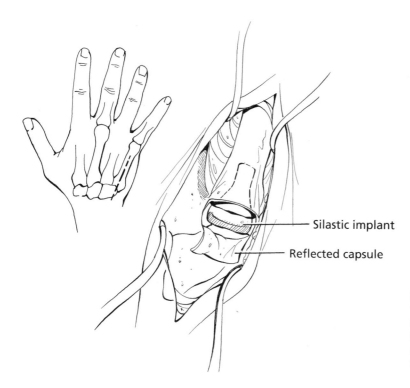

Silastic implant

Reflected capsule

FIGURE 9.5. A silastic prosthesis has been utilized for treatment of fifth CMC arthrosis. A longitudinal incision is utilized. The capsule is incised transversely and preserved. The metacarpal base has been resected and the canal prepared. This has allowed for joint reconstruction by an interposition hemiarthroplasty.

fifth or, more rarely, the fourth and fifth CMC joints in an attempt to preserve motion. No one technique was studied in more than 16 patients.

Tendon Interposition Arthroplasty Technique

For soft-tissue interposition arthroplasty the reader is directed to the study of Gainor et al. in which a rolled autologous tendon spacer is utilized (27). The spacer is constructed from the ipsilateral palmaris longus tendon or a long toe extensor if this tissue is unavailable. A curvilinear incision is utilized. The cutaneous neurovascular structures are identified and protected. A transverse capsular incision is utilized. The ulnar collateral ligament and ECU insertion are preserved. Either the distal articular surface of the hamate or the metacarpal base is resected. Typically 5 mm of the metacarpal base is removed. The donor tendon is rolled into a "cylindrically rolled bolus" (Fig. 9.5). The fifth metacarpal is then stabilized by temporary K-wire fixation through its base to the fourth metacarpal base. The capsule is preserved and closed over the tendon spacer. Immobilization includes the hand and wrist and is reinforced with a plaster splint. This immobilization lasts five weeks.

Tendon Interposition Arthroplasty Results

Ten patients were operated on over a 7-year period. Eight patients were available for follow-up. Average length of fol-

low-up was 60 months with a range of 25 to 103 months. These authors reported a 30% increase in grip strength at an average follow-up of 5 years.

Patients rated their functional capacity as excellent in 50% of the cases. The remainder rated their function as good. No instability was noted in any patients. Of note, on long-term follow-up films a characteristic "egg cup" remodeling of the fifth metacarpal base was noted in half of the patients available for review. Six of the eight patients were noted to have shortening of the fifth ray.

Silicone Interposition Arthroplasty Technique

Ten years earlier than Gainor, Kilgore and Green had described an interposition arthroplasty utilizing Silastic toe prostheses in three patients (28). For their procedure a curvilinear or zigzag approach is utilized. The cutaneous neurovascular structures are identified and protected. The joint capsule is split longitudinally and the capsule/periostium elevated and reflected to each side. Two to 3 mm of bone is removed from the base of the fifth metacarpal. The metacarpal medullary canal is then curetted and sized. A size 0 Silastic great toe prosthesis was used for each of their patients (Fig. 9.6). Satisfactory fit, stability, and motion are then documented. The capsule is preserved and closed over the implant. Nonabsorbable sutures are utilized. The wrist and involved MCP joints are then immobilized in the "functional position" for 7 to 14 days. The authors favored arthroplasty over arthrodesis because of the shorter immo-

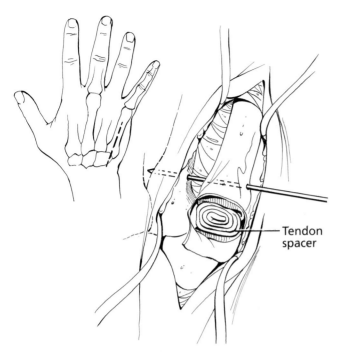

FIGURE 9.6. A rolled tendon spacer provides for a biologic interface at the fifth CMC joint. The fifth metacarpal is stabilized to the fourth metacarpal via K-wire fixation.

bilization period and the avoidance of possible delayed union or nonunion.

Silicone Interposition Arthroplasty Results

Green and Kilgore report three case studies in their paper. Follow-up ranged from 9 to 26 months. They describe one patient as pain free, one with occasional pain (only with shaking hands), and the third as being "happy with her increased functional status." Grip strength was improved in two and decreased in the third.

Partial Resection Arthroplasty Technique

Black et al. reported a partial resection arthroplasty in 16 patients for fifth CMC joint arthrosis (29). Three patients had concomitant fourth and fifth CMC involvement. In their study they describe the shaft healing to the volar fragment, which remains congruent to the hamate. The displaced dorso-ulnar fragment therefore is resected. The joint is then left as an articulation between the palmar-shaft remnant and the hamate. Their surgical procedure involved a transverse incision over the involved joint. The neurovascular structures were then isolated by blunt longitudinal dissection and then retracted. The capsule is incised transversely. The dorsal impingement is then resected with a dental rongeur so that a dorsal void is

formed. This leaves only the reduced volar surfaces in contact. "Early mobilization" is recommended but not specified.

Partial Resection Arthroplasty Results

Of the 16 patients described by Black et al. (28) 10 were pain free. Three had minor discomfort with sports or prolonged activity. The final three had sufficient discomfort that two underwent revision with more extensive resections and one was converted to an arthrodesis.

Carpal Boss Technique

If the discomfort is from a carpal boss, then a simple ostectomy may be performed. In this case the same surgical exposure may be used. The tendons are retracted to either side of the joint. The capsule is split longitudinally and the hypertrophic spurs are removed with osteotomes and/or rongeurs. The joint should be sufficiently debrided so that only normal cartilage interface remains. The resection site should be slightly concave so that the resultant hematoma and scar does not create a resultant "soft-tissue boss." If a concomitant ganglion is discovered, both it and the osteophytes should be removed. In preoperative discussions, the patient must be apprised of the possibility of discovering significant arthrosis. In this instance conversion to a formal arthrodesis may be necessary.

Carpal Boss Results

Sixteen of 30 patients treated surgically for a carpal boss were evaluated by Cuono and Watson (14). Average follow-up was 42 months, ranging from 6 to 72 months. No patients had a recurrence, but one patient who had an incomplete initial resection required two subsequent explorations. All 16 patients returned to full activity. Two patients described aching with cold weather.

COMPLICATIONS

Intra-operative complications include trauma or laceration to either the dorsal cutaneous branch of the ulnar nerve or the superficial sensory branch of the radial nerve. Should a laceration be identified, neurorrhaphy should be performed immediately with the assistance of an operating microscope. Other intra-operative complications included inability to achieve stable fixation of the arthrodesis. In this case, rigid fixation such as that provided by the addition of plates and screws can be sought. Malreduction or malposition of the arthrodesis may be avoided by the use of intra-operative fluoroscopy.

Early postoperative complications include superficial or deep infections. Treatment is with intravenous antibiotics and/or surgical debridement. Stable fixation should not be removed.

The necessity of skin excision and secondary procedures to achieve soft-tissue coverage is left to the surgeon's discretion.

Uncontrolled pain, edema or decreased digital range of motion may cause difficulties during the early postoperative period. Pain must be controlled either with oral or intravenous analgesics. Tapering doses of oral corticosteroids should be considered for refractory edema. Therapy, including active and passive digital range of motion and anti-edema measures, should be initiated early in the convalescence.

Long-term complications include the development of pseudoarthrosis, the presence of painful hardware, extensor tenosynovitis, or adhesions. The development of arthritic changes in adjacent joints, such as the triquetrohamate joint, poses more of theoretical than actual concern.

REHABILITATION

Digital range of motion is encouraged immediately. The dressing and sutures are then removed at two weeks. The patient is then placed in a short arm cast for an additional four to six weeks or until union is documented. K-wires are removed after union is documented (six to eight weeks). A thermoplastic splint is then used for comfort as a graduated motion and strengthening program is initiated.

For arthroplasties the reader is directed to the individual paper describing the chosen technique.

CONCLUSIONS

Arthritis of the lesser CMC joints is an uncommon condition and is often related to previous trauma. In the event that work modification or conservative management does not provide resolution of symptoms, surgical intervention may be indicated. Arthrodesis is the treatment of choice. For lesser CMC joint arthrosis, arthroplasty can also be considered. For arthrodesis the use of bone graft, rigid fixation, and postoperative immobilization are requisite for optimum outcome. A vigorous postoperative rehabilitation program aimed at maintenance of digital motion following surgery is also utilized. The exact etiology of the carpal boss remains unknown. Treatment with aggressive excision of the dorsal osteophytes and any associated ganglia is indicated for the patient refractory to conservative care. If the joint is found to be degenerative or unstable or if symptoms persist following excision, conversion to arthrodesis is warranted.

REFERENCES

1. Dickson RA, Morrison JD. The pattern of joint involvement in the hands with arthritis at the base of the thumb. *Hand* 1979;11: 249–255.
2. Waldron HA. Osteoarthritis of the hands in early populations. *Br J Rheum* 1996;35:1292–1298.
3. El-Bacha A. The carpometacarpal joints (excluding the trapezio-metacarpal). In: Tubiana R, ed. *The hand*, vol 1. Philadelphia: WB Saunders, 1981:158–167.
4. Posner MA, Kaplan EB. The fingers: Osseus and ligamentous structures. In: Spinner M, ed. *Kaplan's functional and surgical anatomy of the hand*, 3rd ed. Philadelphia: JB Lippincott, 1984:29.
5. Gunther SF. The carpometacarpal joints. *Orthop Clin North Am* 1984;15:259–277.
6. Rawles JG. Dislocations and fracture-dislocations at the carpometacarpal joints of the fingers. *Hand Clin* 1988;4:103–112.
7. Markze MW, Markze RF. The third metacarpal styloid process in humans: origin and function. *Am J Phys Anthropol* 1987;73:415–431.
8. Netter FH, Mitchell GAG, Woodburne RT. Anatomy. In: Netter FH, ed. *The Ciba collection of medicalillustrations*, 2nd ed, vol 8. Summit: Ciba-Geigy, 1991:72.
9. Hsu JD, Curtis RM. Carpometacarpal dislocations on the ulnar side of the hand. *J Bone Joint Surg [Am]* 1970;52:927–930.
10. Stevanovic MV, Stark HH. Dorsal dislocation of the fourth and fifth carpometacarpal joints and simultaneous dislocation of the metacarpophalangeal joint of the small finger: A case report. *J Hand Surg* 1984;9A:714–716.
11. Dommisse IG, Lloyd GJ. Injuries to the fifth metacarpal region. *Can J Surg* 1979;22:240–244.
12. Sakuma M, Inoue G. Simultaneous dorsal dislocation of the metacarpophalangeal and carpometacarpal joints of a finger. *Arch Orthop Trauma Surg* 1998;117:286–287.
13. Angelides AC. Ganglions of the hand and wrist. In: Green DP, ed. *Operative hand surgery*, 3rd ed. New York: Churchill Livingstone, 1993:2157–2171.
14. Cuono CB, Watson HK. The carpal boss: Surgical treatment and etiological considerations. *Plast Reconstr Surg* 1979;63:88–93.
15. Mueller JJ. Carpometacarpal dislocation: Report of five cases and review of the literature. *J Hand Surg* 1986;11A:184–188
16. Hartwig RH, Louis DS. Multiple carpometacarpal dislocations: A review of four cases. *J Bone Joint Surg* 1979;61A:906–908.
17. Imbriglia JE. Chronic dorsal carpometacarpal dislocation of the index, middle, ring and small fingers: A case report. *J Hand Surg* 1979;4:343–345.
18. Gurland M. Carpometacarpal joint injuries of the fingers. *Hand Clin* 1992;4(8):733–744.
19. Chen WS. Intratendinous ganglion and the carpometacarpal boss. A report of two cases. *Ital J Orthop Trauma* 1992;18(3):421–425.
20. Bora FW, Didizian NH. The treatment of injuries to the carpometacarpal joint of the little finger. *J Bone Joint Surg* 1974;56A:1459–1463.
21. Kaye JJ, Lister GD. Another use for the Brewerton view. *J Hand Surg* 1978;3:603.
22. Joseph R, Linscheid RL, Dobyns JH, et al. Chronic sprains of the carpometacarpal joints. *J Hand Surg* 1981 6:172–180.
23. Konsens RM, Seitz WH. Posttraumatic arthrosis of the index metacarpal joint. *Orthop* 1987;10:1429–1433.
24. Clendenin MB, Smith RJ. Metacarpo-hamate arthrodesis for posttraumatic arthritis. *Orthop Trans* 1982;6:167–168.
25. Clendenin MB, Smith RJ. Fifth metacarpal/hamate arthrodesis for posttraumatic osteoarthritis. *J Hand Surg* 1984;9A:374–378.
26. Watson HK, Dhillion HS. Intercarpal Arthrodesis. In: Green DP, ed. *Operative hand surgery*, 3rd ed. New York: Churchill Livingstone, 1993:113–130.
27. Gainor BJ, Stark HH, Ashworth CR, et al. Tendon arthroplasty of the fifth carpometacarpal joint for treatment of posttraumatic arthritis. *J Hand Surg* 1991;16A:520–524.
28. Green WL, Kilgore E. Treatment of fifth digit carpometacarpal arthritis with silastic prosthesis. *J Hand Surg* 1981;6:510–514.
29. Black DM, Watson HK, Vender MI. Arthroplasty of the ulnar carpometacarpal joints. *J Hand Surg* 1987;12A:1071–1074.

THE WRIST

LIMITED WRIST ARTHRODESIS

MICHAEL SAUERBIER AND RICHARD A. BERGER

HISTORICAL PERSPECTIVE

Limited wrist arthrodesis is an established and time proven method of treatment for severe carpal pathology maximizing postoperative wrist motion, function, and strength while reducing pain and eliminating instability. It provides (a) a means for load transference across normal residual joints in the wrist, (b) adaptation of preserved intercarpal mobility to compensate for motion pathways lost to fusion, and (c) reasonable assurance of prevention of progressing disease of other wrist joints (1). The experiences of Watson and others encouraged many surgeons to begin various combinations of intercarpal arthrodeses for conditions affecting the wrist, particularly for wrist instabilities (2–4). In clinical series of intercarpal fusions, most authors have reported preserving at least 50% of wrist motion for extension/flexion and ulnar/radial deviation or higher (5,6).

Various groups of wrist disorders, such as scapholunate advanced collapse (SLAC) or scaphoid nonunion advanced collapse (SNAC), patterns of wrist arthrosis, rotary subluxation of the scaphoid, carpal instabilities, degenerative disorders of special carpal units, Kienböck's disease, Preiser's disease, other carpal osteonecroses and congenital synchondrosis can be treated with limited wrist fusions (7–75). Depending on the stage of degenerative arthrosis, different procedures can be considered under the title of limited wrist arthrodesis.

Multiple experimental studies have described the theoretic effects of various limited wrist fusions on wrist motion. Short et al. evaluated the effect of nine different procedures for the treatment of Kienböck's disease (92). Their results after scaphotrapezium-trapezoid (STT) and scaphocapitate (SC) fusion showed successful unloading of the lunate and transferred load to the radioscaphoid joint. Viegas et al. have demonstrated that STT and SC fusions transmitted wrist load disproportionately through the scaphoid fossa of the distal radius (77). Horri et al. showed increased sliding motion of the lunate on the radius after the same fusions (23). Giunta et al. evaluated load transmission and subchondral bone mineralization after midcarpal fusion with computed tomographic osteoabsorbtiometry *in vivo* (78). They found peak mineralization in the radiolunate joint after midcarpal arthrodesis.

The knowledge of causes of degenerative or posttraumatic arthrosis of the wrist has directly paralleled the knowledge concerning the diagnosis, classification, and pathomechanics of traumatic wrist injuries. In one of the classic papers authored by Linscheid et al., it was stated that instability occurs because of either disruption of the ligamentous restraints or changes of the geometry of the osseous links (79). This type of disruption and instability commonly involves the scaphoid and its attachments, which mechanically provide stability to the intercarpal joint (80–82). Carpal collapse can follow both scaphoid fracture and ruptures of the scapholunate interosseous ligament and lead to degenerative arthrosis if not treated (83).

Carpal collapse also occurs in the late stages of Kienböck's disease (Lichtman stage IIIa and IV) and can be treated with limited wrist arthrodesis (84,85). Of course, until the actual etiology of Kienböck's disease is defined, the results of precollapse intervention will be suspect (86,87). STT arthrodesis for the treatment of Kienböck's disease has been recommended as a wrist salvage procedure through the work of Watson et al. (68). Stages IIIa/b and occasionally stage IV of the Lichtman classification are the specific indications for this operative procedure (66). It is considered for providing stable and pain reduced support for wrist load transference through the radioscaphoid joint unloading the radiolunate joint and preserving wrist mobility and adequate grip strength.

The scaphocapitate arthrodesis is based on the same principle as the STT arthrodesis (48). Biomechanically it decompresses the lunate, and the mechanical load is transferred into the radioscaphoid joint.

Other established limited arthrodesis procedures about the wrist include lunotriquetral (LT), radioscapholunate (RSL), radiolunate (RL) and scapholunate (SL) arthrodesis. For lunotriquetral pathologies, LT arthrodesis is a common procedure, especially for significant symptomatic instability. Recent data suggests, however, that residual pain after lunotriquetral arthrodesis is a relatively common phenomenon (88,89). When the articular surfaces of the distal radius, proximal scaphoid, and/or proximal lunate are compromised, the radioscapholunate arthrodesis may be considered as a reasonable option. The loss of wrist motion may be modulated in this instance by resecting the distal pole of the scaphoid, which in effect "unlocks" the midcarpal joint. It should be emphasized, however, that an intact midcarpal joint is a requisite for this procedure. Often used to stabilize the proximal carpal row against ulnar translocation, the RL arthrodesis is also a useful adjunct in the treatment of stage III lunotriquetral dissociation, where the lunate is fixed in a VISI pattern. Finally, for completeness, the SL arthrodesis should be mentioned. Although in theory it would appear that the SL arthrodesis would be an ideal treatment for scapholunate dissociation, in reality it has been a highly unpredictable procedure, with marginal clinical results. It is possible that a combination of factors, including the opposing rotational moments of the scaphoid and lunate as well as the limited surface area available for the fusion to occur, predispose this procedure to nonunion.

Regardless of which limited wrist arthrodesis procedure is being considered, the surgeon should explore the tobacco abuse history of the patient. In a recent study, it was determined that regardless of the mode or dose of tobacco exposure current tobacco abuse increases the risk of nonunion by a factor of 5.3 times that of a nontobacco abuser (90). It is strongly recommended that patients be enrolled in an effective smoking cessation program and all attempts to be tobacco free for a period of at least 3 months should be encouraged prior to committing to an elective limited arthrodesis of the wrist.

The principles and indications of limited wrist arthrodesis in the treatment of posttraumatic or degenerative arthrosis are addressed in this chapter. Limited wrist arthrodeses can be divided into these procedures primarily fusing the midcarpal joint (STT, SC, and four-bone), radiocarpal joint (RSL, RL), or intercarpal joints (SL and LT). This chapter will include discussions on scaphotrapezium-trapezoid, scaphocapitate, four-bone, scapholunate, lunotriquetral, radioscapholunate and radiolunate arthrodeses. Also, several operative techniques, their outcomes, and the authors' preferred techniques will be described and discussed as well. Alternative salvage procedures are discussed and a therapeutic algorithm is presented for different wrist pathologies.

INDICATIONS/CONTRAINDICATIONS

Midcarpal Arthrodesis

Scaphotrapezium-trapezoid (STT) Arthrodesis

The indications for scaphotrapezium-trapezoid, or triscaphe (STT) fusion, are the same as those for the scaphocapitate arthrodesis. Additionally, the biomechanical effects of load transmission to the radiocarpal joint of the STT arthrodesis are similar to those of the SC arthrodesis (23). The STT arthrodesis is indicated by primary arthrosis or instability of the scaphotrapezium-trapezoid joint and scapholunate dissociation. They both can be used for chronic rotatory subluxation of the scaphoid after scapholunate dissociation and

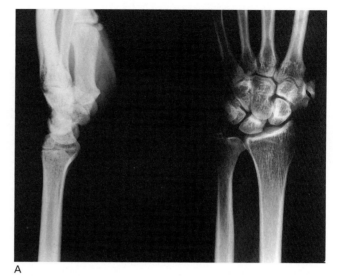

A

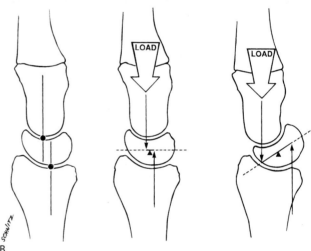

B

FIGURE 10.1. Posteroanterior and lateral wrist radiographs of a patient with static scapholunate dissociation. Note the scapholunate diastasis and foreshortened scaphoid on the PA view, and the increased scapholunate angle on the lateral view. There is no radiographic evidence of degenerative arthrosis.

SLAC wrist stage I combined with a radial styloidectomy (Figs. 10.1 and 10.2). Severe arthrosis in the STT joint and Lichtmann stage IIIa/b of Kienböck's disease are common indications as well (Figs. 10.3–10.6).

Contraindications specific to these procedures would include degenerative arthrosis of either the proximal articular surface of the scaphoid or of the scaphoid fossa of the distal radius and mechanical dissociation of the trapezoid from the hamate in the case of STT arthrodesis or of the capitate and hamate in the case of SC arthrodesis.

Scaphotrapezium-trapezoid Arthrosis

Scaphotrapezium-trapezoid (STT) arthrosis may occur as an isolated phenomenon or in association with other conditions

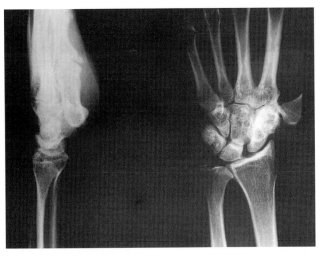

FIGURE 10.2. Posteroanterior and lateral wrist radiographs of the same patient in Figure 10.1 following successful scapho-trapezium-trapezoid (STT) arthrodesis. Note the maintenance of the appropriate radioscaphoid angle.

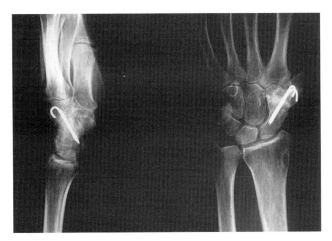

FIGURE 10.4. Posteroanterior and lateral wrist radiographs of the same patient in Figure 10.3 following successful STT arthrodesis. Note the maintenance of the appropriate radioscaphoid angle.

(see Fig. 10.3). As an isolated arthrosis, it is probably most commonly the result of trauma, such as a fracture of the distal articular surface of the scaphoid or disruption of the ligaments stabilizing the joint. It may also result from an inflammatory arthropathy such as rheumatoid arthritis. Additionally, the STT joint may become arthrotic secondary to involvement of another joint associated with the scaphoid or trapezium, such as arthrosis of the first carpometacarpal joint or scapholunate dissociation. The indications and contraindications are otherwise the same as those noted above.

Scapholunate Dissociation

Scapholunate dissociation is by definition a mechanical dissociation of the scaphoid and lunate resulting from injury to

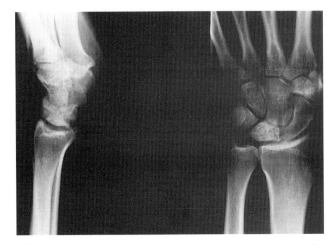

FIGURE 10.5. Posteroanterior and lateral wrist radiographs of a patient with stage IIIa Kienböck's disease.

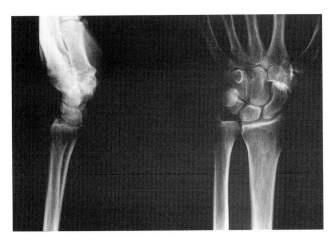

FIGURE 10.3. Posteroanterior and lateral wrist radiographs of a patient with primary arthrosis of the scaphotrapezium-trapezoid (STT) joint.

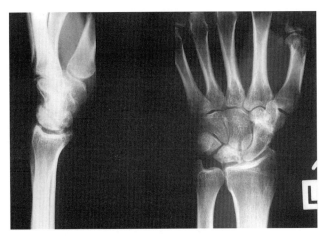

FIGURE 10.6. Posteroanterior and lateral wrist radiographs of the same patient in Figure 10.5 following successful STT arthrodesis. Note the maintenance of the appropriate radioscaphoid angle.

the scapholunate interosseous ligament (91). This dissociation results in a progression of carpal malalignment, including scaphoid palmarflexion, lunate dorsiflexion (DISI deformity), and proximal migration of the capitate (see Fig. 10.1). Left uncorrected, this pattern of carpal malalignment will almost invariably result in degenerative arthrosis involving the radioscaphoid and capitolunate articular surfaces (SLAC wrist) due to changes in the contact area and distribution of forces transmitted through these specific joint surfaces (77,92). Treating scapholunate dissociation soon after the injury is ideal, because it is more likely that the ligament will be amenable to direct repair and the secondary postural changes of carpal alignment will be less fixed. However, it is not uncommon to see these patients at a more protracted stage, already with a fixed DISI deformity. This is felt to represent a relative contraindication to soft-tissue procedures due to legitimate concern over their ability to securely stabilize the carpus against recurrence of the deformity. If the joint has little or no arthrosis, it has been advocated to perform a midcarpal stabilizing procedure such as an STT or SC arthrodesis, thereby controlling the position and orientation of the scaphoid relative to the radius, hence decreasing the likelihood of progressive arthrosis.

Scaphocapitate (SC) Arthrodesis

Due to the perception that a high complication rate was associated with STT arthrodesis, Pisano et al. introduced the technique of scaphocapitate (SC) arthrodesis (49). They reported a lower incidence of nonunion and malunion, as did the report of Kleinman (27). Laboratory studies have verified that the STT and SC arthrodeses behave in an essentially identical manner (23). Some surgeons feel that the potential for attenuation of the trapezocapitate ligament may, over time, improve the range of motion for an STT arthrodesis—a phenomenon that will have no bearing on an SC arthrodesis.

Regardless of the technique (STT or SC arthrodesis), the indications and contraindications are virtually the same. Common sense should intervene when necessary, however, where it would seem much more logical to perform an STT arthrodesis than an SC arthrodesis, in the face of isolated STT arthrosis.

Four-Bone Arthrodesis

A four-bone arthrodesis implies the intentional fusion of the mutually articulating surfaces of the lunate, triquetrum, capitate, and hamate. The most common indications for carrying out a four-bone arthrodesis include advanced degenerative disease involving the radioscaphoid joint, arthrosis involving the ulnar half of the midcarpal joint, and midcarpal instability, each described below. It is often combined with a scaphoidectomy, particularly in a patient with advanced degenerative disease resulting from scapholunate dissociation, scaphoid nonunion, or scaphoid malunion.

Since the entire mass of bones following a four-bone arthrodesis articulates almost entirely through the radiolunate joint, the only constant contraindication for this procedure is radiolunate arthrosis. Kienböck's disease, mechanical dissociation of the radiolunate joint, and extreme positive variance of the ulnar should be considered relative contraindications for the four-bone arthrodesis.

Scapholunate/scaphoid Nonunion Advanced Collapse (SLAC Wrist/SNAC Wrist) Degenerative Disease

Longstanding scaphoid nonunion or scapholunate ligament injury may result in carpal collapse and subsequent arthrosis, termed SLAC-wrist (scapholunate advanced collapse) (83) following scapholunate dissociation and SNAC-wrist (scaphoid nonunion advanced collapse) after failed union of scaphoid fractures are the most common patterns of arthrosis in the wrist (Fig. 10.7). The severity of the degenerative change is classified in three stages (83). The primary signs of SLAC arthrosis appear between the scaphoid and the radial styloid (stage I), later the radioscaphoid joint is narrowed and radiocarpal arthrosis will progress (stage II). In stage III midcarpal joint arthrosis develops between the scaphoid, lunate and the capitate head.

In SNAC (scaphoid nonunion advanced collapse) arthrosis, the pattern differs slightly. As only the distal fragment of the scaphoid flexes, arthrosis arises only between it and the radial styloid (stage I). The proximal fragment, aligned with the lunate and hemispherical in shape, remains congruous with the radius, and thus free of degenerative changes. In SNAC stage II the cartilage between the distal scaphoid and the scaphoid fossa of the radius is involved and occasionally

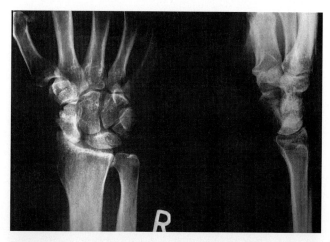

FIGURE 10.7. Posteroanterior and lateral wrist radiographs of a patient with Stage III scapholunate advanced collapse arthrosis, involving degenerative changes in the radioscaphoid and lunocapitate articulations.

scaphocapitate arthrosis between the proximal fragment of the scaphoid and the radial area of the head of the capitate. The presentation depends on the degree of arthrotic process and the amount of carpal instability. Further shift and collapse of the scaphoid occur, resulting in an increasing load on the capitolunate joint. The loaded capitate is driven off the radial side of the lunate between lunate and scaphoid, with shear loading of the capitolunate cartilage resulting in arthrosis in the midcarpal joint, which is termed as stage III. The capitate then migrates proximally toward the scaphoid and lunate. Finally the pathomechanics also lead to advanced carpal collapse (SNAC-wrist) (93).

A correct anatomical and biomechanical linkage of the scaphoid, lunate, and triquetrum is essential for maintaining the equilibrium of forces between the carpal components. Disruption of the proximal row connection upsets the normal balance and results in abnormal shifting of bones. The scaphoid flexes palmarly in scapholunate dissociation, and its proximal pole translates dorsally against the dorsal rim of the radius. The lunate and triquetrum, conversely, extend. Their motion is therefore dissociated from the scaphoid. The capitate migrates proximally and radially toward the scapholunate gap diminishing the carpal height. The extension of the lunate relative to the radius and capitate is termed dorsiflexion intercalated segment instability or DISI (79,94). SNAC or SLAC patterns may cause abnormal contact of the radiolunate and ulnocarpal joint. However, they usually do not lead to arthrosis between the lunate and the radius. Unlike the articulations at the radioscaphoid and capitolunate joint, the corresponding surfaces of the distal radius and lunate are spherical. The loads applied to the lunate remain perpendicular to its radial surface regardless of its rotational stance, and shear forces don't develop. This allows the possibility of preserving wrist mobility even in stage III disease. Ulnar carpal translocation may occur in association with SLAC or SNAC arthrosis. Viegas confirmed that the contact area and pressure increase in the scaphoid fossa and decrease in the lunate fossa of the radius with progressive perilunate instability (77).

In our experience, the procedure of choice for SLAC stage I with arthrosis only between the distal scaphoid and the radial styloid is a radial styloidectomy alone or combined with distal scaphoid fusion (STT or scaphocapitate). For SNAC wrist stage I a scaphoid reconstruction with an interpositional bone graft and a screw fixation should be used. Additionally a total or partial denervation of the wrist can be performed as a pain-relieving and motion-sparing procedure (95–99). In stage II disease a midcarpal arthrodesis (four-bone fusion) with scaphoid excision can be considered (Fig. 10.8). An alternative option to a limited wrist arthrodesis in SLAC stage II may be a proximal row carpectomy (PRC) (100,101). For stage III disease (radioscaphoid and ulnocapitate arthrosis), the procedure of choice is the four-corner fusion with scaphoid excision. A second choice is scaphoid excision and ulnocapitate arthrodesis. Proximal row carpec-

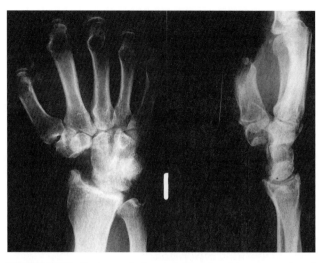

FIGURE 10.8. Posteroanterior and lateral wrist radiographs of the same patient in Figure 10.7 following successful four-bone fusion (lunate-capitate-hamate-triquetrum). Note the proper centering of the capitate on the lunate in the PA view and the correction of the DISI posture of the lunate in the lateral view.

tomy is not appropriate once the head of the capitate has arthrotic involvement.

Midcarpal Instability

Midcarpal instability is generally felt to belong to the so-called nondissociative patterns of carpal instability. This implies that interosseous ligaments connecting mutual bones within each carpal row are intact. Thus, the behavior of each carpal bone within either the proximal or distal row is appropriate relative to the other bones with that row, but the behavior of the entire row of bones as a functional unit is abnormal relative to the other carpal row of the radius. The hallmark clinical sign of midcarpal instability is the "catch-up clunk." This actively generated sign is one where during radial-to-ulnar deviation of the wrist, the proximal carpal row remains palmar-flexed well beyond the point where it would begin to dorsiflex until the extreme of ulnar deviation is reached, at which point the proximal row suddenly shifts into dorsiflexion. This sudden shift is interpreted as a "clunk" and may be quite painful when the maneuver is repeated. The reverse phenomenon has been reported, albeit it is quite rare, where the proximal carpal row suddenly palmar-flexes as the wrist reaches radial deviation. This phenomenon is referred to as a "reverse catch-up clunk." The etiology of midcarpal instability is not understood. It may stem from subtle disruptions of the capsular ligaments and may even have a neurogenic origin. Regardless, Lichtman has advocated a midcarpal fusion as the definitive treatment for midcarpal instability. This could take the form of an STT, SC, or four-bone fusion. Recently, however, attempts to treat this entity with soft-tissue–based procedures has gained popularity.

Capitolunate Arthrodesis

The capitolunate arthrodesis has recently been promoted as a procedure that carries the advantages of the four-bone fusion and minimizes the disadvantages. The principal advantage of the capitolunate arthrodesis compared to the four-bone arthrodesis is in the reduced fusion mass. By eliminating the lunotriquetral and triquetrohamate joints from the arthrodesis requisite, there may be a lower incidence of arthrodesis-related complications such as delayed union, nonunion, hardware failure, and fusion malunion. The indications and contraindications for a capitolunate arthrodesis are the same as for a four-bone arthrodesis. It typically is accompanied by a complete excision of the scaphoid and the triquetrum.

Intercarpal Arthrodesis

Scapholunate (SL) Arthrodesis

The principal reason for attempting a scapholunate arthrodesis is to stabilize the scapholunate joint. The most common cause of scapholunate instability is scapholunate dissociation, followed by a very proximal pole fracture of the scaphoid. The rationale is sound, but unfortunately the success rate of scapholunate arthrodesis is low, regardless of technique. In published series, the rate of nonunion and clinical failure has been unacceptably high (102). Anecdotally, the use of vascularized bone grafts has not resulted in a lower nonunion rate. Although the reason for the high nonunion incidence remains unknown, it may be related to (a) the retrograde interosseous blood flow of the proximal scaphoid; (b) the small surface area available for the fusion; (c) the counter-rotational tendencies of the scaphoid and lunate; and (d) the difficulty in achieving compression across the fusion site without changing the arc of curvature of the midcarpal joint. Thus, without an improvement in the results of this surgery, it will remain relatively contraindicated.

Lunotriquetral (LT) Arthrodesis

Lunotriquetral dissociation is the second most common instability pattern in the wrist following scapholunate dissociation (79,85,94,103,104). The fundamental injury is complete division of the lunotriquetral interosseous ligament, although less severe injuries may be symptomatic as well (105). With the triquetrum dissociated from the remainder of the proximal carpal row, it is unrestrained from dorsiflexion caused by contact with the hamate. If the dorsal radiocarpal ligament is attenuated, the lunate and scaphoid are then allowed to abnormally palmarflex, leading to the classic VISI (volarflexed intercalated segment instability) posture. Lunotriquetral dissociation must be clinically and radiographically distinguished from a lunotriquetral ligament tear. Both may present with the same symptoms; however, the tear may simply represent a degeneration of the proximal region of the LT ligament, perhaps from ulnar abutment syndrome. This condition is mechanically stable and will typically not respond to treatment options used for true lunotriquetral dissociation. There are a number of provocative maneuvers for the demonstration of LT dissociation, including direct tenderness of the LT joint, LT shuck, LT shear, and LT compression. Radiographically, there is no diastasis between the bones as there is in scapholunate dissociation. Rather, the hallmark of LT dissociation is a distal translation of the triquetrum relative to the lunate in a posteroanterior film. In advanced LT dissociation, the VISI deformity of the lunate may be evident in a lateral radiograph. Although many prefer soft-tissue reconstructions for lunotriquetral dissociation, and there is evidence that these techniques are preferable to arthrodesis, many still prefer lunotriquetral arthrodesis (LT arthrodesis). Laboratory studies only demonstrated a slight loss of motion in both flexion-extension and radial-ulnar deviation, validated by the fact that lunotriquetral coalition is the most common developmental abnormality involving this joint. It should be remembered, however, that in the case of a fixed VISI deformity, LT arthrodesis alone will not correct the volarflexed attitude of the lunate. A radiolunate arthrodesis is typically recommended as an augmentation procedure for this condition (106). Other conditions that may warrant an LT arthrodesis include, but are not limited to, primary arthrosis of the LT joint and following bone reconstruction for tumors (20,88,107).

Radiocarpal Arthrodesis

Radioscapholunate/Radiolunate (RSC/RL) Arthrodesis

Ulnar Translocation of the Carpus

Ulnar translocation of the carpus is defined as any condition where the lunate translate ulnarly to such a degree that less than 50% of its proximal articular surface is in contact with the lunate fossa of the distal articular surface of the radius. Of the known causes of ulnar translocation of the carpus, the most common is an inflammatory arthropathy of the wrist, such as rheumatoid arthritis, followed by traumatic disruption of the radiocarpal ligaments. Once identified, radiocarpal arthrodesis is the only reliable means of treating it. Often, a radiolunate arthrodesis is all that is necessary, which has the least significant influence on radiocarpal motion.

Other indications for radiocarpal arthrodesis include painful arthrosis resulting from inflammatory arthropathies such as rheumatoid arthritis and posttraumatic arthrosis resulting from interarticular fractures of the distal radius, scaphoid, and lunate (Fig. 10.9). One relatively rare indication for a radiolunate arthrodesis is in a patient with a fixed flexion deformity resulting from a chronic lunotriquetral dissociation, where soft-tissue correction of the VISI deformity is not likely.

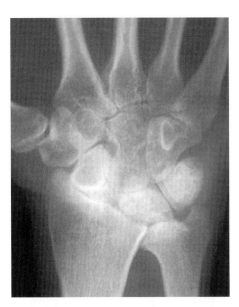

FIGURE 10.9. Posteroanterior wrist radiograph of a patient with marked degenerative changes of the radiocarpal articulation, as well as the distal radioulnar joint. Although it is difficult to judge the degree of arthrosis of the midcarpal joint for this view, supplemental imaging (tomograms, MRI, or arthroscopy) determined that the midcarpal joint articular surfaces were normal.

The principal contraindication for a radiolunate or radioscapholunate arthrodesis is the presence of significant arthrosis of the midcarpal joint.

PREOPERATIVE PLANNING

Common to limited wrist arthrodesis procedures will be several preoperative planning steps. First, the patient needs to have a clear understanding about what to expect from the planned procedure, both in the immediate perioperative period as well as in the long term, and the surgeon must have a clear understanding of what the patient's expectations and demands will be. If the patient is an active tobacco abuser, it is strongly recommended that he undergo a successful smoking cessation program. It has been shown recently that tobacco abuse increases the likelihood of nonunion in wrist arthrodesis procures by a factor of over fivefold, which is unacceptable in light of the elective nature of the procedure (48).

Careful attention must be directed preoperatively to a functional assessment of the entire affected upper extremity, including the hand, forearm, elbow, and shoulder. A careful radiographic analysis of the affected wrist must be made to maximize the familiarity of the surgeon with the principal pathology of the wrist and to detect co-existent conditions (58). It is often helpful to obtain similar imaging of the contralateral wrist to determine what the normal carpal height and angles are, in an attempt to replicate those values as much as possible in the affected wrist.

Scaphotrapezium-trapezoid (STT) Arthrodesis

STT arthrodeses are commonly used for STT arthritis, chronic scapholunate dissociation, and Kienböck's disease stage IIIa/b. After clinical examination plain X-rays are the next step. For SL dissociation, it may be desirable to obtain stress X-rays. It can be useful to perform a wrist arthroscopy to check whether there is radioscaphoid arthrosis or not.

For the late stages of Kienböck's disease a tomogram or CT scan to evaluate the condition of the lunate and the radiolunate joint can be worthwhile. It is also desirable to obtain posteroanterior and lateral radiographs of the contralateral wrist in order to estimate the natural posture of the scaphoid relative to the lunate, capitate, and radius.

The procedure can be performed with regional anesthesia if bone graft from the distal radius is used. If the fusion will be performed using bone graft from the iliac crest, a general anesthesia is required.

Scaphocapitate (SC) Arthrodesis

As an alternative to the STT arthrodesis, Pisano and Peimer first advocated the use of the scaphocapitate arthrodesis (49). Because of the rigidity of the intercarpal articulations of the distal row bones, it was felt that theoretically, the SC arthrodesis would behave mechanically and clinically in the same manner as an STT arthrodesis. The indications and preoperative planning are therefore identical to the STT arthrodesis described above.

Four-Bone Arthrodesis with Complete Scaphoid Excision and Lunocapitate Arthrodesis with Complete Excision of the Scaphoid and Triquetrum

After a careful clinical examination, plain X-rays with pa/lateral view are indicated. The severity of arthrosis and the stage of SLAC or SNAC can be identified easily. If more information about the condition of the radioscaphoid and radiolunate joint is needed, tomograms or a CT scan might be helpful. Usually, wrist arthroscopy is not necessary.

The procedure can be performed with regional anesthesia if bone graft from the distal radius is used. If the fusion will be performed using bone graft from the iliac crest, a general anesthesia is required.

Lunotriquetral Arthrodesis

Preoperative planning for a lunotriquetral (LT) arthrodesis is relatively simple, as the only indications for its use are lunotriquetral dissociation and lunotriquetral joint degenerative disease. One of the major complications of LT arthrodesis is pain resulting from an unrecognized positive variance of the ulna producing an ulnar impaction syndrome. Therefore, standard posteroanterior and lateral radiographs of the wrist must be obtained with careful attention to positioning of the extremity and the x-ray source. From the PA radiograph, an accurate determination of the relative length of the head of the ulna to the lunate fossa of the distal radius can be made. If positive variance of the ulna is encountered, the surgeon may wish to perform an osteotomy of the ulna, using the technique of either Milch or Feldon, to equalize the length of the bones. Additionally, an estimation of the normal arc of curvature of the contralateral midcarpal joint through the lunotriquetral region should be made. The surgeon will need to attempt to either maintain this arc if already normal, or correct it if abnormal. From the lateral radiograph, a determination of the posture of the lunate can be made. If the lunate is palmarflexed in the face of an otherwise neutrally oriented wrist, thus in a VISI (volarflexion intercalated segment instability) position, many would advocate a primary radiolunate arthrodesis. This is due to the difficulty encountered in maintaining a normal radiolunate posture with a static VISI deformity.

Radiolunate and Radioscapholunate Arthrodesis

Careful assessment of the midcarpal joint is necessary prior to performing a radiocarpal joint arthrodesis. This can be carried out with plain radiographs to assess the presence of typical signs of degenerative disease. Also, if a malalignment is present due to either an abnormal angulation of the radius or of the lunate, it is helpful to calculate the degree of correction that will be attempted in the operating room. The normal angles can be determined easily from the contralateral wrist, if uninjured. Plain radiographs will also provide information regarding ulnar variance. It is typically not necessary to obtain further imaging, unless one is concerned about the status of the lunate (e.g., ruling out Kienböck's disease).

TECHNIQUES

Universal Dorsal Approaches to the Wrist

Any number of skin incisions can be utilized, including a longitudinal, curvilinear, or transverse orientation. After clearing the subcutaneous tissue to expose the deep antebrachial fascia and the extensor retinaculum, care is taken to avoid injury to the terminal branches of the superficial radial nerve. The third extensor compartment is incised, allowing radial translocation of the extensor pollicis longus tendon. The fourth and second extensor compartments are elevated on ulnar and radial-based flaps, respectively. After mutual retraction of the digital and wrist extensor tendons, the dorsal wrist joint capsule is exposed.

To expose the midcarpal joint and the radial ⅔ of the radiocarpal joint, a radial-based capsular flap is developed (Figs. 10.10 and 10.11) (108). On the dorsal rim of the distal radius, the midpoint between Lister's tubercle and the dorsal

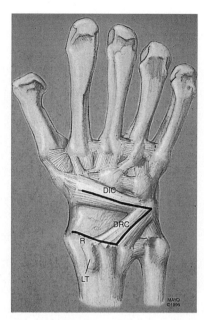

FIGURE 10.10. Drawing of the dorsal wrist outlining the landmarks for the radial-based capsulotomy. The dorsal radiocarpal ligament (DRC) attaches to the distal radius (R) between Lister's tubercle (LT) and the sigmoid notch. Distally, it attaches to the dorsal tubercle of the triquetrum, the same location as the proximal attachment of the dorsal intercarpal ligament (DIC). The bold lines demonstrate the incision lines for splitting the DRC and DIC ligaments, and continuing the proximal capsulotomy along the dorsal rim of the radius to the radial styloid process. (Reprinted with permission from: Berger RA, Bishop AT. A fiber-splitting capsulotomy technique for dorsal exposure of the wrist. *Tech Hand Upper Extremity Surg* 1997;1(1):2–10.)

edge of the sigmoid notch is identified, as is the central point on the dorsal tubercle of the triquetrum and the sulcus of the scaphotrapezium-trapezoid joint. A full thickness incision is made connecting these three points, thereby longitudinally dividing the dorsal radiocarpal and intercarpal ligaments. The flap is further developed by incising the dorsal joint capsule from the dorsal rim of the radius until the distal extent of the radial styloid process is reached. Avoiding injury to the dorsal regions of the scapholunate and lunotriquetral ligaments, the flap is elevated from the carpus on a radial base.

To expose the ulnar ⅓ of the radiocarpal joint, a proximally based capsular flap is developed (Figs. 10.12 and 10.13) (108). On the dorsal rim of the distal radius, the midpoint between Lister's tubercle and the dorsal edge of the sigmoid notch is identified, as is the septum between the fifth and sixth extensor compartments and the central point on the dorsal tubercle of the triquetrum. A full thickness incision is made by connecting the points on the dorsal rim of the distal radius and the triquetrum, and extending the incision proximally until the dorsal radioulnar ligament is encountered. This ligament may be difficult to visualize, but the surgeon will encounter increased resistance to the incision as the ligament is reached. It is also possible to detect the presence

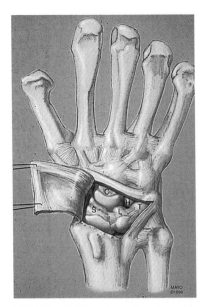

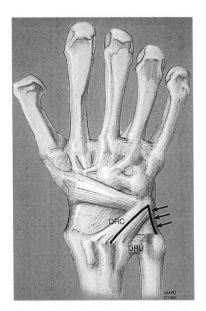

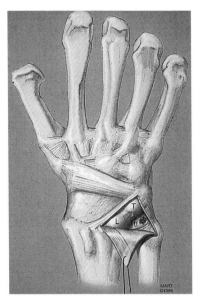

FIGURE 10.11. After elevating the radial-based capsular flap created with the incisions in Figure 10.10, the radial half of the radiocarpal joint and the entire midcarpal joint are exposed, as well as the scaphoid (S), lunate (L), capitate (C), and hamate (H). (Reprinted with permission from: Berger RA, Bishop AT. A fiber-splitting capsulotomy technique for dorsal exposure of the wrist. *Tech Hand Upper Extremity Surg* 1997;1(1):1–12.)

FIGURE 10.12. Drawing of the dorsal wrist outlining the landmarks for the ulnar-based capsulotomy. The dorsal radiocarpal ligament (DRC) attaches to the distal radius between Lister's tubercle and the sigmoid notch. Also at the sigmoid notch, the dorsal radioulnar ligament (DRU) attaches, where it courses ulnarly to attach to the ulna at the fovea. The bold lines demonstrate the incision lines for splitting the DRC ligament, and paralleling the sixth extensor compartment (arrows) in a distal to proximal direction to the level of the DRU ligament. (Reprinted with permission from: Berger RA, Bishop AT. A fiber-splitting capsulotomy technique for dorsal exposure of the wrist. *Tech Hand Upper Extremity Surg* 1997;1(1):2–10.)

FIGURE 10.13. After elevating the ulnar-based capsular flap created with the incisions in Figure 10.10, the ulnar half of the radiocarpal joint as well as the proximal surfaces of the lunate (L) and triquetrum (T) and the distal surface of the triangular fibrocartilage complex (tf) are exposed. (Reprinted with permission from: Berger RA, Bishop AT. A fiber-splitting capsulotomy technique for dorsal exposure of the wrist. *Tech Hand Upper Extremity Surg* 1997;1(1):2–10.)

of this ligament by simply pinching the dorsal joint capsule in various points, where the ligament will feel substantially thicker than the surrounding nonligamentous joint capsule. This capsulotomy effectively splits the dorsal radiocarpal ligament, and is then elevated proximally, with care taken to avoid inadvertent injury to the dorsal region of the lunotriquetral ligament.

Scaphotrapeziotrapezoid (STT) Arthrodesis

Because the STT joint is quite distal and radial to the remainder of the carpus, a smaller, more specific incision may be used. It is also possible to expose the joint through the universal capsulotomy, or even through a volar approach. An S-shaped incision over the STT joint and the second and third extensor compartment is used. Care is taken to preserve the superficial branch of the radial nerve and the dorsal vessels. The extensor retinaculum is then approached. The triscaphe joint resides beneath the crossing of the extensor pollicis longus (EPL), the extensor carpi radialis longus (ECRL), and the extensor carpi radialis brevis (ECRB). The extensor retinaculum is opened distally along the extensor pollicis longus ten-

don and retracted to expose the wrist capsule. The wrist is then entered by a way of a transverse capsular incision placed between the ECRL and the ECRB. Then the posterior interosseus nerve is severed at the base of the fourth compartment.

If absolutely necessary to prevent radial styloid impingement, 5–7 mm of the radial styloid may be removed with a rongeur or, alternatively, with an osteotome. Great care must be taken, however, not to disturb the proximal attachment of the radioscaphocapite ligament. The radioscaphoid joint is inspected for arthrosis. This joint bears the majority of load after STT fusion, and any degenerative change at this joint is destined to progress over time and may lead to a symptomatic wrist. Thus, radioscaphoid arthrosis is a contraindication to STT arthrodesis. After resection of the styloid tip the STT joint is exposed and the articular surfaces of the trapezium, trapezoid, and distal scaphoid are removed with a rongeur or an osteotome down to soft cancellous bone. The articular surfaces between the trapezium and the trapezoid are excised proximally. One 1.5 mm K-wire is inserted into the trapezium and one into the trapezoid in a distal to proximal direction and advanced until they protrude slightly at the proximal area of the bone. Cancellous bone graft is now harvested from the distal radius. A temporary spacer is placed between the trapezoid and the scaphoid. Next the radio-scaphoid angle is established between 41° and 60° (109). The K-wires are forwarded into the scaphoid and the spacer is removed (see Fig. 10.4). The resultant spaces between the scaphoid, trapezium, and trapezoid are then densely packed with the cancellous bone. The K-wires are cut and buried underneath the skin, and the wound is closed in layers.

Scaphocapitate Arthrodesis

The carpus is exposed utilizing the universal approach to expose the radial aspect of the radiocarpal and midcarpal joints, described above. Since laboratory studies have shown that the SC arthrodesis behaves mechanically in a fashion similar to the STT fusion, the same inspection criteria outlined above for the STT arthrodesis apply here as well. If the radioscaphoid joint is clear of significant arthrosis, the mutually articulating surfaces of the scaphoid and capitate are denuded through the subchondral cortical bone to expose the underlying cancellous bone. Next the radioscaphoid angle is established between 30° and 57° and maintained by pinning the scaphocapitate joint with 2 or more 0.045 K-wires (109). If cannulated screws are to be used as the final mode of fixation, the guide wires may be used instead of the K-wires. It is preferable to approach fixation from the lateral (radial) aspect, again taking care to avoid injury to the superficial radial nerve branches. Cancellous bone graft, either autologous or from an allograft source, or a bone substitute is then packed into the recesses of the scaphocapitate joint. Final

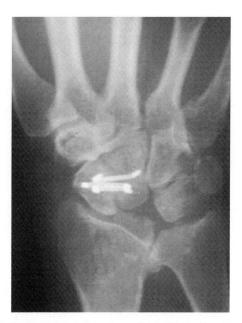

FIGURE 10.15. Posteroanterior wrist radiograph of a patient following scaphocapitate arthrodesis using dorsally placed 3-M® staples.

radiographs should be obtained in the operating room prior to closure of the wounds to check for alignment of the fusion and the status of the hardware. Fixation may be achieved with any number of techniques, including K-wires, screws (Fig. 10.14), staples (Fig. 10.15), or even small plates and screws.

Four-Bone Arthrodesis with Complete Scaphoid Excision

The carpus is exposed utilizing the universal approach to expose the radial aspect of the radiocarpal and midcarpal joints, described above. Great care is taken during resection of the joint surfaces of the capitate, lunate, and triquetrum to completely decorticate the concave distal surface of the lunate. The scaphoid is excised completely while preserving all palmar radiocarpal ligaments. The reduction of the lunate and realignment of the bones can be performed with a K-wire into the lunate as a joystick. If the joint surfaces are removed with an osteotome in a straight direction, a corticocancellous strut can be inserted between the four bones. Two 1.5 mm K-wires are inserted into the capitate in a distal to proximal direction and advanced until they protrude slightly at the head of the capitate, with one in the same direction from the hamate through the capitate. The lunate and capitate are reduced, and perfectly shaped bone graft is inserted between capitate, lunate, hamate, and triquetrum. Inclusion of the triquetrum and hamate in the fusion mass improves the union rates and does not effect ultimate wrist motion (81,82,97).

Corticocancellous chips can be used alternatively, if the cartilage is removed with a rongeur. Care is taken to align the radial borders of the lunate and capitate as well as the lunotri-

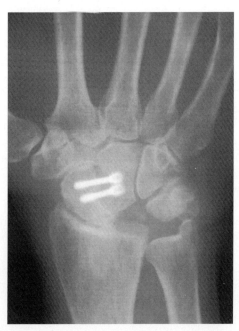

FIGURE 10.14. Posteroanterior wrist radiograph of a patient following a scaphocapitate arthrodesis using Herbert-Whipple® screws.

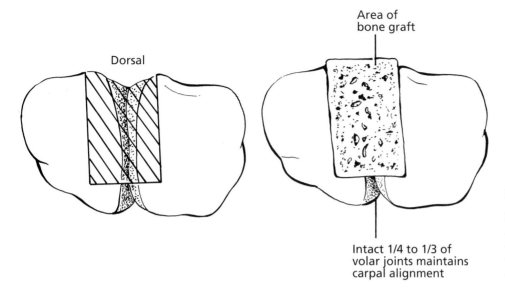

Dorsal

Area of
bone graft

Intact 1/4 to 1/3 of
volar joints maintains
carpal alignment

FIGURE 10.16. When denuding joints to be fused, regardless of the type of fusion being performed, a small amount of the volar joint should be left intact so that carpal alignment is maintained during the fusion procedure.

quetral and the capitohamate joints. Denution of the cartilage and a small amount of subchondral bone should be taken down to at least one-half of the joint depth and can be progressed even further, if desired. A small amount of the joints to be fused should be left intact in the volar-most reaches to maintain carpal alignment (Fig. 10.16). The K-wires are advanced into the proximal row. Another one or two K-wires are inserted to stabilize the hamate to the triquetrum. The correct position of the fusion and inserted K-wires is confirmed with X-rays. After closing the joint capsule, the extensor retinaculum is sutured leaving the EPL subcutaneously.

There are also several other fixation devices for midcarpal arthrodesis, such as screws, staplers, or the recently developed Spider Plate® (KMI, San Diego, CA). The Spider Plate was specifically developed for four-bone arthrodesis, although it has been used for other limited wrist fusions. This novel device is a 3-D, recessed plate that allows circumferential compression and has a central hole for the placement of additional bone graft (Fig. 10.17). A newer mini-Spider Plate has been developed for smaller fusion areas.

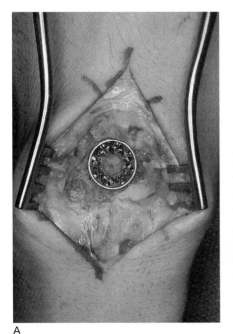

A

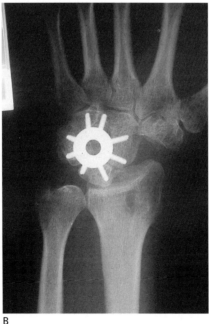

B

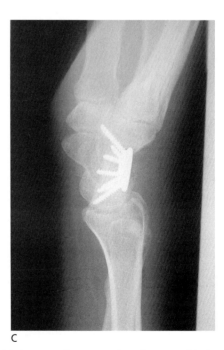

C

FIGURE 10.17. An intra-operative view of the Spider Plate placed in the dorsal wrist with bone graft augmenting the central hole **(A)**. Posteroanterior **(B)** and lateral **(C)** radiographs demonstrate that the plate provides two screw fixations in each of the four bones being fused and is completely recessed below the level of the dorsal carpus, avoiding any impingement with wrist extension postoperatively. (See Color Fig. 10.17.)

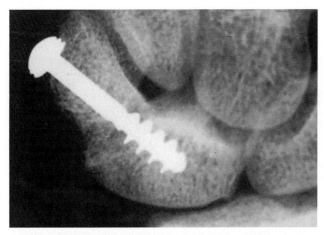

FIGURE 10.18. Posteroanterior radiograph of a wrist following lunotriquetral arthrodesis. A corticocancellous screw with a washer was chosen here, but any number of screw configurations can be utilized. Note the preservation of the arc of curvature of the distal articular surfaces of the proximal row bones.

Lunotriquetral Arthrodesis

Exposure of the lunotriquetral joint may be accomplished using either the radial or ulnar capsulotomy techniques described above. Once the joint is exposed, the residual dorsal and proximal regions of the lunotriquetral ligament should be excised. The mutually articulating surfaces of the lunotriquetral joint are excised until cancellous bone is exposed. Great care must be taken, however, to avoid overcompression of the lunotriquetral joint, as this will change the curvature of the midcarpal joint, leading to a less optimal result. Cancellous bone graft, either autogenous or allograft, or a bone substitute is then packed into the fusion site, which is then fixed with K-wires or screws (Fig. 10.18). Final radiographs should be obtained in the operating room prior to closure of the wounds to check for alignment of the fusion and the status of the hardware. Care must be taken to be certain that the alignment of the lunate relative to the radius is neutral.

Radioscapholunate and Radiolunate Arthrodesis

The universal capsulotomy for exposure of the radial aspect of the wrist is used. Inspection of the midcarpal joint, either through the capsulotomy or arthroscopy, is mandatory to rule out midcarpal arthritic changes. If found, an alternative salvage procedure should be considered. The mutually articulating surfaces of the lunate fossa of the distal radius and the proximal surface of the lunate are debrided to cancellous bone, for a radiolunate arthrodesis, while the scaphoid fossa and proximoradial surface of the scaphoid are added for a radioscapholunate arthrodesis. The resulting void is packed with autologous or allograft cancellous bone or a bone substitute. The ideal angle for the scaphoid relative to the radius should be 50° of flexion, while the lunate should be in neu-

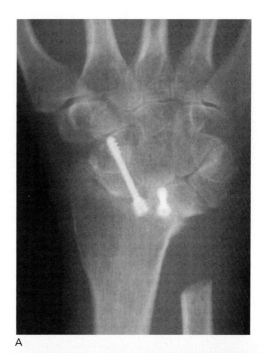

A

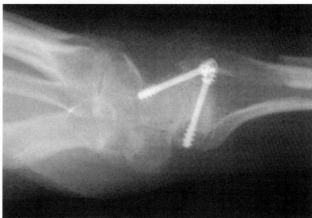

B

FIGURE 10.19. Posteroanterior (**A**) and lateral (**B**) wrist radiographs of a patient following radioscapholunate arthrodesis using Herbert-Whipple screws® oriented from the dorsal rim of the radius proximally into the scaphoid and lunate distally. This patient also suffered from degenerative joint disease involving the distal radioulnar joint, resulting in a Darrach resection of the distal ulna at the same time as the radioscapholunate arthrodesis.

tral extension. Fixation can be achieved with K-wires, distally oriented, obliquely angled screws from the dorsal cortex of the radial metaphysis (Fig. 10.19), proximally oriented obliquely angled screws from the dorsal cortices of the scaphoid and lunate (Fig. 10.20), staples (Figs. 10.21 and 10.22), or even a small plate and screw fixation system (Fig. 10.23). Fixation should be secure regardless of methods, due to the tremendous loading and torque that occurs across the radiocarpal joint. For example, screw purchase through the dorsal cortex of the distal radial metaphysis may prove to be suboptimal, resulting in loss of fixation and failure to unite. As an option

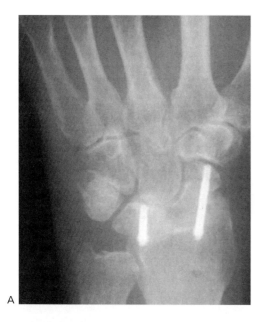

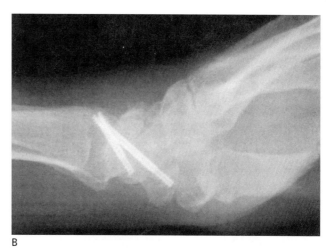

FIGURE 10.20. Posteroanterior (**A**) and lateral (**B**) wrist radiographs of a patient following radioscapholunate arthrodesis using Herbert-Whipple screws® oriented from the dorsal cortex of the scaphoid and lunate distally into the distal radius proximally.

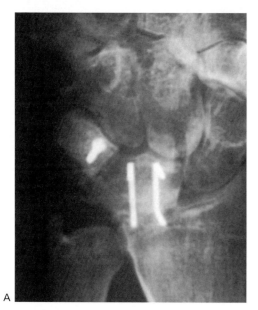

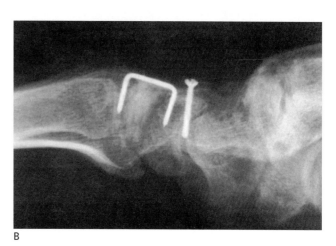

FIGURE 10.21. Posteroanterior (**A**) and lateral (**B**) wrist radiographs of a patient following a radiolunate arthrodesis, stabilized with 3-M staples® from a dorsal approach. The screw was previously placed in the dorsal cortex of the triquetrum as a means of stabilizing a dorsal cortical fracture, independent from the arthrodesis.

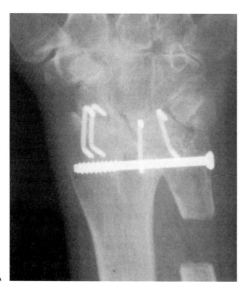

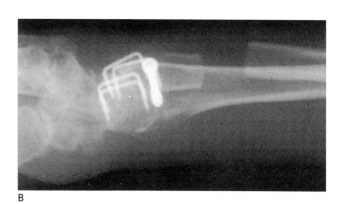

FIGURE 10.22. Posteroanterior (**A**) and lateral (**B**) wrist radiographs of a patient following radioscapholunate arthrodesis, stabilized with 3-M staples® from a dorsal approach. Note that two staples were placed each across the radioscaphoid and radiolunate arthrodesis sites. This patient also underwent a simultaneous Kapandji procedure for degenerative joint disease of the distal radioulnar joint.

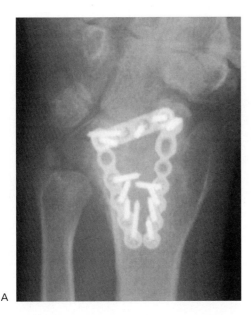

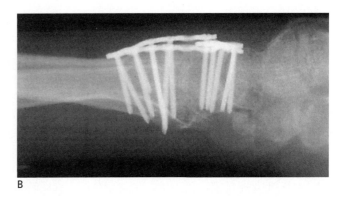

FIGURE 10.23. Posteroanterior **(A)** and lateral **(B)** wrist radiographs of a patient following radioscapholunate arthrodesis, stabilized with multiple Synthes Modular® plates and screws.

with the radioscapholunate arthrodesis, the distal pole of the scaphoid can be excised. This essentially "unlocks" the proximal and distal rows, enhancing midcarpal range of motion.

RESULTS/OUTCOMES FOR EACH TECHNIQUE

A generalization of all limited wrist arthrosis procedures is that they will result in less than normal global wrist ranges of motion (Fig. 10.24). This may or may not lead to a substantial impairment of function, depending on whether the resultant range of motion falls within functional limits (48). However, the conditions leading to the decision to embark upon a limited wrist arthrodesis will more than likely have already imparted such a limitation. Certainly the more bones that are fused, the more restriction in motion that will occur. Generally speaking, fusions carried out within a carpal row will have a minimal impact on motion, such as a capitohamate or lunotriquetral arthrodesis, where those that cross the radiocarpal or midcarpal joint will have a more profound effect on motion. Several laboratory analyses have been carried out to study the effect on range of motion with simulated limited wrist arthrodesis procedures. These proved an excellent foundation for predicting the postoperative range of motion. However, biological factors *in vivo*, such as prolonged immobilization and scar formation, make the laboratory values somewhat optimistic (5,110). A recent study by Minami et al. has shown that overall, the results seen 22 months postoperatively represent a stable point in the postoperative course, with no further deterioration expected (42). However, if the arthrodesis is carried out for changes associated with an inflammatory arthropathy, both the patient and surgeon should be aware that the underlying disease can continue to be active, causing further deterioration of function (111). It

should also be emphasized that few of the studies available for review regarding outcomes of surgery have employed the currently available tools for validated assessment of functional outcome, which will hopefully be rectified in future studies (25,111–113).

STT Arthrodesis

The STT arthrodesis was popularized by Watson et al. but first described by Sutro in 1946 and later by Peterson and Lipscomb in 1967 (4,48). The results of this procedure in the literature are quite satisfactory.

Watson et al. have the most overall experience with STT arthrodesis for all mentioned indications (67,70–72). They report on excellent results with no pain with normal activity levels in 71% of their patients. Watson has modified his technique since the early publication in 1980, choosing to abandon lunate replacement with a silicone prosthesis and adding a radial styloidectomy routinely.

Mean wrist flexion in Watson's last series was 57% and extension was 73% of the opposite unaffected side (72). Mean grip strength was 92% of the contralateral side. Patients in the series of other groups reached at least 55% grip strength of the contralateral side and an average ROM of at least 50% compared to the nonoperated wrist.

The authors have experience with STT arthrodesis on more than 40 patients. Fusion was established in 95% of the patients after an average of 7 weeks. The pain relief rate was significantly high. Grip strength improved to 60% on the opposite side. Active range of motion (AROM) showed 65% of extension/flexion and 50% of radial/ulnar deviation on average, compared to the contralateral hand. Eighty percent of patients were satisfied with the final result and would undergo the operation again.

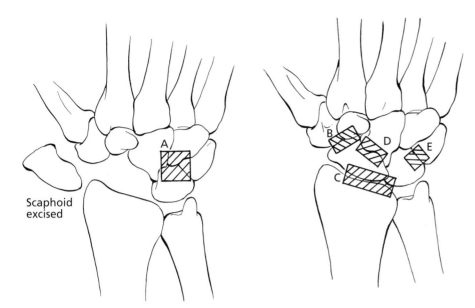

Scaphoid excised

FIGURE 10.24. A schematic diagram of the various limited wrist fusion locations: **A.** four-corner fusion with scaphoid excision, **B.** scaphotrapeziotrapezoid (STT) fusion, **C.** radioscapholunate (RSL) fusion, **D.** scaphocapitate (SC) fusion, **E.** lunotriquetral (LT) fusion.

Scaphocapitate (SC) Arthrodesis

The scaphocapitate arthrodesis is based on the same principle as the STT arthrodesis. Biomechanically, it is designed to decompress the lunate and transfer the load to the radioscaphoid joint. Laboratory studies have demonstrated that the load distribution and kinematics for the STT and SC arthrodesis procedures are similar (23). Moy and Peimer and Pisano et al. report results with good pain relief in a small series of patients (43,49). Sennwald and Ufenast reported a series of 11 patients with complete pain relief following scaphocapitate arthrodesis for the treatment of Kienböcks disease (59).

Midcarpal Arthrodesis with Scaphoid Excision (Four-Bone Fusion)

Scaphoid excision with midcarpal fusion is designed to relieve pain while preserving some measure of wrist mobility. In Watson's series, pain was significantly reduced, range of motion preserved (33% of extension and 37% of flexion) and grip strength improved (3,72,83). After 44 months on average, the results achieved were similar to the observations of Lanz et al. and Krimmer et al. in 31 and 45 patients, respectively (35,36,114). Nagy and Büchler reported the results in 12 patients after four-corner fusion, where the range of motion was adequate and the average grip strength 79% of the opposite hand (46,47). Siegel and Ruby examined 11 patients with midcarpal fusion of a series of 14 operated patients of which 4 underwent total wrist fusion finally due to continued pain (61). Most groups exclude silicone scaphoid implants due to severe problems with silicone-induced synovitis and dislocation of the prosthesis (38). In a recently published series with 31 patients the results of Sauerbier et al. compared favorably with most of these groups (115).

The resection of the proximal row of the carpus (PRC) is another popular operative procedure for treating SLAC or SNAC-wrist (56,73,90,100,101,116). It converts a mechanical link system into a simple hinge. In our opinion PRC may be indicated, if the head of the capitate is normal or near normal as it is in SLAC or SNAC stage II.

Lunotiquetral Arthrodesis

Lunotriquetral arthrodesis has a theoretical advantage of having minimal detrimental effects of the range of motion on the wrist, however, clinical series have shown a particularly high rate of postoperative complications. Included is a rate of nonunion as high as 57% and a high rate of postoperative pain (60). The nonunion rate may be due to the small surface available for fusion between the two bones and problems with adequate fixation. Postoperative pain, however, is much more difficult to decipher. Pain may emanate from the midcarpal joint if the arc of curvature of the proximal carpal row is not returned to normal, and care must be directed to be certain that residual ulnar impaction syndrome does not result from the procedure. Often, surrounding soft-tissue damage resulting from the initial injury leading to the indication for a lunotriquetral arthrodesis may be the source of residual pain.

Radioscapholunate/Radiolunate Arthrodesis

The results of radiocarpal arthrodesis can be very gratifying with the proper indications and surgical technique. All series reviewed demonstrate a very low rate of complications, but also report substantially below normal ranges of motion. Care must be taken, however, in interpreting these resultant ranges of motion, as the preoperative condition leading to the decision to proceed with a radiocarpal arthrodesis is generally severe to impart a substantial loss of motion in the first place. Partial resection of the distal scaphoid in patients undergoing a radioscapholunate arthrodesis may enhance midcarpal motion.

REHABILITATION

Introduction

Any attempt to establish an immutable rule regarding the length of time postoperatively that cast immobilization is used should be avoided. Rather, the decision to remove the cast should be based on definitive radiographic evidence that sufficient bony union across the arthrodesis site has occurred. This may require special radiographic views or tomographic evaluation. Additionally, the decision about which variety of cast immobilization should be applied is dependent on the experience of the surgeon and the reliability of the patient, rather than validated outcome studies, which are lacking in the literature. Torque will be transmitted across the wrist if the forearm is left free, such as with a standard short-arm cast. Therefore, it may be prudent to maintain the patient in a long-arm or Muenster-type cast for the first month, until the arthrodesis site has begun to consolidate. Additionally, for the more radial-sided arthrodeses, inclusion of the thumb is also left to the surgeon's discretion.

Common to all procedures is the necessity to initiate immediate postoperative therapy for finger range of motion and edema control. Additionally, it may be beneficial to include a shoulder range of motion maintenance program.

If pins have been utilized for fixation across the arthrodesis site, they may be removed once an adequate bony consolidation across the arthrodesis is verified. Once bony union has been achieved, all patients may be placed in a removable wrist splint, initiated on range of motion exercises and strengthening programs, liberated to activities as tolerated, and then weaned from the splint, also as tolerated.

COMPLICATIONS

Failure of a limited wrist arthrodesis may occur at several levels (1,53,61,117,118). From a biological standpoint, infection, delayed union, and nonunion may lead to substantial morbidity and less than optimal results (84). The most common complications of limited wrist fusions can be nonunion, hardware failure (Fig. 10.25), persistent pain, and progression of the degenerative patterns. Also pin tract infection, neuralgia following inadvertent injury to a cutaneous nerve passing through the surgical site, and sympathetic reflex dystrophy (SRD) can occur.

In our experience we have found that several of the limited wrist arthrodesis are very effective and predictable. Procedures such as STT fusion, SC fusion, four-corner fusion with complete scaphoid excision, and LT arthrodesis are reliable

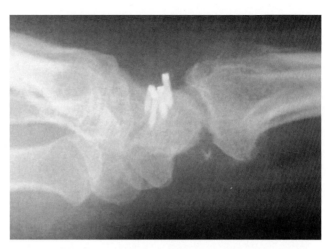

FIGURE 10.25. Lateral wrist radiograph of a patient following attempted scaphocapitate arthrodesis using dorsally placed staples, complicated by hardware failure and ultimate nonunion.

procedures for achieving sufficient pain relief and satisfying AROM. Regarding wrist mobility, performance of activities of daily living and patient's satisfaction make the results of limited wrist arthrodesis superior to total wrist fusion.

SALVAGE PROCEDURES

When contemplating the course of action for treating a failed limited wrist arthrodesis, the clinician should do all that he or she can to determine the cause of the failure. If the cause of failure is persistent pain, the source of the pain should be determined as definitively as possible. For example, if the pain is resulting from a nonunion at the original arthrodesis site, treatment aimed at correcting the nonunion should be carried out, either through the use of further immobilization with or without external stimulation with pulsed electromagnetic fields or high energy ultrasound, or returning to the operating room for a second attempt. It is also important to try to determine what the cause of the nonunion was in order to avoid the frustrating experience of developing a nonunion a second time.

If the pain is due to progressive degenerative disease in a previously unaffected region of the wrist, treatment should be directed to that region. For example, painful degenerative arthritis occurring at the radioscaphoid joint following an STT or SC arthrodesis might be treated with scaphoidectomy and a four-bone fusion. One could also consider performing a total wrist arthrodesis, particularly if the patient would tolerate the loss of motion and is requesting the most reliable and efficacious treatment for wrist pain.

If the patient is complaining of restricted motion, painful or otherwise, revision arthrodesis procedures will not be helpful and may, in fact, make the situation worse. If a patient has pain following a limited wrist arthrodesis but does not want to consider a procedure that will further compromise their motion, consideration might be given for performing a wrist denervation procedure (36,95–97,99,119).

No matter what the underlying source of the patient's complaints are following a limited wrist arthrodesis, an exhaustive trial of conservative management should be considered, as long as the patient's complaints are stemming from a progressive problem that has a solution, or obviously, if the problem is life or limb threatening. Conservative measures should include splinting, anti-inflammatory medications, and activity modifications.

Surgical options after failure of conservative measures might include revision limited arthrodesis, total wrist arthroplasty, total wrist arthrodesis, and partial or complete wrist denervation. Each of these procedures will be discussed in more detail in other chapters.

REFERENCES

1. Meyerdierks EM, Mosher JF, Werner FW. Limited wrist arthrodesis: a laboratory study. *J Hand Surg* 1987;12A:526–529.
2. Palmer AK, Werner FW, Murphy D, Glisson R. Functional wrist motion: a biomechanical study. *J Hand Surg* 1985;10A:39–46.
3. Watson HK, Goodman ML, Johnson TR. Limited wrist arthrodesis. Part II: Intercarpal and radiocarpal combinations. *J Hand Surg [Am]* 1981;6:223–233.
4. Watson HK, Hempton. Limited wrist arthrodesis. I. The triscaphoid joint. *J Hand Surg* 1980;5:320–327.
5. Douglas DP, Peimer CA, Koniuch MP. Motion of the wrist after simulated limited intercarpal arthrodeses: An experimental study. *J Bone Joint Surg* 1987;69A:1413–1418.
6. Gellman H, Kauffman D, Lenihan M, et al. An in vitro analysis of wrist motion: the effect of limited intercarpal arthrodesis and the contributions of the radiocarpal and midcarpal joints. *J Hand Surg* 1988;13A:378–383.
7. Ashmead D, Watson HK, Damon C, et al. Scapholunate advanced collapse wrist salvage. *J Hand Surg [Am]* 1994;19:741–750.
8. Bach AW, Almquist EE, Newman DM. Proximal row fusion as a solution for radiocarpal arthritis. *J Hand Surg* 1991;16A:424–431.
9. Buck-Gramcko D. Die STT-Arthrodese bei karpalen Instabilitäten und bei Mondbeinnekrose. Literaturübersicht und eigene Ergebnisse. *Operat Orthop Traumatol* 1990;2:153–159.
10. Buck-Gramcko D. Die skapholunäre Dissoziation. *Handchir Mikrochir Plast Chir* 1985;17: 194–199.
11. Chamay A, Della Santa. Radiolunate arthrodesis in rheumatoid wrist (21 cases). *Ann Chir Main Super* 1991;10:197–206.
12. Chamay A, Della Santa D, Vilaseca A. Radiolunate arthrodesis. Factor of stability for the rheumatoid wrist. *Ann Chir Main* 1983; 2:5–17.
13. Cooney WP, Bussey R, Dobyns JH, Linscheid RL. Difficult wrist Fractures. *Clin Orthop Rel Res* 1987;213:136–147.
14. Crosby EB, Linscheid RL, Dobyns JH. Scaphotrapezial trapezoidal arthrosis. *J Hand Surg* 1978;3A:223–234.
15. Eckenrode JF, Louis DS, Greene TL. Scaphoid-trapezium-trapezoid fusion in the treatment of chronic scapholunate instability. *J Hand Surg* 1986;11A:497–502.
16. Fischer M, Segmueller G. Lunatummalazie—Indikation und Grenzen der Niveauoperation. *Orthopäde* 1993;22:52–56.
17. Frykman EB, Ekenstam FA, Wadin K. Triscaphoid arthrodesis and its complications. *J Hand Surg* 1988;13A:844–848.
18. Giunta RE, Krimmer H, Krapohl B, et al. Pattern of subchondral bone mineralisation in the wrist after midcarpal fusion. *J Hand Surg* 1999;24A:138–147.
19. Graner O, Lopes BC, Carvalho, Atlas S. Arthrodesis of the carpal bones in the treatment of Kienböck's disease, painful ununited fractures of the navicular and lunate bones with avascular necroses, and old fracture-dislocations of carpal bones. *J Bone Joint Surg* 1966; 48A:767–774.
20. Gross SC, Watson HK, Strickland JW, et al. Triquetral-lunate arthritis secondary to synostosis. *J Hand Surg* 1989;14A:95–102.
21. Hastings DE, Silver RL. Intercarpal arthrodesis in the management of chronic carpal instability after trauma. *J Hand Surg* 1984;9A:834–840.
22. Heymans, Adelmann E, Koebke J. Anatomical bases of the pediculated pisiform transplant and the intercarpal fusion by Graner in Kienböck's disease. *Surg Radiol Anat* 1992;14:195–201.
23. Horri E, Garcia-Elias M, Bishop AT, et al. Effect on force transmission across the carpus in procedures to treat Kienböck's disease. *J Hand Surg* 1990;15A:393–400.
24. Inoue G, Tamura Y. Radiolunate and radioscapholunate arthrodesis. *Arch Orthop Trauma Surg* 1992;111:333–335.
25. Iwasaki N, Genda E, Barrance PJ, et al. Biomechanical analysis of limited intercarpal fusion for the treatment of Kienböck's disease: a three-dimensional theoretical study. *J Orthop Res* 1998;16:256–263.
26. Kirschenbaum D, Schneider LH, Kirkpatrick WH, et al. Scaphoid excision and capitolunate arthrodesis for radioscaphoid arthritis. *J Hand Surg* 1993;18A:780–785.
27. Kleinman WB. Long-term study of chronic scapho-lunate instability treated by scapho-trapezio-trapezoid arthrodesis. *J Hand Surg* 1989;14A:429–445.
28. Kleinman WB. Management of chronic rotary subluxation of the scaphoid by scapho-trapezio-trapezoid arthrodesis. Rationale for the technique, postoperative changes in biomechanics, and results. *Hand Clin* 1987;3:113–133.
29. Kleinman WB, Steichen JB, Strickland JW. Management of chronic rotary subluxation of the scaphoid by scapho-trapezio-trapezoid arthrodesis. *J Hand Surg* 1982;7A:125–136.
30. Krakauer JD, Bishop AT, Cooney WP. Surgical treatment of scapholunate advanced collapse. *J Hand Surg* 1994;9A:358–365.
31. Krimmer H. Der fortgeschrittene karpale Kollaps. Habilitationsschrift der Medizinischen Fakultät der Julius-Maximilians-Universität zu Würzburg. 1998.
32. Krimmer H, Hahn P, Prommersberger KJ, et al. Therapie der skapholunären Dissoziation. *Akt Traumatol* 1996;26:264–269.
33. Krimmer H, Krapohl B, Sauerbier M, Hahn P. Der posttraumatische karpale Kollaps (SLAC und SNAC-Wrist). Stadieneinteilung und therapeutische Möglichkeiten. *Handchir Mikrochir Plast Chir* 1997;29:228–233.
34. Krimmer H, Lanz U. Die mediokarpale Teilarthrodese des Handgelenkes. *Operat Orthop und Traumatol* 1996;8:175–184.
35. Krimmer H, Sauerbier M, Vispo-Seara JL, et al. Fortgeschrittener karpaler Kollaps (Slac-wrist) bei Skaphoidpseudarthrose. Therapiekonzept: mediokarpale Teilarthrodese. *Handchir Mikrochir Plast Chir* 1992;24:191–198.
36. Lanz U, Häusser D, Sauerbier M. Karpale Instabilitäten—Konventionelle Therapie. In: Hempfling H, Beickert R, Bauer K, Ishida A (Hrsg). *Arthroskopie des Handgelenkes*. Landsberg: Ecomed Verlag, 1996:123–136.
37. Lanz U, Krimmer H, Sauerbier M. Advanced carpal collapse: Treatment by limited wrist fusion. In: Büchler U (Hrsg). *Wrist instability*. London: M. Dunitz, 1996:139–145.
38. Lichtman DM, Bruckner JD, Culp RW, Alexander CE. Palmar midcarpal instability: results of surgical reconstruction. *J Hand Surg* 1993;18:307–315.
39. Lin HH, Stern PJ. "Salvage" procedures in the treatment of Kienböck's disease. Proximal row carpectomy and total wrist arthrodesis. *Hand Clin* 1993;9:521–526.

40. Linscheid RL, Dobyns JH. Radiolunate arthrodesis. *J Hand Surg* 1985;10A:821–829.

41. Minami A, Ogino T, Minami M. Limited wrist fusions. *J Hand Surg* 1988;13A:660–667.

42. Minami A, Kato H, Iwasaki N, Minami M. Limited wrist fusions: comparison of results 22 and 89 months after surgery. *J Hand Surg* 1999;24A:133–137.

43. Moy JO, Peimer CA. Scaphocapitate fusion in the treatment of Kienböck's disease. *Hand Clin* 1993;9:501–504.

44. Minami A, Kimura T, Suzuki K. Long-term results of Kieböck's disease treated by triscaphe arthrodesis and excisional arthroplasty with a coiled palmaris longus tendon. *J Hand Surg* 1994;19A:219–228.

45. Nagy L, Büchler U. Ist die Panarthrodese der Goldstandard der Handgelenkchirurgie? *Handchir Mikrochir Plast Chir* 1998;30:291–297.

46. Nagy L, Büchler U. Long term results of radioscapholunate fusion following fractures of the distal radius. *J Hand Surg* 1997;22B:705–710.

47. Nakamura R, Horii E, Watanabe K, et al. Proximal row carpectomy versus limited wrist arthrodesis for advanced Kienböck's disease. *J Hand Surg* 1998;23B: 741–745.

48. Peterson HA, Lipscomb PR. Intercarpal Arthrodesis. *Arch Surg* 1967;95:127–134.

49. Pisano SM, Peimer CA, Wheeler DR, Sherwin F. Scaphocapitate intercarpal arthrodesis. *J Hand Surg* 1991;16A:328–333.

50. Posner MA. Scapholunate dissociation: Treatment by intercarpal fusion. *Techniques Orthop* 1992;7:35–41.

51. Rayhack JM, Linscheid RL, Dobyns JH, Smith JH. Posttraumatic ulnar translation of the carpus. *J Hand Surg* 1987;12A:180–189.

52. Rittmeister M, Kandziora F, Rehart S, Kerschbauer F. Radiolunäre und Mannerfelt-Arthrodes bei rheumatoider Arthritis. *Handchir Mikrochir Plast Chir* 1999;31:266–273.

53. Rotman MB, Manske PR, Pruitt DL, Szerzinski J. Scaphocapitolunate arthrodesis. *J Hand Surg* 1993;18A:26–33.

54. Rozing PM, Kauer JM. Partial arthrodesis of the wrist. An investigation in cadavers. *Acta Orthop Scand* 1984;55:66–68.

55. Saffar P, Fakhoury B. Resection de la premiere rangee contre arthrodese partielle des os du carpe dans les instabilites du carpe. *Ann Chir Main Memb Super* 1992;11:276–280.

56. Sauerbier M, Bickert B, Tränkle M, et al. Operative Behandlungsmöglichkeiten bei fortgeschrittenem karpalen Kollaps (SNAC-/SLAC-Wrist). *Unfallchir* 2000;103:564–571.

57. Sauerbier M, Tränkle M, Erdmann D, Germann G. Functional outcome with scapho-trapezio-trapezoid arthrodesis in the treatment of Kienböck's disease stage III. *Ann Plast Surg* 2000;44:618–625.

58. Schmitt R, Lanz U, Lucas D, et al. Computertomographie der Hand: Untersuchungstechnik, Normalanatomie, Indikationsgebiete. *Handchir Mikrochir Plast Chir* 1989;21:89–96.

59. Sennwald GR, Fischer M, Mondi P. Lunotriquetral arthrodesis. A controversial procedure. *J Hand Surg* 1995;20B:755–760.

60. Sennwald GR, Ufenast H. Scaphocapitate arthrodesis for the treatment of Kienböck's disease. *J Hand Surg* 1995;20A:505–510.

61. Siegel JM, Ruby LK. A critical look at intercarpal arthrodesis: review of the literature. *J Hand Surg* 1996;21A:717–723.

62. Stanley JK, Boot DA. Radiolunate arthrodesis. *J Hand Surg* 1989;14B:283–287.

63. Viola RW, Kiser PK, Bach AW, et al. Biomechanical analysis of capitate shortening with capitate hamate fusion in the treatment of Kienböck's disease. *J Hand Surg* 1998;23A:395–401.

64. Voche P, Merle M. Arthrodesis of 4 bones of the wrist. Study of 12 follow-up cases. *Rev Chir Orthop Reparatrice Appar Mot* 1993;79:456–463.

65. Voche P, Bour C, Merle M. Scapho-trapezio-trapezoid arthrodesis in the treatment of Kienböck's disease. A study of 16 cases. *J Hand Surg* 1992;17B:5–11.

66. Watson HK, Ryu J, DiBella A. An approach to Kienböck's disease: Triscaphe arthrodesis. *J Hand Surg* 1985;10A:179–187.

67. Watson HK, Fink JA, Monacelli DM. Use of triscaphe fusion in the treatment of Kienböck's disease. *Hand Clin* 1993;9:493–499.

68. Watson HK, Monacelli DM, Milford RS, Ashmead D. Treatment of Kienbock's disease with scaphotrapezio-trapezoid arthrodesis. *J Hand Surg* 1996;21A:9–15.

69. Watson HK, Ryu J. Evolution of arthritis of the wrist. *Clin Orthop* 1986;201:57–67.

70. Watson HK, Ryu J, Akelman E. Limited triscaphoid intercarpal arthrodesis for rotatory subluxation of the scaphoid. *J Bone Joint Surg* 1986;68A:345–349.

71. Watson HK, Ryu J, DiBella A. An approach to Kienböck's disease: Triscaphe arthrodesis. *J Hand Surg* 1985;10A:179–187.

72. Watson HK, Weinzweig J, Guidera PM, et al. One thousand intercarpal arthrodeses. *J Hand Surg* 1999;24B:307–315.

73. Yajima, Tamai S, Ono H. Partial radiocarpal arthrodesis. *Nippon Seikeigeka Gakkai Zasshi* 1994;68:847–853.

74. Zdravkovic V, Sennwald GR. Scaphocapitate Fusion. *Atlas Hand Clin* 1999;4:135–143.

75. Sauerbier M, Tränkle M, Linsner G, Bickert B, Germann G. Midcarpal arthrodesis with complete scaphoid excision and interposition bone graft in the treatment of advanced carpal collapse (SNAC/SLAC Wrist): Operative technique and outcome assessment. *J Hand Surg* 2000;25B:341–345.

76. Shin AY, Battaglia MJ, Bishop AT. Lunotriquetral instability: diagnosis and treatment. *J Am Acad Orthop Surg* 2000;8:170–179.

77. Viegas SF, Patterson RM, Peterson PD, et al. Evaluations of the biomechanical efficacy of limited intercarpla fusions for the treatment of scapholunate dissociation. *J Hand Surg* 1990;15A:120–128.

78. Giunta R, Rock C, Löwer N, et al. Über die Beanspruchung des Handgelenks bei Mondbeinnekrose—Eine morphologische Untersuchung am Lebenden. *Handchir Mikrochir Plast Chir* 1998;30:158–164.

79. Linscheid RL, Dobyns JH, Beabout JW. Traumatic instability of the wrist. Diagnosis, classification and pathomechanics. *J Bone Joint Surg* 1972;54A:1612–1632.

80. Berger RA, Blair WF, Crowninshield RD, Flatt AE. The scapholunate ligament. *J Hand Surg* 1982;7A:87–91.

81. Berger RA, Kauer JM, Landsmeer JM. Radioscapholunate ligament: a gross anatomic and histologic study of fetal and adult wrist. *J Hand Surg* 1991;16A:350–355.

82. Berger RA, Landsmeer JM. The palmar radiocarpal ligaments: a study of adult and fetal human wrist joints. *J Hand Surg* 1990;15A:847–854.

83. Watson HK, Ballet FL. The SLAC wrist: scapholunate advanced collapse pattern of degenerative arthritis. *J Hand Surg [Am]* 1984;9:358–365.

84. Lichtman DM, Alexander AH, Mack GR, Gunther SF. Kienböck's disease—update on silicone replacement arthroplasty. *J Hand Surg* 1982;7:343–347.

85. Lichtmann DM, Martin RA. Introduction to the carpal instabilities. In: Lichtmann DM (Hrsg). *The wrist and its disorders*. Philadelphia: WB Saunders, 1988:244–250.

86. Gelberman RH, Bauman TD, Menon J, Akeson WK. Vascularity of the lunate bone and Kienböck's disease. *J Hand Surg* 1980;5:272–278.

87. Gelberman RH, Salamon PB, Jurist JM, Posch JL. Ulnar variance in Kienböcks disease. *J Bone Joint Surg* 1975;57A:674–676.

88. Ambrose L, Posner MA. Lunate-triquetral and midcarpal joint instability. *Hand Clin* 1992;8:653–668.

89. Sauerbier M, Kania NM, Kluge S, et al. Erste Ergebnisse mit der neuen AO-Handgelenk-Arthrodesenplatte. *Handchir Mikrochir Plast Chir* 1999;31:260–265.

90. Ortiz, J, Berger RA. The effects of tobacco abuse on wrist arthroses. Presented at the 51st annual meeting of the American Society for Surgery of the Hand, Baltimore, MD, 1999.

91. Berger RA. The gross and histologic anatomy of the scapholunate interosseus ligament. *J Hand Surg* 1996;21:170–178.

92. Short WH, Werner FW, Fortino MD, Palmer AK. Distribution of pressures and forces on the wrist after simulated intercarpal fusion and Kienböck's disease. *J Hand Surg* 1992;17A:443–449.

93. Vender MI. Watson HK, Wiener BD, Black DM. Degenerative change in symptomatic scaphoid nonunion. *J Hand Surg* 1987; 12A:514–519.

94. Linscheid RL, Dobyns JH, Beckenbaugh RD, et al. Instability patterns of the wrist. *J Hand Surg [Am]* 1983;8:682–686.

95. Berger RA. Partial denervation of the wrist: a new approach. *Tech Hand Upper Ext Surg* 1998;2:25–35.

96. Buck-Gramcko D. Wrist denervation in the treatment of Kienböck's disease. *Hand Clin* 1993;9:517–520.

97. Buck-Gramcko D. Denervation of the wrist joint. *J Hand Surg* 1977;2A:54–61.

98. Lanz U. Indikation zur Denervation. In: Hempfling H (Hrsg). *Die Arthroskopie am Handgelenk.* Stuttgart: Wissenschaftliche Verlagsgesellschaft, 1992:141–145.

99. Wyrick JD, Stern PJ, Kiefhaber TR. Motion-preserving procedures in the treatment of scapholunate advanced collapse wrist: proximal row carpectomy versus four-corner arthrodesis. *J Hand Surg [Am]* 1995;20:965–970.

100. Neviaser RJ. On resection of the proximal carpal row. *Clin Orthop* 1986;202:12–15.

101. Tomaino MM, Delsignore J, Burton RI. Long-term results following proximal row carpectomy. *J Hand Surg* 1994;19A:694–703.

102. Hom S, Ruby LK. Attempted scapholunate arthrodesis for chronic scapholunate dissociation. *J Hand Surg* 1991;16A:334–339.

103. Lichtman DM, Noble WH III, Alexander CE. Dynamic triquetrolunate instability: case report. *J Hand Surg* 1984;9A:185–188.

104. Mathoulin C, Saffar P, Roukoz S. Lunar-triquetral instability. *Ann Chir Main Memb Super* 1990;9:22–28.

105. Ritt, MJ, Linscheid RL, Cooney WP III, et al. The lunotriquetral joint: kinematic effects of sequential ligament sectioning, ligament repair, and arthrodesis. *J Hand Surg* 1998;23A:432–445.

106. Halikis MN, Colello-Abraham K, Taleisnik J. Radiolunate fusion. The forgotten partial arthrodesis. *Clin Orthop* 1997;341:30–35.

107. Louis DS, Hankin FM, Braunstein EM. Giant cell tumor of the triquetrum. *J Hand Surg* 1986;11B:279–280.

108. Berger RA, Bishop AT, Bettinger PC. New dorsal capsulotomy for the surgical exposure of the wrist. *Ann Plast Surg* 1995;35:54–59.

109. Minamikawa Y, Peimer CA, Yamaguchi T, et al. Ideal scaphoid angle for intercarpal arthrodesis. *J Hand Surg* 1992;17A:370–375.

110. Saffar P. Radiolunate arthrodesis for distal radial intraarticular malunion. *J Hand Surg* 1996;21A:14–20.

111. Della Santa D, Chamay A. Radiological evolution of the rheumatoid wrist after radiolunate arthrodesis. *J Hand Surg* 1995;20B:146–154.

112. Amadio PC. Outcomes assessment in hand surgery. What's new? *Clin Plast Surg* 1997;24:191–194.

113. Germann G, Wind G, Harth A. Der DASH Fragebogen—Ein neues Instrument zur "Outcome" Evaluation an der oberen Extremität. *Handchir Mikrochir Plast Chir* 1999;31:149–152.

114. Larsen CF, Jacoby RA, McCabe SJ. Nonunion rates of limited carpal arthrodesis: a meta-analysis of the literature. *J Hand Surg* 1997;22A:66–73.

115. Sauerbier M, Bickert B, Kluge S, et al. Mittelfristige Resultate nach STT-Arthrodese zur Behandlung der aseptischen Lunatumnekrose im Stadium IIIa/b. *Langenbecks Arch Chir Suppl II (Kongreßbericht)* 1998:1274–1278.

116. Begley BW, Engber WD. Proximal row carpectomy in advanced Kienböck's disease. *J Hand Surg* 1994;19A:1016–1018.

117. McAuliffe JA, Dell PL, Jaffe R. Complications of intercarpal arthrodesis. *J Hand Surg* 1993;18A:1121–1128.

118. Rogers WD, Watson HK. Radial styloid impingement after triscaphe arthrodesis. *J Hand Surg* 1989;14A:297–301.

119. Wilhelm A. Die Gelenkdenervation und ihre anatomischen Grundlagen. Ein neues Behandlungskonzept in der Handchirurgie. Zur Behandlung der Spätstadien der Lunatummalazie und Navicularepseudarthrose. *Hefte Unfallheilkd* 1966;86:1–109.

LIMITED WRIST ARTHROPLASTY

THOMAS B. HUGHES, JR., AND MARK E. BARATZ

INTRODUCTION

Wrist fusion sacrifices mobility for durability and pain relief, while total wrist arthroplasties sacrifice durability for mobility and increased function. Limited wrist arthroplasties provide a means to combine durability and pain relief with a functional arc of motion. This chapter reviews the evolution, indications, surgical technique, and outcomes of limited wrist arthroplasties.

HISTORICAL PERSPECTIVES

Surgical management of wrist arthritis has been an evolutionary process that includes total wrist arthrodesis, intercarpal arthrodesis, resection arthroplasty, carpal implant arthroplasty, and a combination of resection arthroplasty and intercarpal fusion. In 1910, Ely described the use of total wrist arthrodesis to treat tuberculous arthritis (1). Thornton described a mid-carpal arthrodesis performed for a chronic perilunate dislocation in 1924 (2). The first proximal row carpectomy (PRC) is usually attributed to Stamm in 1939 (3); however, a series published by Inglis and Jones in 1937 is the first to describe a proximal row carpectomy (4). In 1945, Waugh and Reuling (5) reported on the use of a vitallium scaphoid prosthesis in the treatment of scaphoid nonunion. Since then, many materials have been used as carpal arthroplasties including acrylic (6,7), titanium (8), fascia (9,10), silastic (11–13), and costo-osteochondral allografts (10,14). Watson described the sequence of wrist degeneration in patients with scapholunate advanced collapse (SLAC) (Fig. 11.1), and recommended scaphoid excision with capitolunate-triquetralhamate (four-bone) fusion (12,15). Watson had initially recommended replacing the excised scaphoid with a silicone scaphoid until it became apparent that silicone implants could fragment and lead to a silicone-induced wrist synovitis (16–23). Others have treated the SLAC wrist with PRC or with interpositional arthroplasty (9,24).

Limited arthroplasties are used to treat SLAC wrist, scaphoid nonunion, and radioscaphoid arthritis following scaphoid fracture, Keinböck's disease, and other intercarpal arthroses (e.g., pisotriquetral arthritis). We will review a spectrum of limited wrist arthroplasties ranging from radial styloidectomy to PRC.

RESECTION ARTHROPLASTY AND PROSTHETIC IMPLANTS

Indications

Isolated resection of the scaphoid has been performed in the past for scaphoid nonunion, but it is a procedure of historical interest only (25–29). The addition of a fascial graft following partial scaphoid excision was initially described by Qvick in 1980 (30). Eaton et al. reported on 20 patients treated for scaphoid nonunion, radioscaphoid arthritis, or irreducible transcaphoid perilunate dislocations with scaphoid fascial hemireplacement arthroplasty. Nine years after arthroplasty, patients had an average 140° arc of motion and 95% had significant pain relief (9). This procedure is no longer considered a desirable option, because it fails to control the wrist instability that is likely to develop following scaphoid resection.

Swanson performed the first silicone scaphoid arthroplasty in 1967 and reported his 58-month follow-up results in 1986 (11). At that time no implant failures were identified. However, over the long term, silicone implants have been prone to failure (8,16–23,31). Early reports noted implant migration and subluxation (32–34). Peimer described a reactive synovitis that presented with swelling, erosive osteolysis, implant failure, and pathologic fracture (19,21). The term "silicone synovitis" has been coined to describe the proliferative inflammatory synovitis that is characterized by multinucleated giant cells that contain microparticles (2–80 μm) of silicone wear debris. These cells release inflammatory mediators that lead to an aggressive synovitis that is responsible for the erosive osteolysis (8,18,21,22). Carter et al. reported that the incidence of these complications following silicone carpal arthroplasty ranged from 55% to 75% (22). Because of the long-term complications of silicone arthroplasty of the wrist and the poor results following simple resection arthroplasty, these treatment modalities cannot be recommended.

In 1942, Waugh and Reuling performed the first vitallium scaphoid implants in an effort to improve the results of simple resection arthroplasty (5,35). The results were marginal

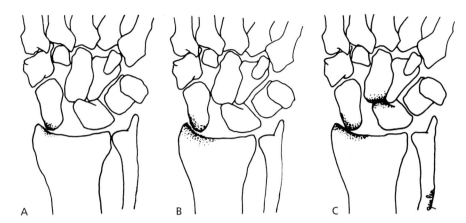

FIGURE 11.1. Scapholunate advanced collapse (SLAC) wrist as described by Watson et al. **A.** In stage 1 disease, there is wear of the radial styloid and distal radial scaphoid. **B.** Stage II shows degeneration extending into the scaphoid fossa of the radius. **C.** Stage III SLAC wrists develop deepening of the radiolunate joint and loss of the capitate-lunate joint space. In stage IV, the capitate migrates proximally between scaphoid and the lunate. (Reproduced with permission from Divelbiss BJ, Baratz ME. The role of arthroplasty and arthrodesis following trauma to the upper extremity. *Hand Clin* 1999;15:335–345.)

and the techniques were abandoned until the 1980s. Complications arising from silicone replacements prompted a renewed interest in titanium implants. Indications for titanium scaphoid replacement proposed by Swanson et al. (8) include acute scaphoid fractures with small proximal fragments, SLAC wrist with scaphoid arthritis, and for revision, implant arthroplasties. Indications for lunate replacement arthroplasty included Keinböck's disease, localized osteoarthritis, chronic perilunate or lunate dislocations, and revision implant arthroplasty. Contraindications to both procedures include diffuse arthritis not limited to a single carpal bone, inadequate bone stock to support the implants, and severe carpal instability.

While Swanson et al. reported good results with both scaphoid and lunate titanium implant arthroplasty (8), we cannot recommend this procedure in light of the results obtained with PRC and intercarpal arthrodesis. We feel that these other alternatives yield better results with fewer risks and complications.

RADIAL STYLOIDECTOMY

Indications

Kitchin first described radial styloidectomy as a treatment for nonunion of the scaphoid in the 1940s (36). Series published since have confirmed the value of styloidectomy in patients with scaphoid nonunion and early radioscaphoid arthritis (36,37). Currently, radial styloidectomy is rarely performed as an isolated procedure, as the underlying pathology of the wrist is not addressed. It is usually performed in conjunction with another procedure, such as intercarpal arthrodesis or PRC.

Siegel and Gelberman studied the anatomical affects of three types of styloidectomy (38). They described a short oblique osteotomy, a vertical oblique osteotomy, and a horizontal/transverse osteotomy (Fig. 11.2). The horizontal osteotomy is most likely to lead to scaphoid instability and ulnar translation of the carpus, as it involves sectioning 100% of the radial collateral ligament, 95% of the radioscaphocapitate ligament, 50% of the dorsal radiocarpal ligament, and

46% of the radiolunotriquetral ligament. Scaphoid instability was also noted by Linscheid et al. (39) following sectioning of the radioscaphocapitate ligament. The short oblique osteotomy, in contrast, involves primarily the radial collateral ligament (92% removed on average) and spares 91% of the radioscaphocapitate ligament. There have been no reported adverse effects of radial collateral ligament sectioning, and short oblique styloidectomy is well tolerated.

Candidates for radial styloidectomy will usually complain of dorsoradial wrist pain and swelling. Radiographs should be obtained in maximum radial deviation to assess impingement of the scaphoid on the radial styloid. The ideal patient for a radial styloidectomy without concurrent wrist reconstruction is the individual with arthritis limited to the radial half of the scaphoid fossa. This corresponds to Watson's stage I SLAC or scaphoid nonunion advanced collapse (SNAC) wrist. In practice, degeneration limited to the radial half of the scaphoid fossa is usually seen in arthritis due to SNAC. The distal pole of the fracture scaphoid rotates into a flexed position creating wear on the opposing surface of the scaphoid fossa. The patient with stage I arthritis due to SNAC may opt for styloidectomy alone as an approach that permits a short period of immobilization and a potentially quick recovery (40,41). Since the scaphoid nonunion is not addressed these patients must be warned about the risk of persistent symptoms.

The use of radial styloidectomy in conjunction with PRC has been evaluated extensively (3,4,42–49). Many authors recommend styloidectomy to prevent the trapezium from impinging on the radial styloid (3,4,42,44,46,47,49). However, others have stated that results are no better following PRC combined with radial styloidectomy and do not recommend that the styloidectomy be performed on a routine basis (4,43,45,48). Imbriglia et al. (47) demonstrated the relationship of the trapezium to the styloid after PRC using three-dimensional computer tomography. They found that the trapezium lies palmar to the styloid and is unlikely to cause impingement. In their series, a radial styloidectomy was performed only if the trapezium appeared to impinge on the radial styloid when the wrist was placed in radial deviation and moved through the flexion-extension arc. Each case must

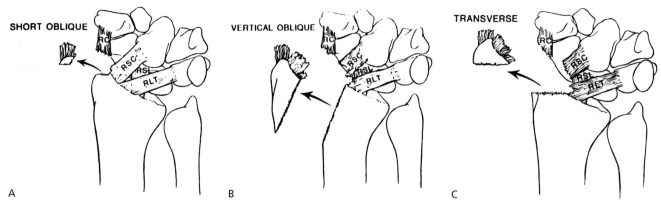

FIGURE 11.2. Ligamentous injury with radial styloidectomy. **A.** The short oblique osteotomy involves removal of most of the radial collateral ligament (RC), preservation of most of the radioscaphocapitate ligament (RSC), and preservation of all of the radioscapholunate (RSL) and radiolunocapitate (RLT) ligaments. **B.** The vertical oblique osteotomy removes most of the RC and RSC ligaments, as well as a portion of the RLT ligament. **C.** The transverse osteotomy is similar to the vertical except that a greater portion of the RLT ligament, along with a small portion of the RSL ligament, are removed. (Reproduced with permission from Siegel DB, Gelberman RH. Radial styloidectomy: An anatomical study with special reference to radiocarpal intracapsular ligamentous morphology. *J Hand Surg* 1991;16A:40–44.)

be evaluated individually depending on the specifics of each patient's anatomy.

Technique and Rehabilitation

Axillary block combined with an intravenous sedative or general anesthesia is preferred. This is supplemented with 0.5% bupivocaine in the skin and subcutaneous tissue, to minimize postoperative pain. The patient is supine with the arm on a hand table. A tourniquet is used and is released prior to closure to ensure hemostasis.

Radial styloidectomy can be done through a small transverse or longitudinal dorsal incision centered on the radial styloid. The procedure can also be done via a radial approach between the extensor pollicis longus and the abductor pollicis brevis, or it can be performed arthroscopically (see below). Sharp dissection is taken down through the skin only. The subcutaneous tissues are bluntly dissected to identify and protect branches of the superficial radial nerve. In the radial approach care should be taken to protect the radial artery. Using the information provided by Siegel et al. (38), the short oblique osteotomy preserves the largest portion of the palmar carpal ligaments. If this technique does not remove the involved segment, failure is likely.

When performed in conjunction with a PRC, the standard dorsal approach for PRC can be used. Following resection of the proximal carpal row, place the wrist in radial deviation and put it through a range of flexion and extension. If the trapezium impinges on the radial styloid, a short oblique radial styloidectomy may be beneficial. Preservation and/or repair of the radial collateral ligament may help prevent the development of scaphoid instability.

Postoperatively, the patient is placed in a palmar splint for 10 to 14 days, at which time the splint is discontinued and

the sutures removed. Finger motion is encouraged immediately postoperatively, and gentle wrist motion is begun at the time of splint removal. Formal physical therapy is reserved for those that fail to regain their preoperative range of motion and grip strength.

Results

Early studies demonstrated good results with isolated radial styloidectomy, with 81% of patients having excellent results (36,37). However, the development of wrist reconstruction procedures that address the underlying pathologic processes has decreased the indications for radial styloidectomy alone.

The use of radial styloidectomy in combination with PRC has been discussed in reports on PRC, but there appears to be little consensus on its role (3,4,42–49). Culp et al. (45) reported better radial deviation following styloidectomy (14° compared to 4° for PRC without radial styloidectomy), but wrist scores showed no difference and they concluded that radial styloidectomy is not necessary in most cases.

ARTHROSCOPIC RADIAL STYLOIDECTOMY
Indications

Advances in wrist arthroscopy combined with the decreased morbidity and stiffness of arthroscopic procedures has increased the interest in expanding the use of the arthroscope in the treatment of wrist arthritis (40,41,50–52). Arthroscopic radial styloidectomy is currently being studied.

The indications for arthroscopic radial styloidectomy are similar to those for open radial styloidectomy (Fig. 11.3A). Ruch et al. (51) recommend arthroscopic styloidectomy and excision of the proximal pole of the scaphoid in stage I SNAC

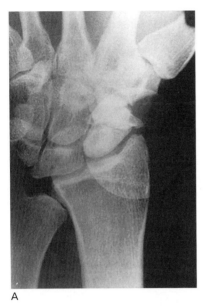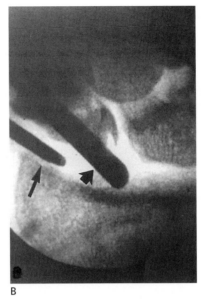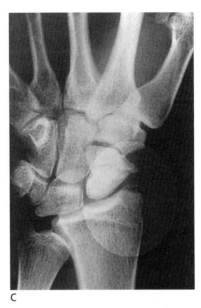

A   B   C

FIGURE 11.3. Arthroscopic radial styloidectomy in a patient with stage I SNAC wrist. **A.** Preoperative radiographs show signs of degeneration between the distal pole of the scaphoid and the radial styloid. **B.** Intraoperative fluoroscopy of the wrist. The arthroscope (broad arrow) is used to visualize the shaver (thin arrow) performing the styloidectomy. **C.** Radiograph of the wrist following styloidectomy. (Reproduced with permission from Atik TL, Baratz ME. The role of arthroscopy in wrist arthritis. *Hand Clin* 1999;15:489–494.)

wrist where bone grafting and internal fixation of the nonunion is not indicated. They described the advantages of this technique as being minimal morbidity, relief of mechanical pain, and improved motion. As with any arthroscopic procedure, poor intra-operative visualization is an indication to convert to an open procedure.

Technique and Rehabilitation

Instruments required for the procedure include a 2.9 mm shaver, a 4.0 mm bur, and a 2.7 mm arthroscope. General or regional anesthesia can be employed, and a tourniquet is used for hemostasis. The hand is suspended in fingertraps and a mechanical pump is used to provide constant water pressure. All portals are made with superficial skin incisions followed by blunt dissection of the subcutaneous tissues.

The radiocarpal and midcarpal joints are inspected to confirm the location and extent of wrist arthritis. The radiocarpal joint is inspected through a 3–4 portal. The midcarpal joint is examined via a portal 1 cm distal to the 3–4 portal. Arthrosis in the midcarpal joint, the ulnar half of the scaphoid fossa, or in the radiolunate joint may be an indication to abort the arthroscopic styloidectomy and consider a different reconstructive procedure.

Prior to beginning the radial resection, the radioscaphocapitate ligament and radiolunotriquetral ligaments must be identified and protected (40). Synovectomy is performed, if required, with the shaver through the 1–2 portal. The bur is then used through the 1–2 portal to resect the radial styloid (Fig. 11.3B). A Freer elevator can be placed in the

radioscaphoid joint to protect the articular surface. A small osteotome can also be used to assist with styloidectomy. Adequate resection should be confirmed arthroscopically in radial deviation through a flexion-extension arc. Fluoroscopic or radiographic confirmation can also be helpful in determining adequacy of resection (Fig. 11.3C). Do not be discouraged if a dramatic change in the contour of the styloid is not apparent on a plain radiograph. A 2-mm resection of the radial half of the styloid will probably effect a decompression but will not be easily apparent on a plain radiograph.

Postoperatively, patients are placed in a palmar splint. At two weeks, the splint and sutures are removed, and gentle motion is started. Strengthening is advanced as tolerated.

Results

Several authors have reported good results with arthroscopic styloidectomy, but the volume of cases and length of follow-up is limited (40,41,51,52). Ruch et al. reported the results of three arthroscopic styloidectomies with proximal scaphoid resection (51). Two of the patients were laborers and returned to their work two and four weeks postoperatively. They were all highly satisfied, without pain or mechanical symptoms, and had increased wrist extension and radial deviation postoperatively. If adequate styloidectomy can be performed, it would seem reasonable that arthroscopic techniques would lend themselves to decreased morbidity, decreased recovery periods, and increased motion. The ability to effectively perform this procedure safely and efficiently must be studied further.

Complications and Salvage of Radial Styloidectomy

Complications of radial styloidectomy include radial sensory nerve neuropraxia, persistent pain, progression of wrist arthritis, and scaphoid instability. Salvage procedures include PRC, wrist arthrodesis, or intercarpal arthrodesis.

Complications following wrist arthroscopy are uncommon. Bain reported an incidence of less than 8% (53), with the most common being reflex sympathetic dystrophy (3.7%). Complications specifically related to arthroscopic radial styloidectomy include radial sensory nerve neuropraxia, inadequate styloid resection, and chondral injury to the surrounding carpus, excessive operative time, and injury to the palmar wrist ligaments. Evaluation of the best method of salvage for these procedures is limited. While repeat arthroscopic styloidectomy may be possible if inadequate resection or progressive impingement is suspected, it is probably wiser to proceed with an open reconstructive procedure with or without an open radial styloidectomy.

PROXIMAL ROW CARPECTOMY

Indications

Proximal row carpectomy is a time-honored treatment for advanced stages of Keinböck's disease and posttraumatic arthritis (3,4,24,42–48,54–56). Common causes of posttraumatic arthritis include scaphoid nonunion, perilunate dislocations, and SLAC wrist. Proximal row carpectomy has also been used in the treatment of wrist flexion deformities in processes such as arthrogryposis multiplex congenita, cerebral palsy, cerebral vascular accidents, and arthritis mutilans of psoriasis (57–59). Proximal row carpectomy has not been shown to be effective in the treatment of the rheumatoid wrist (45,60).

Common complaints from patients with wrist arthritis include pain, weakness, and decreased motion (4). They may relate a history of previous trauma, but frequently the initiating injury is unknown.

Radiographs of the wrist of patients with posttraumatic arthritis will usually demonstrate radioscaphoid degeneration as well as some possible signs of the inciting injury. Wrist arthritis arising from scapholunate advanced collapse (SLAC) or scaphoid nonunion advanced collapse (SNAC) follows a predictable pattern of articular degeneration (12). In stage I, typical of early SNAC, arthritis is found in the radial half of the scaphoid fossa and the reciprocal surface of the scaphoid. In stage II, seen in early SLAC, wear involves the entire scaphoid fossa. Stage III arthritis, common to both SNAC and SLAC, occurs when the pattern of wear extends to the mid-carpal joint involving the head of the capitate. Finally in stage IV, there is widening diastasis between the scaphoid and lunate with proximal migration of the capitate.

Patients with Keinböck's disease are managed according to the severity of their symptoms and the radiographic appearance of the lunate. The stages of Keinböck's disease were described by Stahl and later modified by Lichtman (Fig. 11.4) (61). In stage I disease, radiographs are normal, but avascular necrosis can be identified with magnetic resonance imaging. In stage II disease, radiographs show sclerosis, but no lunate collapse (Fig. 11.5A). Stage IIIa is characterized by collapse of the lunate. In stage IIIb lunate collapse progresses to the extent that there is proximal migration of the distal carpal row (Fig. 11.5B). To accommodate this loss of carpal height the scaphoid rotates into a palmar-flexed position. Stage IV Keinböck's disease is characterized by carpal arthrosis, including the lunate fossa.

We feel that the ideal candidate for PRC in Keinböck's disease is in stage IIIb disease where there is lunate collapse and carpal malalignment. In stage IV disease, many surgeons would avoid using PRC since this stage is characterized by degeneration of the lunate fossa. In older or debilitated patients with stage II and IIIa Keinböck's disease, we have used PRC instead of radial shortening to avoid prolonged immobilization and the risk of nonunion.

When PRC is being considered, specific attention should be focused on the lunate fossa of the radius and the proximal capitate. Historically, degenerative arthrosis at

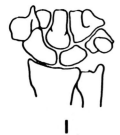 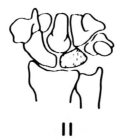 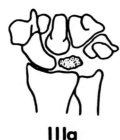 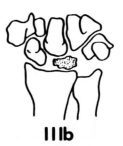 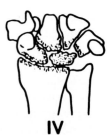

I **II** **IIIa** **IIIb** **IV**

FIGURE 11.4. Classification of Keinböck's disease. Stage I: Radiographically normal, but avascular necrosis evident with magnetic resonance imaging. Stage II: Lunate sclerosis. Stage IIIa: Lunate collapse. Stage IIIb: Lunate collapse with proximal migration of the distal carpal row. Stage IV: Carpal arthrosis. (Reproduced with permission from Weiss et al. Radial shortening for Keinböck's disease, *JBJS* 1991;73-A:384–391.)

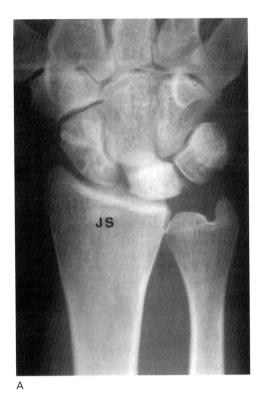
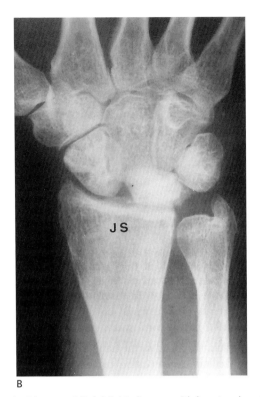

FIGURE 11.5. Progressive Keinböck's disease. **A.** The patient presented with stage II Keinböck's disease, with lunate sclerosis, but no collapse. The patient was offered a radial shortening at that time, which he choose to decline. **B.** The patient returned to the office eight months later with stage IIIb Keinböck's. Note the proximal migration of the distal carpal row and the rotation of the scaphoid.

these sites has been a contraindication to PRC (42,43, 47,48,56,62). Culp et al. (45) classified radiolunate and capitolunate degeneration as mild if there was decreased joint space only, moderate if joint space narrowing was accompanied by subchondral sclerosis, and severe if there were collapse and cyst formation. They found, as have other authors, that PRC is unsuccessful in patients with mild capitolunate and radiolunate arthritis (44–46,48,55). The debate continues concerning how much radiocapitate degeneration is acceptable at the time of PRC.

Proximal row carpectomy performed on patients with inflammatory arthritis has shown uniformly poor results, and therefore should be considered a contraindication to PRC (45,60). Some authors have suggested that PRC is not an appropriate treatment for manual laborers (45). However, many other studies have shown that most laborers are able to return to their previous occupations (43,46–48,55).

Taking all of these factors into consideration, it would appear that the best candidates for PRC would be non-rheumatoid patients with stage I, II, or III SLAC disease with minimal capitolunate or radiolunate degeneration, and patients with Stage IIIb Keinböck's disease. It is important to select each patient carefully and fully educate them to the treatment alternatives.

Technique and Rehabilitation

Axillary block combined with an intravenous sedative or general anesthesia is preferred. This is supplemented with 0.5% bupivocaine in the skin and subcutaneous tissue, to minimize postoperative pain. The patient is supine with the arm on a hand table. A tourniquet is used and is released prior to closure to ensure hemostasis.

A dorsal approach is used to expose the carpus and distal radius. The procedure has been described through both a transverse and longitudinal incision. The advantage of the transverse incision is the appearance of the resulting scar. The advantage of the longitudinal incision is the ability to better visualize the radius, the midcarpal joint, and the distal carpal row. The longitudinal incision is easier to work through and the scar is acceptable to most patients. The incision is made through the skin and subcutaneous tissue and the dorsum of the extensor retinaculum is identified. The extensor pollicis longus is released from the third dorsal wrist compartment and retracted radially. The fourth extensor compartment is identified and elevated off the radius as a unit and retracted ulnarly.

The capsule is then elevated off the dorsal lip of the radius and a large u-shaped distally based capsular flap is then cre-

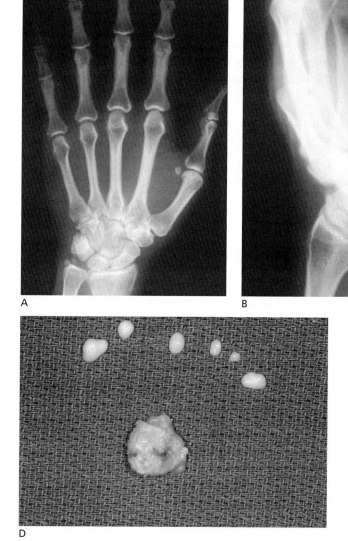

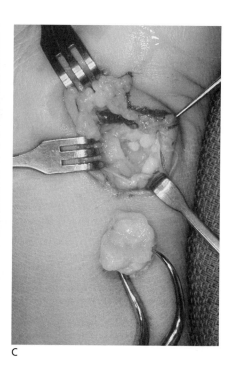

FIGURE 11.14. Pisotriquetral arthritis. **A.** Anteroposterior and **B.** 45° supinated views of the wrist. In addition to the presence of the calcified mass proximal to the pisiform, the supinated view demonstrates narrowing of the pisotriquetral joint distally. **C.** Intra-operative photograph demonstrating the multiple loose bodies found in the joint, as well as the worn undersurface of the pisiform. **D.** The loose bodies excised from the joint as well as the resected pisiform. The patient was diagnosed with synovial chondromatosis. (See Color Fig. 11.14.)

pisiform. The superficial palmar fascia and abductor digiti minimi are split longitudinally to reveal the ulnar nerve and artery proximally. Distally, the pisiform-hamate ligament is divided to open Guyon's canal. This releases the ulnar nerve if the patient has had ulnar neuropathy symptoms preoperatively, it allows greater nerve retraction and protection, and it prevents ulnar nerve symptoms from developing with postoperative edema. The ulnar nerve and artery are retracted radially.

A longitudinal incision is made on the palmar surface of the pisiform, in line with the fibers of the flexor carpi ulnaris. The pisiform is then dissected subperiosteally and removed, leaving the tendon intact. The longitudinal rent in the tendon and periosteum is repaired. The skin is closed in an interrupted fashion with nylon suture.

The wrist is immobilized postoperatively in a plaster splint for 7–10 days. The sutures are then removed, and the patient is started on gentle range of motion exercises. Since the insertion of the flexor carpi ulnaris tendon is preserved, wrist strength is rarely decreased and active motion may begin as soon as patient comfort allows. Full return to activities without pain can usually occur within 2 to 3 months postoperatively.

Results

Palmieri reported the results of medical and surgical treatment for pisotriquetral pain (75). For pisotriquetral arthritis, they initially attempted conservative treatment with a soluble steroid injection into the joint and two weeks of immobilization. If symptoms persisted at one week, a second injection was given. Forty percent of patients had significant relief with this regimen. If a pisiform nonunion was present in addition to the arthritis, only 28% were successfully treated conservatively. Twenty-one patients were treated with pisiform excision. All patients with pisotriquetral arthritis had relief of pain, returned to work, and regained their preoperative wrist motion.

Belliappa reported 12 patients with pisotriquetral arthritis, of which 11 underwent pisiform excision (76). Conservative measures were usually only temporarily effective. Seventy-eight percent had pain relief and full motion, and all returned to racquet sports and golf; usually within eight weeks. Ulnar nerve symptoms had been present in four patients preoperatively, and these symptoms resolved following pisiform excision.

Complications and Salvage of Pisotriquetral Resection Arthroplasty

Complications related to excision of the pisiform include damage to the flexor carpi ulnaris, ulnar nerve, or ulnar artery. Excessive fraying or transection of the flexor carpi ulnaris demands primary tendon repair. Some weakness may result if significant damage to the tendon is caused at the time of pisiform excision. Care must be taken throughout the procedure to protect the ulnar artery and nerve, as they are intimately opposed to the pisiform in this region.

The most frequent complication following pisiform excision is persistent pain. In most cases, this can be attributed to incorrect diagnosis. The various etiologies of ulnar-sided wrist pain are difficult to differentiate. The presence of radiographic changes in the pisotriquetral joint alone is not enough to determine the cause of ulnar-sided wrist pain, and precise examination of the wrist is required to accurately diagnose pisotriquetral arthritis. Therefore salvage usually is related to determining the true cause of pain.

REFERENCES

1. Ely LW. A study of tuberculosis. *Surg Gyn Obstr* 1910;10:561–572.
2. Thornton L. Old dislocation of os magnum; open reduction and stabilization. *South Med J* 1924;17:433–434.
3. Stamm TT. Excision of the proximal row of the carpus. *Proc R Soc Med* 1944;38:74–75.
4. Inglis AE, Jones EC. Proximal row carpectomy for diseases of the proximal row. *J Bone Joint Surg* 1977;59A:460–463.
5. Waugh RL, Reuling L. United fractures of the carpal scaphoid: preliminary report on the use of vitallium replicas as replacements after excision. *Am J Surg* 1945;67:184–200.
6. Agner O. Treatment of nonunion navicular fractures by total excision of the bone and insertion of an acrylic prosthesis. *Acta Orthop Scand* 1960;32:235.
7. Agerholm JC, Lee ML. The acrylic scaphoid prosthesis in the treatment of ununited carpal scaphoid fracture. *Acta Orthop Scand.* 1966;37:67–76.
8. Swanson AB, Swanson G, DeHeer, et al. Carpal bone titanium implant arthroplasty: 10 years' experience. *Clin Orthop* 1997;342:46–58.
9. Eaton RG, Akelman E, Eaton BH. Fascial implant arthroplasty for treatment of radioscaphoid degenerative disease. *J Hand Surg* 1989;14A:766–774.
10. Osterman AL, Mikulics M. Scaphoid nonunion. *Hand Clin* 1988;14:437–455.
11. Swanson AB, Swanson G, Maupin BK, et al. Scaphoid implant resection arthroplasty: Long-term results. *J of Arthroplasty* 1986;1:47–61.
12. Watson HK, Ballet FL. The SLAC wrist: Scapholunate advanced collapse pattern of degenerative arthritis. *J Hand Surg* 1984;9A:358–365.
13. Kaarela OI, Raatidainen TK, Torianen PJ. Silicone replacement arthroplasty for Keinböck's disease. *J Hand Surg* 1998;23B:735–740.
14. Sandow MJ. Proximal scaphoid costo-osteochondral replacement arthroplasty. *J Hand Surg* 1998;23B:201–208.
15. Watson HK, Goodman ML, Johnson TR. Limited wrist arthrodesis: II. Intercarpal and radiocarpal combinations. *J Hand Surg* 1981;20A:223–233.
16. Gordon M, Bullough PG. Synovial and osseous inflammation in failed silicone-rubber prosthesis. *J Bone Joint Surg* 1982;64A:574–580.
17. Worsing RA, Engber WD, Lange TA. Reactive synovitis from particulate silastic. *J Bone Joint Surg* 1982;64A:581–585.
18. Minamikawa Y, Peimer CA, Ogawa R, et al. In vivo experimental analysis of silicone implants on bone and soft tissue. *J Hand Surg* 1994;19A:575–583.
19. Peimer CA, Talesnik J, Sherwin FS. Pathologic fractures: a complication of microparticulate synovitis. *J Hand Surg* 1991;16A:835–843.
20. Peimer CA. Long-term complications of trapeziometacarpal silicone arthroplasty. *Clin Orthop* 1987;220:86–98.
21. Peimer CA, Medige J, Eckert BS et al. Reactive synovitis after silicone arthroplasty. *J Hand Surg* 1986;11A:624–638.
22. Carter PR, Benton LJ, Dysert PA. Silicone rubber carpal implants: A study of the incidence of late osseous complications. *J Hand Surg* 1986;11A:639–644.
23. Stanley JK, Tolat AR. Long-term results of Swanson silastic arthroplasty in the rheumatoid wrist. *J Hand Surg* 1993;18B:381–388.
24. Krakauer JD, Bishop AT, Cooney WP. Surgical treatment of scapholunate advanced collapse. *J Hand Surg* 1994;19A:751–759.
25. Codman EA, Chase HM. The diagnosis and treatment of the carpal scaphoid and dislocation of the semilunar bone. *Ann Surg* 1905;41:321–332.
26. Davidson AJ, Horowitz MT. An evaluation of excision in the treatment of ununited fractures of the carpal scaphoid bone. *Ann Surg* 1938;108:291–295.
27. Edelstein JM. Treatment of ununited fractures of the carpal navicular. *J Bone Joint Surg* 1939;21:902–911.
28. Dwyer FC. Excision of the carpal scaphoid for ununited fracture. *J Bone Joint Surg* 1949;31B:572–577.
29. Graner O, Lopes EI, Carvalho BC, et al. Arthrodesis of the carpal bones in the treatment of Keinböck's disease: painful ununited fractures of the navicular and lunate bones with avascular necrosis, and old fracture-dislocations of carpal bones. *J Bone Joint Surg.* 1966;48A:767–774.
30. Qvick LI. Tendon interposition arthroplasty after resection of necrotic carpal bones. *Aust NZ J Surg* 1980;50:272–277.
31. Swanson AB, de Groot Swanson G. Failed carpal bone arthroplasty: Causes and treatment. *J Hand Surg* 1989;14A (part2):S417–424.
32. Bjornsson HA, Gestsson J, Ekelund L et al. Silastic scaphoid implants in osteoarthritis of the radioscaphoid joint. *J Hand Surg* 1984;9B:177–180.
33. Keinert JM, Stern PJ, Lister GD et al. Complications of scaphoid silicone arthroplasty. *J Bone Joint Surg* 1985;67A:422–427.
34. Kleinert JM, Lister GD. Silicone implants. *Hand Clin* 1986;2:271–290.
35. Leslie BM, O'Malley M, Thibodeau AA. A forty-three-year follow-up of a vitallium scaphoid arthroplasty. *J Hand Surg.* 1991;16A:465–468.
36. Smith L, Friedman B. Treatment of ununited fracture of the carpal navicular by styloidectomy of the radius. *J Bone Joint Surg* 1956;38A:368–376.

37. Barnard L, Stubbins SG. Styloidectomy of the radius in the surgical treatment of nonunion of the carpal navicular. *J Bone Joint Surg* 1948;30A:98–102.

38. Siegel DB, Gelberman RH. Radial styloidectomy: An anatomical study with special reference to radiocarpal intracapsular ligamentous morphology. *J Hand Surg* 1991;16A:40–44.

39. Linscheid RL, Dobyns JH, Beaubout JW, et al. Traumatic instability of the wrist. Diagnosis, classification, and pathomechanics. *J Bone Joint Surg* 1972;54A:1612–1632.

40. Osterman AL. Wrist arthroscopy: operative procedures. In: Green DP, Hotchkiss RN, Pederson WC, eds. *Green's operative hand surgery*, 4th ed. Philadelphia: Churchill Livingston, 1999:207–222.

41. Atik TL, Baratz ME. The role of arthroscopy in wrist arthritis. *J Hand Clin* 1999;15:489–494.

42. Crabbe WA. Excision of the proximal row of the carpus. *J Bone Joint Surg* 1964;46B:708–711.

43. Jorgensen EC. Proximal row carpectomy: an end result study of twenty-two cases. *J Bone Joint Surg* 1969;51A:1104–1111.

44. Neviaser RJ. Proximal row carpectomy for posttraumatic disorders of the carpus. *J Hand Surg* 1983;8A:301–305.

45. Culp RW, Osterman AL, Talsania JS. Arthroscopic proximal row carpectomy. In: *Techniques in hand and upper extremity surgery*. Philadelphia: Lippincott-Raven, 1997:116–119.

46. Tomaino MM, Delsignore J, Burton RI. Long-term results following proximal row carpectomy. *J Hand Surg* 1994;19A:694–703.

47. Imbriglia JE, Broudy AS, Hagberg WC, et al. Proximal row carpectomy: clinical evaluation. *J Hand Surg* 1990;15A:426–430.

48. Wyrick JD, Stern PJ, Kiefhaber TR. Motion preserving procedures in the treatment of scapholunate advanced collapse wrist: proximal row carpectomy versus four-corner arthrodesis. *J Hand Surg* 1995;20A:965–970.

49. Green DP. Proximal row carpectomy. 1987;3:163–168.

50. Bain GI, Roth JM. The role of arthroscopy in arthritis: "ectomy procedures." *J Hand Clin* 1995;11:51–58.

51. Ruch DS, Chang DS, Poehling GG. The arthroscopic treatment of avascular necrosis of the proximal pole of the scaphoid following scaphoid nonunion. *J Arthroscopic Rel Surg* 1998;14:747–752.

52. Nagle DJ. Laser-assisted wrist arthroscopy. *Hand Clin* 1999;15:495–499.

53. Bain GI, Richard RS, Roth JM. Arthroscopy of the wrist: Introduction and indications. In: McGinty JB, Caspari RB, Jackson RW, Poehling GG, eds. *Operative arthroscopy*, 2nd ed. Philadelphia: Lippincott-Raven, 1996:897–904.

54. Tomaino MM, Miller RJ, Cole I, et al. Scapholunate advanced collapse wrist: proximal row carpectomy or limited wrist arthrodesis with scaphoid excision? *J Hand Surg* 1994;19A:134–142.

55. Begley BW, Engber WD. Proximal row carpectomy in advanced Kienbock's disease. *J Hand Surg* 1994;19A:1016–1018.

56. Salomon GD, Eaton RG. Proximal row carpectomy with partial capitate resection. *J Hand Surg* 1996;21A:2–8.

57. Mennen U. Early corrective surgery of the wrist and elbow in arthrogryposis multiplex congenita. *J Hand Surg* 1993;18B:304–307.

58. Omer, GE, Capen, DA. Proximal row carpectomy with muscle transfers for spastic paralysis. *J Hand Surg* 1976;1A:197–204.

59. Blair WF, Kilpatrick WC. Proximal row carpectomy: an unusual indication. *Clin Orthop* 1980;153:223–225.

60. Ferlic DC, Clayton ML, Mills MF. Proximal row carpectomy: review of rheumatoid and nonrheumatoid wrists. *J Hand Surg* 1991;16A:420–424.

61. Lichtman DM, Mack GR, MacDonald RI, et al. Keinbock's disease: The role of silicone replacement arthroplasty. *J Bone Joint Surg* 1977;59A:899.

62. Fitzgerald JP, Peimer CA, Smith RJ. Distraction resection arthroplasty of the wrist. *J Hand Surg* 1989;14A:774–781.

63. Nakamura R, Horii K, Nakao E, et al. Proximal row carpectomy versus limited wrist arthrodesis for advanced Keinböck's disease. *J Hand Surg* 1998;23B:741–745.

64. Stahl F. On lunatomalacia (Keinböck's disease): A clinical and radiographic study, especially on its pathogenesis and the late results of immobilization treatment. *Acta Chir Scand* 1947;126:123.

65. Lin HH, Stren PJ. "Salvage" procedures in the treatment of Keinböck's disease: Proximal row carpectomy and total wrist arthrodesis. *Hand Clin* 1993;9:521–526.

66. Inoue G, Miura T. Proximal row carpectomy in perilunate dislocations and lunatomalacia. *Acta Orthop Scand* 1990;61:449–452.

67. Rhee SK, Kim HM, Bahk WJ, Kim YW. A Comparative study of the surgical procedures to treat advanced Keinböck's disease. *J Korean Med Sci* 1996;11:171–178.

68. Eaton RG. Excision and fascial interposition arthroplasty in the treatment of Kienbock's disease. *Hand Clin* 1993;9:513–516.

69. Eaton RG. Proximal row carpectomy and soft tissue interposition arthroplasty. *Techniques Hand Upper Extremity Surg* 1997;1:248–254.

70. Roth JH, Poehling GG. Arthroscopic "-ectomy" surgery of the wrist. *Arthroscopy* 1990;6:140–147.

71. Louis DS, Hankin FM, Bowers WH. Capitate-radius arthrodesis: an alternative method of radiocarpal arthrodesis. *J Hand Surg* 1984;9A:165–169.

72. Richards RS, Roth JH. Simultaneous proximal row carpectomy and radius to distal carpal row arthrodesis. *J Hand Surg* 1994;19A:728–732.

73. Buterbaugh GA, Brown TR, Horn PC. Ulnar sided wrist pain in athletes. *Clin in Sports Med* 1998;17:567–583.

74. Green DP. Pisotriquetral arthritis: A case report. *J Hand Surg* 1979;4:465–467.

75. Palmieri TJ. Pisiform area pain treated by pisiform excision. *J Hand Surg* 1982;7:477–480.

76. Belliappa PP, Burke FD. Excision of the pisiform in piso-triquetral osteoarthritis. *J Hand Surg Br* 1992;17B:133–136.

TOTAL WRIST ARTHRODESIS

KAVI SACHAR AND HILL HASTINGS, II

HISTORICAL PERSPECTIVE

The human wrist is one of the most dynamic joints in the human body. This "joint" in fact is not a single joint but a complex relationship between eight carpal bones, two forearm bones, and five metacarpals. It provides a circular range of motion that is arbitrarily divided into flexion, extension, radial deviation, and ulnar deviation. For all of its versatility, the wrist most importantly functions as a stabilizer, allowing the hand to perform both intricate and forceful activities.

With the demands placed upon the wrist, it is not surprising that it is susceptible to traumatic conditions. In addition, systemic arthritis and conditions such as spasticity have a predilection for involving this joint.

Numerous reconstructive options exist to try to maintain either all or a component of the wrist's arc of motion. These consist of ligamentous repair, limited intercarpal fusion, and joint replacement. When these procedures fail and the wrist becomes painful, its stabilizing function is lost. Without stability, the wrist is unable to effectively generate strength and the hand is unable to easily perform tasks.

Arthrodesis of the radiocarpal and midcarpal joints, otherwise known as total wrist fusion, serves as an important surgical procedure for providing stability to the hand-forearm axis.

The earliest wrist fusions were performed as an alternative to wrist joint resection or amputation in tuberculosis (1). In 1920 Ely published a technique for wrist fusion in tuberculosis using a block mortise iliac crest bone graft (1). Other early indications for wrist fusion included correction of deformity in poliomyelitis and spasticity as described by Steindler in 1918 (2). Subsequently, it was used to correct deformity in severe Volkman's ischemic contracture (3). Today, total wrist arthrodesis is most commonly performed in cases of posttraumatic arthritis, osteoarthritis, rheumatoid arthritis, and other conditions where a stable, painless wrist is necessary (3–33).

Total wrist arthrodesis has traditionally been labeled as a "salvage" procedure. It is, however, one of the most reliable surgical procedures utilized by hand surgeons. When performed for the correct indications and with proper technique, it remains the gold standard by which all other limited wrist procedures must be judged.

INDICATIONS

Posttraumatic Arthritis

Total wrist arthrodesis is most commonly performed for posttraumatic arthritis involving the radiocarpal and midcarpal joints. The end result of a scapholunate ligament tear is a scapholunate advanced collapse deformity that results in pancarpal arthritis (34,35). Scaphoid nonunions often follow a similar pattern resulting in pancarpal arthritis. Malunited distal radius fractures with excessive dorsal angulation can result in midcarpal followed by pancarpal arthritis. Intra-articular distal radius fractures that heal with a significant articular step-off or involve a significant impaction injury can go on to require total wrist arthrodesis. Other posttraumatic examples include perilunate and lunate dislocations.

In the posttraumatic wrist, numerous factors must be considered in determining whether total wrist arthrodesis is indicated. Radiographs should be studied carefully to determine which joints are involved. If only the midcarpal or radiocarpal joints demonstrate arthritic changes, limited wrist fusion should be considered. Four quadrant fusion and proximal row carpectomy are excellent alternatives to total wrist arthrodesis in the early SLAC wrist (36–41). Radioscapholunate fusion is also an alternative in arthritis following intra-articular distal radius fractures. Limited wrist fusions are less predictable than total wrist fusions but allow for the preservation of some motion.

Failed previous procedures consisting of either ligament reconstructions or limited fusions are another common indication for total wrist arthrodesis. In a series of total wrist fusions by Hastings et al., an average of 2.3 previous procedures were performed prior to total wrist arthrodesis (42). In this scenario, total wrist arthrodesis truly serves as a salvage procedure for failed attempts at motion sparing operations. Motion is typically severely limited and further attempts at maintaining movement are futile.

If preoperative motion of extension/flexion is less than 30° in the posttraumatic wrist, total wrist arthrodesis should be strongly considered. Limited fusions or ligament reconstructions will further restrict motion leaving a nonfunctional range and most likely residual pain (15). Figure 12.1 outlines this treatment algorithm.

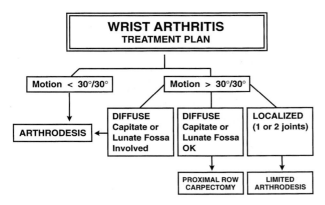

FIGURE 12.1. Decision tree of surgical decision making in the arthritic wrist.

Systemic Arthritis

Total wrist arthrodesis is indicated in any systemic arthritis, such as rheumatoid arthritis, lupus or pigmented vilonodular synovitis, for pain relief, instability, to correct deformity, and to prevent further deformity (44–53).

The rheumatoid wrist commonly undergoes joint destruction resulting in pain. Because of the pancarpal nature of this disease, limited procedures are rarely indicated. There are occasions when only the radiocarpal joint is involved and radioscapholunate fusion is an option. In addition, in cases of ulnar translocation, radiolunate fusion may be used to correct deformity.

The rheumatoid wrist must be stable and without the typical volar subluxation radial deviation pattern in order for distal reconstructive procedures such as metacarpophalangeal implant arthroplasty to be performed (54). Without stabilization and correction of the wrist deformity, distal realignment procedures will go on to early failure. Poor wrist positioning in a flexed position results in weakness of grasp and may contribute to attritional tendon rupture. For these reasons, total wrist arthrodesis must be considered as a foundation upon which to work when performing any procedures on the rheumatoid hand.

Total wrist arthroplasty is a motion preserving option in the rheumatoid wrist (91). In the failed total joint arthroplasty, total wrist fusion is an excellent option to eliminate pain and achieve stability.

Miscellaneous

In severe traumatic bone loss resulting in the loss of carpal bones or distal radius, total wrist arthrodesis may be considered to maintain length and stability.

Tumors that result in en bloc resection of either radius or carpus may require reconstruction with either vascular or nonvascular bone graft and subsequent arthrodesis (55,56).

Cerebral palsy often results in a wrist flexion deformity. Tendon transfers as described with or without proximal row carpectomy can often rebalance the spastic wrist. When the deformity cannot be maintained with soft-tissue and motion-preserving procedures, wrist fusion is indicated to better position the hand (57).

Contraindications

The most obvious contraindication to total wrist fusion is the patient who is unwilling to lose wrist motion. In the laborer or young patient, limited intercarpal fusion or procedures such as wrist denervation should be considered with the understanding that pain may persist (58). In the nondominant hand of an elderly patient or the rheumatoid wrist, total wrist arthroplasty may be considered.

Wrist fusion is contraindicated in tetraplegics or quadriparetics who use wrist motion for modified tenodesis grasp and transfer techniques. Additionally, it is contraindicated in the insensate wrist.

Active infection is a relative contraindication to internal fixation techniques. However, appropriate medical management of the infection and external fixation techniques may be an option.

Preoperative Planning

The decision to proceed with wrist fusion is based on the patient's underlying disease process, pattern of arthritic or traumatic changes as determined through imaging modalities, and the patient's understanding of the surgical procedure.

Minimum necessary preoperative imaging studies include anteroposterior (AP), lateral, and oblique views. In addition, baseline AP and lateral views of the opposite wrist should be obtained to determine if arthritic changes are present. If so, the prospect of bilateral total wrist fusions in the future must be weighed. If basic radiographs do not adequately identify the arthritic joints, more advanced modalities should be considered. These consist of tomograms and/or computerized tomography (CAT scan). Both modalities will allow evaluation of the critical radiolunate and capitolunate joints. Additionally, wrist arthroscopy is a direct way to further quantitate the location of cartilage loss. These modalities allow the physician to determine if salvage procedures are an option and which joints, such as the triquetrohamate and capitohamate, should be included in the fusion. All of the information gathered adequately allows the physician to present objective parameters to the patient so an appropriate clinical decision can be made.

The physical exam should consist of inspection of previous surgical or traumatic scars. Adequate soft-tissue coverage is essential if internal fixation is to be used. In traumatic soft-tissue loss, soft-tissue coverage can be performed at the same time as wrist fusion.

Extensor tendon rupture is often found in the rheumatoid wrist. This is most commonly due to attritional rupture in the caput ulnae syndrome or rupture of the extensor policis longus at Lister's tubercle. Tendon transfers can be performed at the same time as wrist fusion.

Distal radioulnar joint (DRUJ) arthritis or instability also must be evaluated in the rheumatoid and posttraumatic wrist. Zero rotation radiographs CAT scan can be used to evaluate this joint. Surgical options include complete or hemiresection of the distal ulna, triquetrum excision, or the Suave-Kapanji procedure (59).

The incidence of concomitant carpal tunnel syndrome in patients undergoing wrist fusion is 5%. In addition, the incidence of carpal tunnel syndrome following wrist fusion is between 4% and 10% (42). Therefore, adequate preoperative assessment of carpal tunnel syndrome must be performed. This should consist of clinical tests such as Tinel's sign, Phalen's test, and the median nerve compression test. Neurodiagnostic testing should be performed if indicated. Carpal tunnel release can be performed either concurrently or prior to wrist fusion.

Preoperative range of motion and grip strength should be recorded and the patient should have a full understanding of the procedure. Trial cast immobilization in the position of fusion should be offered so that the patient fully realizes his or her motion limitations.

Surgical Techniques

Certain basic principles apply to all surgical techniques of wrist fusion. Although the surgical approaches and fixation techniques vary, the goal of the procedure is a solid fusion from the radius to the midcarpal joint and/or the metacarpals (60–72).

Position of Fusion

Several authors have studied the functional arc of motion required to perform activities. Swanson et al. believed that most activities could be performed between 10° of flexion and 10° of extension (73). Brumfield and Champoux found most activities of daily living could be performed between 10° of flexion and 35° of extension (74). Palmer et al. determined the functional range to be between 10° of flexion, 30° of extension, 10° of radial deviation, and 15° of ulnar deviation (75).

Weiss et al. found a 64% task completion rate in the Jebsen Hand Function Test in the fused wrist compared to 78% in the normal wrist when the wrist was fused between 18° of flexion and 24° of extension with 8° of ulnar deviation (76). They concluded that people could perform most tasks but in a modified fashion.

There are various recommendations as to what position to fuse the wrist. Pryce (77) and Colonna (11) recommended slight extension and ulnar deviation to maximize power grip.

Weiss and Hastings recommend 10° to 15° of dorsiflexion and slight ulnar deviation (78). Kraft and Detels recommend avoiding flexion because of the diminished grip strength (79). Sennwald recommends fusion in neutral flexion-extension and 10° of ulnar deviation (80). He states that fusions in extension make working on flat surfaces like tables clumsy. Most authors believe the rheumatoid wrist should be fused in the neutral position with bilateral fusions both placed in the neutral position (81).

There is no ideal position for wrist fusion but we recommend placing them between 0° and 15° of extension and 5° of ulnar deviation. This allows for power grip and is cosmetically acceptable and functionally practical. In bilateral wrist fusions one may consider placing one wrist in slight extension and the other in neutral to maximize the functions that can be performed. Individual patient functions must be considered because some occupations and recreational activities require varying degrees of flexion and extension.

Joints to Be Fused

Total wrist fusion always includes the radiolunate joint and capitolunate joint except in cases of tumor resection or traumatic bone loss where this may not be an option. In rheumatoid arthritis all articular surfaces should be included to avoid continued synovitis. Whether other joints are included in the fusion mass is dependent on evidence of arthrosis in those joints. If the capitotriquetrohamate joint is arthritic, it should be included in the fusion. If it is not arthritic, leaving the ulnar bones out of the fusion will maintain some supple motion on the ulnar side of the wrist. With fixation techniques that span the index or middle carpometacarpal (CMC) joints, opinions vary as to whether or not to include these joints. Abbott et al. recommended against fusion of the CMC joints because of their importance in flexion and power grip (5). Haddad and Riordan and Brittain included the index and middle CMC joints in the fusion mass (8,14). Bolano and Green and Louis et al. found subsequent degenerative changes in these joints when they were not included in the fusion (38,61). With the use of plate fixation that spans the CMC joint, Weiss and Hastings recommend incorporating the middle CMC joint in the fusion (15,78,82). The only absolute indication for incorporation of the index and middle CMC joints in the fusion is, if upon inspection, these joints are degenerative.

Pin Fixation Technique (Rheumatoid Patients)

Mannerfelt popularized a simple technique of fixation in rheumatoid patients undergoing total wrist arthodesis (22). After dorsal wrist exposure, denution of the remaining cartilage, and placement of autogenous bone graft, large Steinman pins can be advanced from between the index/middle and/or

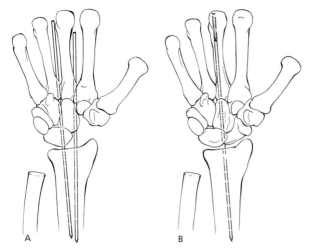

FIGURE 12.2. A schematic illustration of the technique for pin fixation in rheumatoid patients. One or two large Steinman pins may be used (**A**) or a single pin passed via an intramedullary approach through the third metacarpal head (**B**).

the middle/ring metacarpal heads through the carpus and into the radius intramedullary canal providing fixation of the entire construct. Alternatively, a single Steinman pin can be advanced through the third metacarpal head, down the intramedullary canal of the third metacarpal, through the carpus, and into the radius intramedullary canal (Fig. 12.2).

Carrol and Dick Technique

Carrol and Dick utilized a dorsal approach and entered the wrist between the third and fourth compartments (Fig. 12.3A) (9). The joint is entered with an I-shaped capsular incision and the creation of osteoperiosteal flaps, which they believe help decrease the potential for extensor tendon adhesions (Fig. 12.3B). The medullary canals of the second metacarpal, third metacarpals, and distal radius are excavated to later receive the slots of the bone graft. The dorsal half of the carpal bones are then removed with rongeurs, bone biters, and power drills if necessary (Fig. 12.3C).

Iliac crest bone graft is utilized with a 3 by 5 cm portion of outer crest being harvested. The wrist is fused in 15° to 20° of wrist extension with the metacarpals longitudinally aligned with the radius. This allows for 5° to 7° of ulnar deviation. The graft is then trimmed in a rabbit ear configuration and locked into the slots with K-wires being utilized only if necessary (Fig. 12.3D). Additional corticocancellous bone graft is placed and the capsular flaps are closed (Fig. 12.3E).

Rayan has described a modification of this technique with a hexagonal type bed being prepared from the radius across the midcarpal joint (82a). A corresponding portion of the inner iliac crest is then fashioned to fit in the defect and secured with four 4.0 mm cancellous screws (Fig. 12.4).

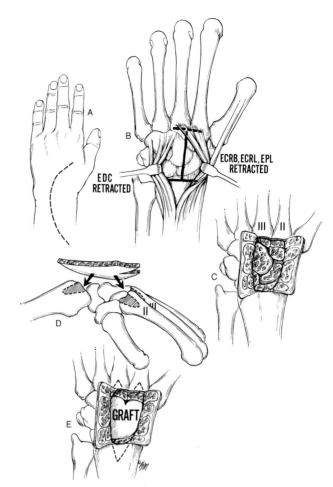

FIGURE 12.3. Carrol and Dick technique for total wrist arthrodesis. **A.** Curvilinear incision for dorsal approach. **B.** Retraction of second and fourth compartments and I-shaped capsular incision. **C.** Osteoperiosteal flaps developed. **D.** Corticocancellous inlay graft with rabbit ear configuration. **E.** Closure of osteoperiosteal flap over graft. (Reprinted with permission from Green D. *Green's Operative Hand Surgery.* New York: Churchill Livingstone, 1999: 131–146.)

Capitate-Radius Technique

In certain situations it is advantageous to combine proximal row carpectomy with wrist fusion. This may be necessary in cases of severe wrist flexion contractures to correct deformity. Other indications include a failed previous proximal row carpectomy, Kienböck's disease, and previous carpal fractures and dislocations with an avascular lunate. Richards and Roth believe the theoretical advantages of this technique include removal of avascular bone that may not incorporate easily into the fusion, arthrodesis of fewer joint surfaces, technically easier wrist positioning, and less ulnar impaction (83).

Louis et al. initially described this technique through a dorsal longitudinal incision (37). The entire lunate and triquetrum are removed along with the proximal 80% of the scaphoid. A cup-in-cone type technique is used between the radius and capitate. Fixation is achieved with K-wires or sta-

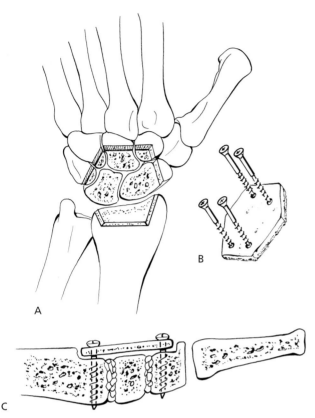

FIGURE 12.4. Rayan modification of Carrol technique with internal fixation. **A.** Cancellous bed is made by removing dorsal cortex of the radius and carpal bones. **B.** An inner table iliac corticocancellous bone graft is shaped similar to the decorticated bed, drilled, and tapped for interfragmentary screw fixation. **C.** The graft is fixed with four 4.0 mm cancellous screws and the spaces are filled with cancellous bone graft. (Reprinted with permission from Ryan GM. Wrist arthrodesis. *Journal of Bone and Joint Surgery* 1986;11A:356–364.)

ples. Only local bone graft is utilized (Fig. 12.5). Richards et al. remove the entire proximal row, utilize iliac crest bone graft and achieve fixation with an AO compression plate.

In Richards' series, patients were immobilized in a short arm cast for six weeks. Union rate was 100% and grip strength was felt to be comparable to standard wrist fusions.

Haddad-Riordan Technique

Haddad and Riordan described a radial approach to wrist fusion (14). They described utilizing a block iliac crest graft that spanned the radius to metacarpals. They believed the dorsal approach had a high likelihood of causing extensor tendon adhesions.

A J-shaped skin incision is utilized extending from 3–4 centimeters proximal to the radial styloid curving over the second metacarpal base. The capsular incision is placed between the first and second dorsal compartments after retracting the radial sensory nerve volarly. Exposure is achieved by retracting the abductor pollicis brevis (APL), extensor pollicis brevis (EPB), wrist extensors and finger extensors. The extensor carpi radialis longus (ECRL) is sectioned with a stump being left distally for repair. The extensor carpi radialis brevis (ECRB) does not have to be sectioned for exposure. A section of the capsule is then removed exposing the radiocarpal, intercarpal, and second CMC joint. The dorsal carpal branch of the radial artery is ligated. Decortication is then performed. An inner table iliac crest graft is harvested measuring 1.5 by 1 in. A corresponding slot is then cut into the carpus with the wrist in 15° of extension using a power saw and avoiding the distal radioulnar joint. The second and third CMC joints are included. The graft is then placed as a mortise and K-wires are only used if necessary (Fig. 12.6). Patients are maintained in a long arm cast until union, which may be up to 12 weeks.

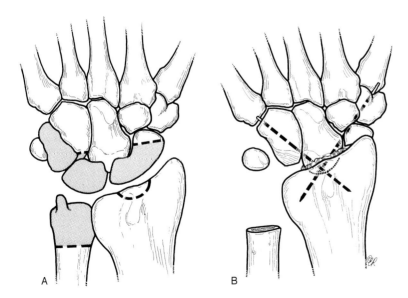

FIGURE 12.5. Louis technique of proximal row carpectomy and wrist fusion. Kirschner wires are used for fixation (Reprinted with permission from Green D. *Green's Operative Hand Surgery*. New York: Churchill Livingstone, 1999:131–146.)

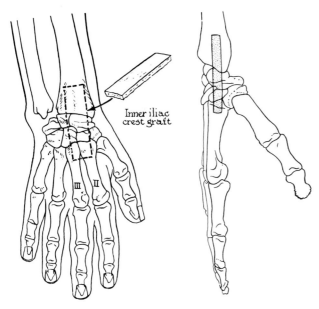

FIGURE 12.6. Radial approach for wrist fusion. (Reprinted with permission from Green D. *Green's Operative Hand Surgery*. New York: Churchill Livingstone, 1999:131–146.)

Compression Plate Fixation

Wrist fusion with plates and screws was introduced by the AO group in the German literature in 1969 and was translated into English in 1970. In 1974, the AO Hand Study Group recommended compression plate fixation for wrist fusion. Larson, in 1974, describes a consecutive series of 23 patients who underwent compression plate fixation utilizing the AO method (19). Since that time there have been numerous studies describing wrist fusion using a dynamic compression plate (84–89).

Authors' Preferred Technique

Surgery can be performed under either an axillary block or general anesthetic. If iliac crest bone graft is necessary, a brief general can be combined with an axillary block. A single perioperative does of a first generation cephalosporin is used as prophylaxis. The procedure is performed under tourniquet control.

A 10 cm straight longitudinal incision is made from the index middle interosseous space passing proximally over Lister's tubercle to lie on the distal radius adjacent to the APL muscle (Fig. 12.7). Supraretinacular flaps are then raised incorporating radial and ulnar sensory nerve branches in the flaps. Larger veins are clamped and tied. Once the retinaculum is exposed, gelpe retractors are used. The third dorsal compartment is entered and the extensor pollicis longus (EPL) tendon is transposed radially. Full transposition requires release of the sheath distal to the retinaculum (Fig. 12.8).

The distal radius is exposed subperiosteally raising the undisturbed second and fourth compartments. The excision

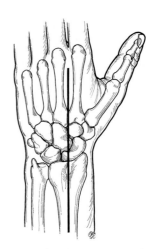

FIGURE 12.7. A 10 cm dorsal incision is made centered over Lister's tubercle. (Reprinted with permission from Green D. *Green's Operative Hand Surgery*. New York: Churchill Livingstone, 1999: 131–146.)

is extended distally over the carpus to the third metacarpal. Subperiosteal dissection of the third metacarpal is carried out, and the insertion of the ECRB is subperiosteally elevated and retracted in a radial direction. The intrinsic musculature on either side of the third metacarpal is not disturbed. The carpus is exposed using sharp dissection raising capsule directly off bone and staying deep to the second and fourth compartments. The distal radioulnar joint is left undisturbed unless distal ulna resection is to be performed.

The joints to be included in the fusion are exposed and decorticated. This includes the third carpometacarpal joint, scaphocapitate joint, capitolunate joint, radioscaphoid joint,

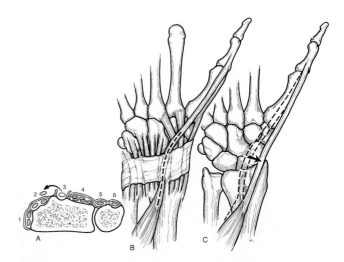

FIGURE 12.8. Dorsal exposure for radiocarpal fusion. **A.** The EPL tendon is identified and released from its compartment. **B, C.** The EPL tendon is transposed, allowing for subperiosteal dissection between the second and fourth compartments. (Reprinted with permission from Green D. *Green's Operative Hand Surgery*. New York: Churchill Livingstone, 1999:131–146.)

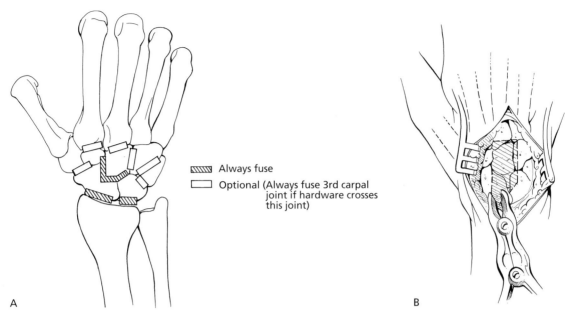

FIGURE 12.9. A. A rigid fusion column from the radius, through the carpus, to the metacarpal must coincide with the plate placement. All joints spanned directly by the plate should be fused. Adjacent joints may be fused if desired. (Reprinted with permission from Weiss, APC, Hastings H, II. Wrist arthrodesis for traumatic conditions: a study of plate and local bone graft application. *J Hand Surg* 1995:20A:50–56.) **B.** Osteotomes and a ronguer should be used to denude the cartilage and subchondral bone from the joints to be fused.

and radiolunate joint. The ulnar midcarpal joint is left undisturbed to preserve supple motion of the ulnar hand unless degenerative changes are noted on inspection. Other joints are included if indicated on preoperative evaluation (Fig. 12.9).

Decortication is primarily performed with the use of osteotomes. The third CMC joint is exposed by shaving the CMC boss while preserving the volar ligaments to prevent rotation with plate application. The carpus and Lister's tubercle are similarly sequentially decorticated removing up to 20% of the anteroposterior diameter. The overall height of the carpus is maintained by preserving the volar cartilage and carpal relationships (Fig. 12.10A).

When only the central column is to be fused, local bone graft is sufficient. The dorsal shavings can be used as bone graft and additional graft can be harvested from the distal radius. This is done through a cortical window radial to the intended plate position leaving the distal 1.5 cm of radial metaphysis untouched.

If additional bone graft is necessary, it may be harvested from the olecronon, Gurdy's tubercle in the tibia, or the iliac crest. Only cancellous bone graft is necessary, therefore, iliac crest graft can be harvested through a central window without stripping musculature or violating the inner and outer table.

A titanium, low contact, dynamic compression plate has been designed by the AO Hand Study Group and produced by Synthes (Paoli, PA) specifically for this operation (Fig. 12.10B). This plate has 3.5 mm screws proximally in the radius and 2.7 mm screws distally in the capitate and metacarpal. The plate is designed with tapered edges and recessed screw heads to avoid prominence. Three versions are

available: one has a short precontoured bend, the second a larger precontoured bend, and the third is a straight plate. The short bend plate is used in smaller wrists and when a proximal row carpectomy is performed. The larger bend is used in most individuals. The straight plate is useful when a corticocancellous intercallary bone graft is needed. The plate is precontoured with 10° of dorsiflexion. Alternatively, a CMC-sparing total wrist fusion plate (Cobra Plate, KMI, San Diego, CA) may be utilized. This plate provides carpal fixation with three capitate, one scaphoid, and one lunate cancellous screws.

In the absence of these plates, a straight plate is chosen and contoured to the desired position of fusion. In most individuals, a 3.5 mm LC-DCP plate is chosen. This plate does have 3.5 mm holes over the metacarpal, which are often prominent. In smaller individuals, a 3.5 mm reconstruction plate or one-third tubular plate may be used.

All joints to be fused are packed with bone graft prior to plate application. The plate is then centered over the third metacarpal and radius. It is important that all three metacarpal holes are directly over the center of the metacarpal. The distal-most hole is marked with a marking pen. The plate is removed and this hole is drilled with a 2.0 mm drill bit, being sure to stay centered within the metacarpal and in a straight anteroposterior direction. If this screw is not placed precisely, the plate will lie oblique to the frontal plane and rotate the metacarpal when the plate is fixed to the radius. The distal hole is then measured, tapped with a 2.7 mm tap, and a 2.7 mm screw is placed through the plate. The alignment of the plate is checked and the proximal metacarpal

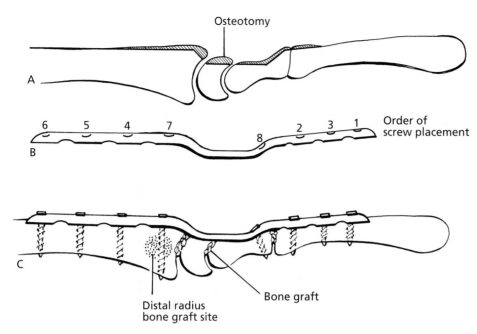

FIGURE 12.10. A. The dorsal osteotomy is achieved with osteotomes, providing a contoured smooth surface for the plate. **B.** Synthes contoured wrist fusion plate with sequence of screw placement. **C.** Bone graft is harvested from the distal radius and packed in the radiocarpal and third CMC joints. (Reprinted with permission from Weiss, APC, Hastings H, II. Wrist arthrodesis for traumatic conditions: a study of plate and local bone graft application. *J Hand Surg* 1995:20A:50–56.).

hole is drilled and an additional 2.7 mm screw is placed. The central metacarpal screw is then placed.

The hand is next aligned with the forearm allowing for some ulnar deviation. Manual compression is performed and the second most distal radius screw is placed. This is accomplished with the 2.5 mm drill bit in compression mode and 3.5 mm cortical screw. Drilling is performed eccentrically away from the wrist joint and away from the bone graft harvest site in the radius. The remaining radius holes are fixed with cortical screws (Fig. 12.10C).

A 2.7 mm screw is placed in the capitate. If the capitate is against the plate, the measured depth screw can be used. If the capitate is away from the plate, a shorter screw can be used to pull the capitate up to the plate. If strong purchase cannot be obtained, this hole can be left empty.

Wound closure is performed over a suction drain. Marcaine-soaked gelfoam can be placed in the bone graft site from the radius to diminish bleeding and help with pain. The capsule is closed over the plate, and often periosteum can be used to cover the distal plate. The now nonfunctional extensor carpi radialis brevis tendon can be fanned out to cover the plate. The EPL tendon is left transposed radially.

Postoperatively, the drain is removed at 24 hours. Elevation and digital motion are encouraged immediately. The volar splint applied in the operating room is removed after 10 to 14 days when sutures are removed. A light compressive dressing or elastic sleeve is applied with a thermoplast molded splint as a protective reminder to use the hand only for light activities. The splint is discontinued at 6 weeks and full use is allowed at 10 weeks. Radiographs typically demonstrate union by 8 to 10 weeks.

Results

The goal of wrist fusion is to accomplish solid bony union, eliminate pain, and preserve function.

The union rate using the AO plate technique ranges between 96% and 100% (43). Weiss and Hastings demonstrated a 100% union rate in 28 consecutive patients using the AO wrist fusion plate and only local bone graft (78). Overall, union rates are higher utilizing the AO technique. Hastings compared AO and non-AO techniques in a closely matched group undergoing total wrist fusion (15). Solid fusion occurred on the first surgical attempt in 98.5% of patients using the AO technique compared to 73.5% using non-AO techniques. In a series by Clendenin and Green, the union rate in the Carrol and Dick technique was 72.5%, in the Riordan and Haddad technique 80%, and in the Nalebuff technique, 91.7% (54a).

Pain relief after wrist fusion is also uniformly good (90). Overall, approximately 85% of patients report excellent relief of preoperative pain. Hastings compared two evenly matched groups of patients undergoing either total wrist fusion or motion-preserving procedures. He found wrist fusion patients had better pain relief (85% versus 66%), more overall satisfaction (91% versus 83%) an equal willingness to have the procedure again (96% versus 96%), and more eagerness to have the procedure done sooner (91% versus 83%) (16).

Weiss et al. evaluated the functional outcome in 23 patients undergoing wrist fusion (91). Fifteen of the 23 patients returned to their original jobs, and all patients were able to perform most tasks but often in a modified fashion. The patients had a 64% task completion rate compared to

78% in the normal wrist in the Jebsen Hand Function Test. The most difficult tasks to perform were perineal care and manipulating the hand in tight spaces. Maximum improvement in function following arthrodesis averaged 14.5 months.

Hastings demonstrated that patients were able to complete 85% of activities of daily living normally. The most difficult tasks included fastening clothes, combing hair, opening jars, and sitting down where the patients axially loaded their wrists with their body weight. Sixty-five percent of patients returned to their original jobs, 25% returned to less strenuous work, and 10% did not return to work for various reasons (15).

Rayan et al. evaluated the result after bilateral wrist fusions in rheumatoid arthritis. They found that 7 of 18 patients had an improvement if hand function compared to their preoperative state and 2 of 18 patients had no change in function. They concluded that bilateral wrist arthrodesis does not adversely affect function of the upper extremity (81).

REHABILITATION

The goal of rehabilitation after a wrist fusion is to maintain digital motion until union is achieved and then to regain strength. Once wound healing has occurred, patients are placed in a removable volar thermoplast splint. This does not serve a protective function but serves as a reminder that a procedure was performed. The splint is discontinued at 6 weeks and full use of the hand is typically allowed at 10 weeks. Union is confirmed on radiographs. Patients typically need only a short course of therapy for strengthening, job simulation, and modification of some activities.

COMPLICATIONS

Total wrist fusion is a major operative procedure. For this reason, complications do occur. Modifications in the surgical techniques, types of implants, and use of local bone graft have decreased the incidence of complications (92).

The advantage of AO plating with regard to union was discussed in the results section. If a nonunion is suspected, imaging modalities such as tomograms and a CAT scan should be utilized to determine which joints have not united. The most common location for nonunion is the third CMC joint. We emphasize the importance of decorticating 80% of the joint at the time of fusion. If a nonunion should occur at the CMC joint, it may cause persistent symptoms and may warrant treatment. If the wrist is fused, the plate should be removed and repeat fusion of the CMC joint should be performed. Additional bone graft will be necessary and the index CMC joint is typically included to increase the fusion mass. Typically, Kirschner wires are utilized, and the wrist is immobilized until fusion is achieved. Using the CMC-sparing

Cobra wrist fusion plate would eliminate this particular complication, but may leave the CMC joint susceptible to increased load and later degenerative changes.

Plate tenderness with standard AO 3.5 mm plates occurred in 19% of patients warranting removal in 12% (15). The new low profile plate, however, has a lower incidence of plate tenderness. If the plate does become tender, we recommend removal anytime after union is achieved. The wrist should be protected from heavy activities for 4 to 6 weeks after plate removal to allow remodeling of the screw holes.

Extensor or flexor tendon adhesions may occur from prominent screw heads or excessively long screws. If a long screw may be causing flexor tendon adherence, it should be removed. In extensor tendinitis, a trial at immobilization and corticosteroid injection should be attempted. If this fails, the plate should be removed once union is achieved and a tenolysis performed at that time.

Carpal tunnel syndrome occurs between 3.6% and 10% of the time after wrist fusion (15). Some of this may represent poorly documented preoperative carpal tunnel syndrome. For this reason, we emphasize a careful preoperative carpal tunnel evaluation. Wrist fusion itself does not significantly change the size of the carpal canal but may cause flexor tenosynovitis leading to clinical symptoms. Nerve studies should be obtained, a trial corticosteroid injection should be performed, and if the symptoms do not resolve, a carpal tunnel release should be performed. We recommend using an open technique and careful isolation of the nerve since the nerve may be adherent to the transverse carpal ligament from the edema and fibrosis associated with the previous procedure.

Distal radioulnar joint symptoms are uncommon after wrist fusion. In most instances these occur because of preexisting pathology. Wrist fusion itself unloads the distal radioulnar joint and should not increase symptoms. The DRUJ must be evaluated critically prior to wrist fusion and if it is contributing to the symptoms, it should be addressed at the time of the index operation. If DRUJ arthritis is discovered after wrist fusion, it can be addressed with standard surgical options such as hemiresection or total resection of the distal ulna (19,93).

Wound healing problems and infection are possibilities after any major surgical procedure. In one series there was a 7% incidence of wound healing problems that resolved without treatment. If a deep infection should occur, surgical debridement is necessary. An attempt should be made to maintain the fixation until fusion is achieved. Appropriate intravenous antibiotics should be utilized.

Although wrist fusion is considered the final procedure for wrist pain, there are occasions where pain may persist. This is most often seen in patients who have undergone multiple procedures previously, all with limited success, and in patients with secondary gain issues. In this instance, selective nerve blocks may be used to determine if wrist denervation is an option. All of the above-mentioned complications should be critically ruled out as causes for underlying persistent pain.

REFERENCES

1. Ely LW. An operation for tuberculosis of the wrist. *JAMA* 1920; 75:1707–1709.
2. Steindler A. Orthopaedic operations on the hand. *JAMA* 1918;17: 1288–1291.
3. Dick HM.. Wrist and intercarpal arthrodesis. In: Green DP, ed. *Operative hand surgery.* New York: Churchill Livingstone, 1982: 127–139.
4. Abbott LC, Saunders JBDM, Bost FC. Arthrodesis of the wrist with the use of grafts of cancellous bone, *J Bone and Joint Surg* 1942;24: 883–898.
5. Albee FH. *Bone graft surgery in disease, injury and deformity.* New York: Appleton-Century-Crofts, 1940.
6. Allende BT. Wrist arthrodesis. *Clin Orthop* 1979;142:164–167.
7. Benkeddache Y, Gottesman H, Fourrier P. Multiple stapling for wrist arthrodesis in the non-rheumatoid patient. *J Hand Surg* 1984;9A:256–261.
8. Brittain HA. *Architectural principles in arthrodesis*, 2nd ed. London: E and S Livingstone, 1952:145–160.
9. Carroll RE, Dick HM. Arthrodesis of the wrist for rheumatoid arthritis. *Bone and Joint Surg* 1971;53A:1365–1369.
10. Clayton ML, Ferlic DC. Arthrodesis of the arthritic wrist. *Clin Orthop* 1984;187: 89–93.
11. Colonna PC. A method for fusion of the wrist. *Southern Med J* 1944;37:195–199.
12. Dupont M, Vainio K. Arthrodesis of the wrist in rheumatoid arthritis: A study of 140 cases. *Ann Chir Gynaecol* 1968;57:513–519.
13. Evans DL. Wedge arthrodesis of the wrist. *J Bone Joint Surg* 1955; 37B:126–134.
14. Haddad Jr RJ, Riordan DC. Arthrodesis of the wrist. A surgical technique. *J Bone Joint Surg* 1967;49A:950–954.
15. Hastings H. Arthrodesis of the osteoarthritic wrist. In: Gelberman RH, ed. *The wrist.* New York: Raven Press, 1994:345–360.
16. Hazewinkel J. Arthrodesis of the radiocarpal joint. A surgical technique. *J Int Coll Surg* 1962;38:137–140.
17. Hastings II H, Weiss APC, Quenzer D, et al. Arthrodesis of the wrist for post-traumatic disorders. *J Bone and Joint Surg* 1996;78A: 897–902.
18. Larsson SE. Compression arthrodesis of the wrist. A consecutive series of 23 cases. *Clin Orthop* 1974; 99:146–153.
19. Learmonth ID, Grobler G, Jeffe R, et al. Arthrodesis of the wrist for inflammatory arthritis. In: Simmen BR, Hagena FW, eds. *The wrist in rheumatoid arthritis.* Basel, Switzerland: Karger, 1992:122–126.
20. Straub LR, Ranawat CS. The wrist in rheumatoid arthritis. Surgical treatment and results. *J Bone Joint Surg* 1969;51(1):1–20.
21. Liebolt FL. Surgical fusion of the wrist joint. *Surg Gynecol Obstet* 1938;66:1008–1023.
22. Mannerfelt L. Total arthrodesis of the wrist. In: Simmen BR, Hagena FW, eds. *The wrist in rheumatid arthritis.* Basel, Switzerland: Karger, 1992:116–121.
23. Meuli HC. Reconstructive surgery of the wrist joint. *Hand* 1972;4:88–90.
24. Mikkelsen OA. Arthrodesis of the wrist joint in rheumatoid arthritis. *Hand* 1980;12:149–153.
25. Millender LH, Terrono Al, Feldon PG. Arthrodesis of the rheumatoid arthritic wrist. In: Gelberman RH, ed. *The wrist.* New York: Raven Press, 1994:287–300
26. Robinson RF, Kayfetz DO. Arthrodesis of the wrist. Preliminary report of a new method. *J Bone Joint Surg.* 1952;34A:64–70.
27. Ross WT. Arthrodesis of the wrist joint. An analysis of 48 operations. *S Afr Med J* 1950;24:755–757.
28. Salenius P. Arthrodesis of the carpal joint. *Acta Orthop Scan*, 1966; 37:288–296.
29. Sovio OM, Gropper PT. Wrist arthrodesis. *Orthop Trans* 1985;9: 561–562.
30. Stein I. Gill turnabout radial graft for wrist arthrodesis. *Surg Gynecol Obstet* 1958;106:231–232.
31. Thomas DF. A method of arthrodesis of the wrist. *Lancet* 1950;1: 808–809.
32. Urbaniak JR. Arthrodesis of the hand and wrist. In: McCollister Evarts C, ed. *Surgery of the musculoskeletal system*, vol. 1. New York: Churchill Livingstone, 1983;2:371–372,386.
33. Epstein S. Arthrodesis for flail wrist. *Am J Surg* 1930;8:621–622.
34. Ashmead IV D, Watson HK, Damon C, et al. Scapholunate advanced collapse wrist salvage. *J Hand Surg* 1994;19A:741–750.
35. Krakauer JD, Bishop AT, Cooney W. Surgical treatment of scapholunate advanced collapse. *J Hand Surg* 1994;19A:751–759.
36. Siegel JM, Ruby LK. Midcarpal arthrodesis. *J Hand Surg* 1996; 21A:179–182.
37. Louis DS, Hankin FM, Bowers WH. Capitate-radius arthrodesis: An alternative method of radiocarpal arthrodesis. *J Hand Surg* 1984;9A:365–369.
38. Minami A, Ogino T, Minami M. Limited wrist fusions, *J Hand Surg* 1988;13A:660–667.
39. Taleisnik J. Subtotal arthrodeses of the wrist joint. *Clin Orthop* 1984;187: 81–88.
40. Watson HK, Goodman ML, Johnson TR. Limited wrist arthrodesis. Part II: intercarpal and radiocarpal combination, *J Bone Joint Surg* 1981;6:223–233.
41. Wyrick JD, Stern PJ, Kiefhaber TR. Motion-preserving procedures in the treatment of scapholunate advanced collapse wrist: Proximal row carpectomy versus four-corner fusion arthrodesis, *J Hand Surg* 1995;20A:965–970.
42. Hastings H, 2nd, Weiss APC, Quenzer D, et al. Arthrodesis of the wrist for post-traumatic disorders. *J Bone Joint Surg* 1996;78A:897–902.
43. Hastings H, Weiss APC, Strickland JE. Arthrodesis of the wrist. Indications technique and functional consequences for the hand and wrist. *Orthop* 1993;22:89–91.
44. Clayton ML. Surgical treatment at the wrist in rheumatoid arthritis. A review of thirty-seven patients. *J Bone Joint Surg* 1965;47A: 741–750.
45. Lee DH, Carroll RE. Wrist arthrodesis: A combined intramedullary pin and autogenous iliac crest bone graft technique. *J Hand Surg* 1994;19A:733–740.
46. Kulick RG, De Fiore JC, Straub LR, et al. Long-term results of dorsal stabilization in the rheumatoid wrist. *J Hand Surg* 1981;6: 272–280.
47. Mannerfelt L, Malmsten M. Arthrodesis of the wrist in rheumatoid arthritis. A technique without external fixation. *Scand J Plast Reconstr Surg* 1971;5:124–130.
48. Millender LH, Nalebuff EA. Arthrodesis of the rheumatoid wrist. An evaluation of sixty patients and a description of different surgical techniques. *J Bone Joint Surg* 1973;55A:1026–1034.
49. Papaioannou T, Dickson RA Arthrodesis of the wrist in rheumatoid disease. *Hand* 1982;14:12–16.
50. Pipkin G. Medullary nailing of the wrist to the radius as a mechanical guide to ensure optimum position for wrist arthrodesis. *Clin Orthop* 1968;57:179–189.
51. Kobus RJ, Turner RH. Wrist arthrodesis for treatment of rheumatoid arthritis. *J Hand Surg* 1990;15A:541–546.
52. Ryu J, Watson HK, Burgess RC. Rheumatoid wrist reconstruction utilizing a fibrous nonunion and radiocarpal arthrodesis. *J Hand Surg* 1985;10A:830–836.
53. Straub LR, Ranawat CS. The wrist in rheumatoid arthritis. Surgical treatment and results. *J Bone Joint Surg* 1969;51A:1–20.
54. Millender LH, Philips C. Combined wrist arthrodesis and metacarpophalangeal joint arthroplasty in rheumatoid arthritis. *Orthop* 1978; 1:43–48.

54a. Clendenin MB, Green DP. Arthrodesis of the wrist—complications and their management. *J Hand Surg* 1981;6:253–257.

55. Murray JA, Schlafly B. Giant-cell tumors in the distal end of the radius. Treatment by resection and fibular autograft interpositional arthrodesis. *J Bone Joint Surg* 1986;68A:687–694.

56. Szabo RM, Thorson EP, Raskin JR. Allograft placement with distal radioulnar joint fusion and ulnar osteotomy for treatment of giant cell tumors of the distal radius. *J Hand Surg* 1990;15A:922–929.

57. Nissen KL. Symposium on cerebral palsy (orthopaedic section). *Proc R Soc Med* 1951;44:87–90.

58. Buch-Gramcko D. Denervation of the wrist joint, *J Hand Surg* 1977;2:54–61.

59. Darrach W. Partial excision of lower shaft of ulna for deformity following Colles' fracture. *Ann Surg* 1913;57:764–765.

60. Bolano LE, Green DP. Wrist arthrodesis in post-traumatic arthritis: A comparison of two methods. *J Hand Surg* 1993;18A:786–791.

61. Butler AA. Arthrodesis of the wrist joint: Graft from inner table of ilium. *Am J Surg* 1949;78:625–630.

62. Campbell CJ, Keokarn T. Total and subtotal arthrodesis of the wrist. Inlay technique. *J Bone Joint Surg* 1964;46A:1520–1533.

63. Lenoble E, Ovadia H, Goutallier D. Wrist arthrodesis using an embedded iliac crest bone graft. *J Hand Surg* 1993;18B:595–600.

64. Mittal RL, Jain NC. Arthrodesis of the wrist by a new technique. *Int Orthop* 1990;14:213–216.

65. Murray PM. Current status of wrist arthrodesis and wrist arthroplasty. *Clin Plast Surg* 1996;23:385–394.

66. Nagy L, Buchler U. Advances in arthrodesis of the hand and wrist. *Curr Opin Orthop* 1994;5(4):51–61.

67. Skak SV. Arthrodesis of the wrist by the method of Mannerfelt. A follow up of 10 patients. *Acta Orthop Scand* 1982;53:557–559.

68. Smith-Petersen MN. A new approach to the wrist joint. *J Bone Joint Surg* 1940;22:122–124.

69. Stanley JK, Gupta SR, Hullin MG. Modified instrument for wrist fusion. *J Hand Surg* 1986;11B:245–249.

70. Vabvanen V, Tallroth K. A follow-up study of forty-five consecutive cases. *J Hand Surg* 1984;9A:531–536.

71. Wickstrom JK. Arthrodesis of the wrist: Modification and evaluation of the use of split rib grafts. *South Med J* 1954;47:968–971.

72. Wood MB. Wrist arthrodesis using dorsal radial bone graft, *J Hand Surg* 1987;12A:208–212.

73. Swanson AB, Swanson GD, Goran-Hagert C. Evaluation of impairment of hand function. In: Hunter JM, Maekin BJ, Callahan AD, eds. *Rehabilitation of the hand: Surgery and therapy*, 4th ed. St. Louis: CV Mosby, 1995:1839–1896.

74. Brumfield RH, Champoux JA. A biomechanical study of normal functional wrist motion. *Clin Orthop* 1984;187:23–25.

75. Palmer AK, Werner FW, Murphy D, et al. Functional wrist motion: A biomechanical study. *J Hand Surg* 1985;10A:39–46.

76. Weiss APC, Wiedmeman G. Jr, Quenzer D, et al. Upper extremity function after wrist arthrodesis. *J Hand Surg* 1995;20A:813–817.

77. Pryce JD. The wrist position between neutral and ulnar deviation that facilitates the maximum power grip strength. *J Biomech* 1980;13:505–511.

78. Weiss, APC, Hastings H, II. Wrist arthrodesis for traumatic conditions: a study of plate and local bone graft application. *J Hand Surg* 1995;20A:50–56.

79. Kraft GH, Detels PE. Position of function of the wrist. *Arch Phys Med Rehabil* 1972;53:272–275.

80. Sennwald GR, Zdraukovic V. Wrist joint arthrodesis. In: Peimer CA, ed. *Surgery of the hand and upper extremity*. New York: McGraw-Hill, 1996:Ch. 33.

81. Rayan GM, Brentlinger A, Purnell D, et al. Functional assessment of bilateral wrist arthrodesis. *J Hand Surg* 1987;12A:1020–1024.

82. Green D. *Green's operative hand surgery.* New York: Churchill Livingstone, 1999:131–146.

82a. Rayan GM. Wrist arthrodesis. *J Hand Surg* 1986;11A:356–364.

83. Richards RS, Roth JH. Simultaneous proximal row carpectomy and radius to distal carpal row arthrodesis. *J Hand Surg* 1994;19A: 728–732.

84. Buck-Gramcko D, Lohmann H. Compression arthrodesis of the wrist. In: Tubiana R, ed. *The hand*, vol. 2. Philadelphia: WB Saunders, 1985:723–729.

85. Heim U, Pfeiffer KM. *Small fragment set manual: Technique recommended by the ASIF (Swiss Association for the Study of internal Fixation) group,* 2nd ed. New York: Springer, 1982:53–54,133–134, 143,160–161.

86. O'Bierne J, Boyer MI, Axelrod TS. Wrist arthrodesis using a dynamic compression plate. *J Bone Joint Surg [Br]* 1995;77-B:700–4.

87. Manetta P, Tavani L. Arthrodesis of the wrist with a compression plate. *Italian J Orthop Trauma* 1975;1:219–224.

88. Ragerman SD, Palmar AK. Wrist arthrodesis using a dynamic compression plate. *J Hand Surg* 1996;21B:437–441.

89. Wright CS, McMurtry RY. AO arthrodesis in the hand. *J Hand Surg* 1983;8:932–935.

90. Weiss APC, Wiedeman Jr G, Quenzer D, et al. Upper extremity function after wrist arthrodesis. *J Hand Surg* 1995;20A:813–817.

91. Vicar AJ, Burton R. Surgical management of the rheumatoid wrist—fusion or arthroplasty. *J Hand Surg* 1986;11A:790–797.

92. Field J, Herbert TJ, Prosser R. Total wrist fusion: A functional assessment. *J Hand Surg* 1996;21B:429–433.

93. Zachary SV, Stern PJ. Complications following AO/ASIF wrist arthrodesis. *J Hand Surg* 1995;20A:339–344.

94. Trumble TE, Easterling KJ, Smith RJ. Ulnocarpal abutment after wrist arthrodesis. *J Hand Surg* 1988;13A:11–15.

were associated with failure. Because loosening of the distal component has been a particular problem, custom, long-stemmed, multipronged modifications for insertion into multiple metacarpal canals have been used for patients with poor bone stock and for revision arthroplasty (26).

Several other prosthesis have been developed in an effort to reduce complications and reduce the need for cement. The Hamas implant had single proximal and distal stems similar to the redesigned Volz and a ball and socket articulation like the Meuli. Although the device demonstrated improved balance, distal component migration and loosening remained a problem (27). The Guepar total wrist, available in France, is an ellipsoidal design similar to the Biaxial with an offset proximal polyethelene component and a distal metal component fixed with screws into the index and long metacarpals (28). The CFV designed by Clayton, Ferlic, and Volz has an ellipsoidal proximal component with variable-sized surfaces and a distal concave metal-backed polyethylene component. The device was designed for insertion without cement. Early results were mixed, with problems of loosening, and imbalance (29). In Germany, Radmer introduced an hydroxyapatite coated device to improve implant fixation. The results have been similar to other stem designs (30).

The persistent problem of distal component loosening that was plaguing previous prostheses prompted Menon to design the Universal total wrist (31). Introduced in 1980, the

prosthesis has a unique method of fixation for the distal component (Figs. 13.4–13.7). Previous designs have relied on fixation in the metacarpal canals, typically with cement, and are associated with a high incidence of loosening, metacarpal erosion, and implant penetration. The distal component of the Universal prosthesis is fixed by a short central stem into the capitate and two deep-threaded screws into the radial and ulnar aspects of the carpus. The fixation is combined with an intercarpal arthrodesis to provide long-term, solid bony support. Because the distal component supports the entire carpus, proximal migration of the first and fifth rays is prevented. The articular surface of the distal component is ellipsoidal and closely matches the contour of the proximal carpal row. The radial component is inclined 20° to replicate the slope of the normal distal radius. Soft-tissue balancing can be adjusted by variations in polyethylene sizes. These design features offer better wrist balance and more normal load transfer. The oblique osteotomy of the radius and the proximal osteotomy through the carpus results in minimal bone resection and allows preservation of the wrist capsule. Because the resection is limited, adequate bone stock is available to salvage the wrist by arthrodesis if the prosthesis fails. The long-term performance of this prosthesis, which is described further below, has shown dramatic improvements in the longevity of wrist implant fixation compared to previous prosthetic designs.

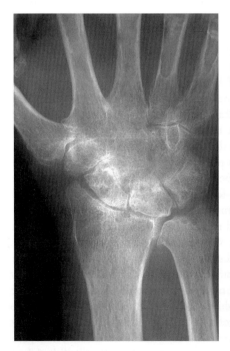

FIGURE 13.4. Preoperative radiographs of patient with rheumatoid arthritis.

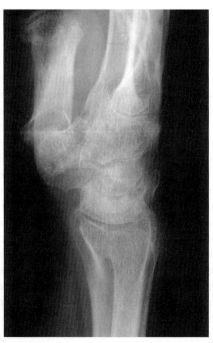

FIGURE 13.5. Preoperative radiographs of patient with rheumatoid arthritis.

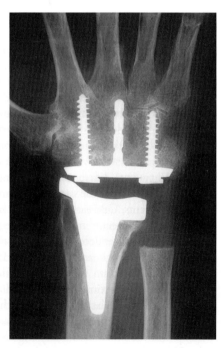

FIGURE 13.6. Universal Total Wrist arthroplasty functionally well at 3 years postoperative.

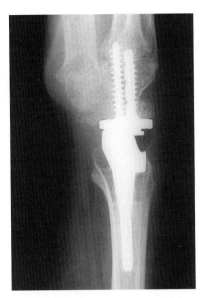

FIGURE 13.7. Universal Total Wrist arthroplasty functionally well at 3 years postoperative.

INDICATIONS/CONTRAINDICATIONS

Although wrist arthrodesis effectively relieves pain and corrects deformity, the sacrificed motion may significantly impair function, especially when the shoulder, elbow, and hand are also affected by arthritis. The impact of lost wrist motion is also magnified when bilateral wrist arthritis is present. Patients who have had wrist fusion on one side and arthroplasty on the other side prefer wrist arthroplasty to fusion (32–34). The motion provided by a total wrist arthroplasty eases the performance of simple daily activities as well as avocations, which are very important to the well-being of an individual afflicted by severe arthritis. In a report by Kobus and Turner on wrist fusion, all unsatisfied patients had an arthroplasty on the opposite wrist (34). Patients with an arthrodesis often have significant difficulties with activities of daily living, including fastening buttons, combing hair, opening a jar, and writing (35). Perineal care is also difficult, especially if multiple joints are involved by rheumatoid arthritis (35). Similar complaints were found in other studies (36–38). Swanson observed that just a few degrees of wrist motion increases finger reach by 6 cm (7). In his comprehensive monograph, Van Gemert reported that only 42% of patients achieved the expected outcome with fusion (39). He concluded that motion should be preserved in at least one wrist. Some people with severe osteoarthritis or posttraumatic arthritis who are not engaged in regular strenuous activities would also choose joint replacement and permanent activity restriction in favor of fusion to retain better dexterity.

Thus, total wrist replacement should be considered an option for certain individuals with specific needs or desires for motion, provided the surgeon and patient clearly understand the risks and benefits. New developments in prosthetic design have provided definite improvements in the functional performance and durability of wrist replacement. When performed technically well in properly selected patients, total wrist arthroplasty provides a functional and durable wrist with high patient satisfaction.

Contraindications for total wrist arthroplasty include a minimally functional hand, recent infection, and lack of wrist extension power due to ruptures of the extensor carpi radialis brevis and longus tendons or a radial nerve palsy. Severe wrist laxity due to highly active synovitis is a relative contraindication because it increases the risk of prosthetic instability. An additional trial of medical control can be attempted before proceeding with surgery; however, these patients are probably best treated by an arthrodesis. Patients with severe bone loss or osteopenia that would prevent adequate implant fixation are not indicated for arthroplasty. The risk of prosthetic loosening and breakage is too high for younger or very active patients with high physical demands. Intercarpal arthrodeses and proximal row carpectomy are more reliable motion-preserving operations for this type of patient.

PREOPERATIVE PLANNING

A majority of the patients undergoing total wrist arthroplasty will have long-standing rheumatoid arthritis. Thus, a careful preoperative assessment of their general health and other orthopedic conditions is necessary. Cervical spine stability should be evaluated with flexion-extension radiographs. If hip or knee arthritis is indicated for joint replacement, these should be done first to obviate weight-bearing on the wrist arthroplasty. Wrist replacement may be done before or after shoulder or elbow replacement but should be done before hand surgery to improve hand balance and to optimize rehabilitation of the digits. A recent rheumatoid flare should be controlled before surgery and current medicines regulated. Our preference is to discontinue methotrexate for approximately one month prior to surgery and for about one month after surgery. Decreasing the dosage or eliminating the use of nonsteroidal anti-inflammatory drugs for 10 days prior to surgery and for 5 days following the operation is recommended to reduce the risk of postoperative bleeding complications. Possible additional requirements for corticosteroids during the perioperative time must be considered.

A preoperative discussion among the surgeon, patient, and therapist will help the patient prepare for rehabilitation. Preoperative assessment of the radiographs for bone quality and erosions, carpal collapse, carpal ulnar translation, volar wrist subluxation, and the condition of the distal radioulnar joint will prepare the surgeon for potential technical difficulties. Implant size and alignment within the bones can be predicted using radiographic templates. Because total wrist arthroplasty is a highly technical procedure, appropriate instruments, power tools, and fluoroscopic imaging are mandatory. Operating personnel familiar with both hand surgery and total joint replacement will improve operative efficiency.

OPERATIVE TECHNIQUE

Although the technique for Universal total wrist arthroplasty will be described, the basic principles apply to other total wrist arthroplasties. The appropriate size of implant is estimated preoperatively using x-ray templates. The operation is performed under general or axillary regional anesthesia and an arm tourniquet is used. A dorsal longitudinal incision is made over the wrist in line with the third metacarpal, extending proximally from its midshaft. The skin and subcutaneous tissue are elevated from the extensor retinaculum and held with retraction sutures. The ECU compartment is opened along its volar margin and the entire retinaculum is elevated radially to the septum between the first and second extensor compartments (Fig. 13.8). Each septum is divided carefully when raising the retinaculum to avoid creating rents, especially at Lister's tubercle, which may need to be osteotomized. An extensor tenosynovectomy is performed and the tendons are examined for damage. The ECRB must be intact or reparable (preferably the ECRL is also functional). A one-fourth-inch Penrose tubing is used to retract the third and fourth compartment tendons.

A distally based rectangular flap of joint capsule is raised over the dorsal wrist. The sides of the flap are made along the far medial and lateral aspects of the wrist. The proximal capsule is raised in continuity with the periosteum over the distal 1 to 1.5 cm of the radius to create a longer flap for closure over the prosthesis (see Fig. 13.8). The distal ulna is resected with an oscillating saw at the level of the proximal aspect of the sigmoid notch (approximately 1.5 cm). The head is saved

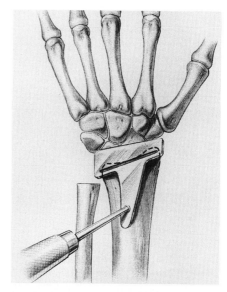

FIGURE 13.9. Distal margin of the radius is resected using a template.

for possible use as bone graft. The brachioradialis and the tendons of the first dorsal compartment are elevated subperiosteally from the styloid. The wrist is flexed and retractors are placed on each side of the radius to expose its end and to protect the tendons. The radial cutting guide is applied to the dorsal aspect of the radius and aligned with its anatomic contours (Fig. 13.9). Using a small oscillating saw, only the dorsal lip and radial articular surface are resected. Additional bone will be removed later if necessary.

The carpal osteotomy is made with an oscillating saw. The line of the osteotomy passes through the proximal aspect of the capitate (Fig. 13.10). If the carpus is subluxed palmarly, traction is applied to the hand to bring the carpal bones out from under the radius. Positively identify the capitate prior to

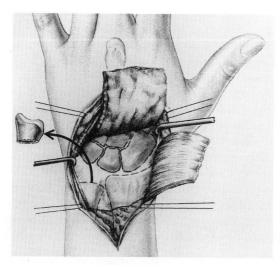

FIGURE 13.8. Exposure for wrist arthroplasty. The retinaculum is reflected radially and the joint capsule raised distally. Distal ulna is resected.

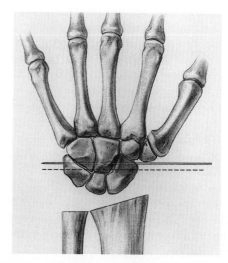

FIGURE 13.10. Carpal osteotomy level is shown by the dotted line. Temporary fixation of the carpus with a wire facilitates the osteotomy and carpal preparation.

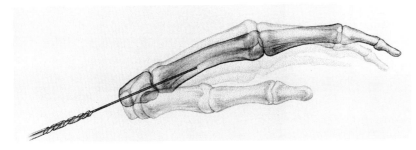

resection. The plane of the osteotomy is perpendicular to the capitate and third metacarpal in both the coronal and sagittal planes. A portion of the scaphoid and triquetrum remain intact along with the distal carpal bones. When the carpal bones are loose or malaligned from chronic synovitis and erosion, the osteotomy and later carpal preparation are greatly facilitated by first temporarily pinning the scaphoid and triquetrum to the capitate and hamate in more reduced positions. A guide pin or Kirschner wire is inserted just beneath the dorsal cortices of the carpal bones to avoid interfering with the carpal osteotomy and the insertion of the carpal component stem and fixation screws (see Fig. 13.10). Two or more Kirschner wires, separately fixing the scaphoid and triquetrum, may be necessary or easier than using one. The pin or pins are left in place until after the true carpal components are implanted.

To align the carpal component, a guide wire for a 3.5 mm cannulated drill bit is inserted into the center of the capitate (Fig. 13.11). The wire should lie in the long axis of the capitate in both the coronal and sagittal planes. Advance the pin into the base of the third metacarpal and check the position using an image intensifier. In most cases, it is better to align the carpal component with the capitate rather than the third metacarpal to achieve the best overall component position. Using the cannulated drill bit, drill a hole to a depth just longer than the carpal component stem. The opening of the hole is slightly widened to accommodate the shoulder of the component stem. Trial components are inserted to determine the correct implant size. The implant should cover the carpus but not extend more than 2 mm beyond the margins of the bones.

A drill hole is made through the radial hole in the carpal plate through the remaining scaphoid, the trapezoid, and across the second CMC joint into the base of the second metacarpal using a 2.5 mm drill bit. To achieve this position, the hole must be drilled at an angle slightly off perpendicular to the carpal component; the screw heads and carpal component are designed to accommodate this oblique angle. Confirm the drill bit's position and estimate its depth with fluoroscopy. A 4.5 mm self-tapping screw of appropriate length, typically 30 to 35 mm, is inserted. If possible, the screw should cross the carpometacarpal joint into the base of the second metacarpal to increase fixation strength (Fig. 13.12). The ulnar screw is inserted in a similar manner through the ulnar hole of the carpal plate. This screw, usually 20 mm in length, should engage the remaining triquetrum and the hamate but does not cross the normally mobile fourth or fifth carpometacarpal joint unless it is necessary for better purchase. Screw positions and lengths are checked with fluoroscopy.

To prepare the radial canal, the surgeon should sit at the end of the hand table to have an end-on view of the distal radius. The medullary canal of the radius is identified with a curette and its position confirmed with the image intensifier. The canal is opened first with the starter broach and then progressively enlarged to the appropriate size using the selection of small, medium, and large broaches (Fig. 13.13). Implant size is based on the best overall fit in both the carpus and radius. The broaches are inserted parallel to the volar cortex of the radius to avoid malrotation (Fig. 13.14), and at a valgus angle (radial tilt) to reduce the tendency for an ulnar deviation deformity (Fig. 13.13). Also, insert the broaches somewhat dorsal in the metaphysis to avoid tracking along the volar

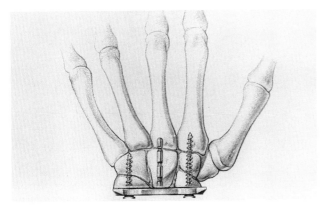

FIGURE 13.12. A trial carpal component with a central stem and two deep-threaded screws is inserted.

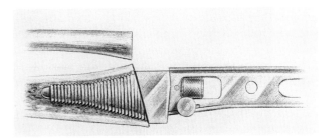

FIGURE 13.13. Radius is prepared beginning with the starter broach and progressively enlarging the canal to the appropriate size with a selection of broaches.

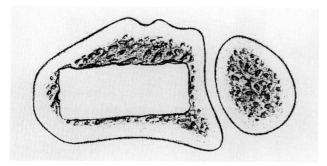

FIGURE 13.14. Proper positioning of the broaches, as shown, is important to avoid malalignment of the radial component.

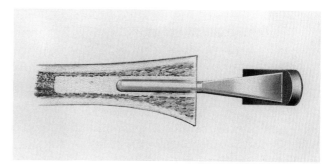

FIGURE 13.15. The radial component should be aligned with the long axis of the radius to avoid volar tilting of the implant.

metaphyseal flare, which will create volar tilting of the radial component and reduce prosthetic stability. The final position of the broach is checked with fluoroscopy. The second radial cutting guide is placed over the broach and the radius trimmed slightly to match the sloping contour of the radial component.

A trial radial component is pressed into the medullary canal of the radius. A trial polyethylene component is slid on the carpal component and the joint reduced. The wrist should rest in a neutral position and a balanced state. A step-cut tendon lengthening of the flexor carpi ulnaris and occasionally the flexor carpi radialis may be required to achieve proper balance and motion. If the joint is too tight, additional bone is removed from the radius. However, a loose joint must be avoided to prevent prosthetic instability. Any defects in the volar capsule are repaired and its proximal edge is sutured to the volar margin of the radius through small drill holes if it was detached during the dissection. Trial polyethylene components of greater thickness can also be tried to further improve prosthetic stability. After the appropriate sizes are determined, the trial components are removed (the same screws will be used for final implantation).

The wound is thoroughly irrigated with pulsed lavage and dried, including the capitate hole and radial canal. If the medullary canal has not been closed off by the broaching process, insert a plug prepared from a resected piece of bone. Two to three sutures are placed through small drill holes along the dorsal margin of the distal radius for later capsule closure. A small amount of bone cement is injected into the hole in the capitate using a 12 cc syringe (slightly widen the syringe opening with a hemostat). The stem of the carpal component is inserted and the implant is pressed flush with the carpal bones. Remove excess cement, especially from the intercarpal spaces. Insert the radial and ulnar carpal screws and tighten. Inject cement into the medullary canal of the radius. The radial implant is pressed into the canal and excess cement is removed. Care is taken to insert the implant into the center of the canal and in correct alignment, avoiding malrotation, varus and palmar tilting (Fig. 13.15). Apply the trial polyethylene to the carpal component and reduce the joint. Apply an axial load across the joint until the cement has hardened. Remove the temporary fixation pin(s) from the

carpus. Using the trials, make a final determination of correct polyethylene thickness to optimize motion and stability. Slide the true polyethylene component in place and lock home using the polyethylene inserter (Fig. 13.16).

Staying dorsal to the carpal fixation screws, the intercarpal articular surfaces of the triquetrum, hamate, capitate, scaphoid, and trapezoid are removed using a curette or bur. Cancellous chips from previously resected bone are packed into the spaces. The capsule over the resected ulna is closed tightly to stabilize the distal ulna. The dorsal capsule of the radiocarpal joint is reattached to the distal margin of the radius using the previously placed sutures. If the capsule is deficient, the extensor retinaculum is divided in line with its fibers and one-half is placed under the tendons to cover the prostheses coverage. Meticulous closure of the capsule is mandatory to ensure postoperative stability and to protect the tendons from irritation. The remaining retinaculum is

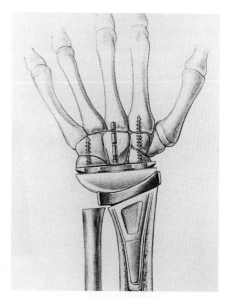

FIGURE 13.16. Universal Total Wrist prosthesis in place. Minimal bone resection is required. The entire carpus is supported by the carpal component, which does not rely on fixation in the metacarpal canals.

repaired over the extensor tendons to prevent bowstringing. The extensor carpi ulnaris tendon is brought dorsally over the ulna and held in place with a sling made from the retinaculum. The wrist is immobilized in a bulky gauze dressing and long arm plaster splint with the wrist in neutral and the forearm in supination. The sutures are removed after 10 days. A new long arm splint is applied for an additional 3 to 4 weeks. An X-ray is taken in the splint to confirm joint reduction. A wrist splint is used for the following month as hand use is gradually increased.

RESULTS/OUTCOMES

Wrist arthroplasty consistently provides good pain relief and an acceptable range of motion. In fact, pain relief after arthroplasty is equal to or better than fusion. Field et al. reported that 10 of 20 patients had mild to moderate pain after fusion (40). The main criticism of wrist arthroplasty has been the relatively early failures, with the primary modes being implant breakage, wrist imbalance, and prosthetic loosening. Breakage occurred primarily with the silicone Swanson implant but has not been a substantial problem with subsequent implants. Although wrist imbalance may occur with any type of prosthesis, especially if a severe preoperative wrist deformity was present, the ball and socket designs are much more prone to this complication than the newer prosthetic designs with an ellipsoidal articulation such as the Biaxial and Universal prostheses. Loosening has continued to be a major problem with most designs and is typically more common on the distal side. The most common method of distal component fixation relies on a stem cemented into the medullary canal of the third metacarpal. This design often requires excision of much of the central carpus resulting in less bony support for the component. As the arthritis progresses there may be further shift of the remaining carpus with motion developing at the carpometacarpal joint resulting in toggling and eventual loosening of the implant. The positive experience with the distal component fixation of the Universal prosthesis is in sharp contrast with nearly all reports on other prosthesis (31). The Universal wrist arthroplasty preserves more of the carpus including nearly the entire capitate and does not rely on metacarpal fixation. The carpal component supports the full width of the carpus and fixation is achieved at three sites within the carpus. An intercarpal arthrodesis is performed to provide solid bony support for the component and it prevents further destruction by synovitis. The wrist is essentially converted into a two-bone joint, which reduces the complexity of the arthroplasty, making it similar to other total joint arthroplasties. Loosening of the carpal component has not been a problem with the Universal wrist arthroplasty.

In Menon's first report of 37 Universal prostheses with a mean follow-up of 6.7 years (range 4 to 10 years), none of the cases demonstrated distal component loosening on radiographs (31). In a further follow-up study that included 57 implants, there was again no evidence of carpal component loosening (41). Radial component loosening occurred in 2 cases in which the component was placed uncemented. These components were reinserted using cement 2 and 3 years after the initial surgery with excellent results. Subsidence of the radial component has been observed but has not been progressive or symptomatic. Similar to other prosthesis, the Universal prosthesis provided consistently good pain relief (>90%) and a functional range of motion. Average postoperative motion was 41° flexion, 36° extension, 7° radial deviation, and 13° ulnar deviation. Dislocation has been the most common complication with this unconstrained prosthesis, with 5 occurring in Menon's first 37 cases and a total of 6 among all 57 cases in the later follow-up (31,41). The early higher incidence of dislocation can be partly attributed to the lack of availability of different implant sizes and thicknesses of polyethylene inserts at that time. In addition, Menon criticized himself for excessive bone resection in the earlier cases (41). Modularity of the polyethylene insert and multiple implant sizes have helped reduce the incidence of dislocation.

In the senoir author's experience with 31 implants, patients have generally been very satisfied with the Universal wrist arthroplasty and express appreciation for a painless and stable but also natural feeling wrist and the ability to perform activities of daily living without having to make physical accommodations due for their wrist. Three patients have chosen bilateral wrist arthroplasty after undergoing Universal wrist arthroplasty on one side. There has been no evidence of prosthetic loosening. Two patients with preoperative, highly active synovitis and severe joint laxity required open reduction, capsular imbrication, and prolonged immobilization for a late dislocation. One of these patients also had a concurrent revision of the carpal component to improve implant position. Both wrists recovered stability and satisfactory motion. Because the prosthesis is unconstrained and depends on capsular reconstitution for stability, patients with active synovitis and excessive joint laxity are not good candidates for the Universal prosthesis. However, radiocarpal joint subluxation or deformity by itself is not a contraindication. Patients with a subluxed but stiff wrist have done well and are among the most satisfied patients, achieving a stable wrist with functional motion.

REHABILITATION

Rehabilitation following Universal wrist arthroplasty follows many of the principles of wrist joint surgery involving ligament repair. A balance must be reached between motion and stability. The duration of postoperative immobilization will depend on the prosthetic stability observed by the surgeon at the time of the operation, but typically ranges from 2 to 4 weeks. If there is any tendency toward instability, increasing the duration of immobilization is recommended. Longer periods of immobilization have not appeared to cause long-term stiffness in rheumatoid patients. Immobilizing the wrist in neutral flexion-extension will allow the volar and dorsal portions of the capsule to heal with equal lengths. Initially placing the forearm in supination will help decrease tension on the volar capsule and reduce the risk of early volar dislocation of the prosthesis. Because the procedure may be associated with substantial postoperative swelling, strict elevation of the hand and immediate active finger motion are extremely important.

After the cast is removed, the patient is placed in a removable well-molded wrist splint for an additional 2 to 4 weeks during which time an active range of motion program for the wrist is performed. The amount of involvement by a therapist varies but is generally recommended when motion is initiated. Active flexion-extension and pronation-supination exercises are performed 4 times daily but passive motion is discouraged for the first 8 weeks postoperatively. After 8 weeks, strengthening exercises are added to the program. If needed, gentle passive range of motion may be performed at this time. Unrestricted use of the hand and wrist is allowed after 3 months. Although long-term activity restrictions are not well-defined for patients with a total wrist arthroplasty, impact loading and repetitive forceful movements should be discouraged.

COMPLICATIONS

The complications associated with total wrist arthroplasty are similar to other joint replacements, including the incidence of infection, which is approximately 1% to 2% (25,41). Perioperative antibiotics and closed suction drainage for 48 hours should be used. The upper extremity may be more prone than the lower extremity to develop a regional pain syndrome. Measures to prevent excessive swelling and appropriate pain management including the use of regional anesthesia may help reduce this risk. Fracture of the radius during broaching and malpositioning of the prosthesis are among possible technical complications. Preoperative assessment of the radiographs for bone quality, wrist deformity, and implant size will help the surgeon prepare for technical difficulties. Unconstrained prostheses carry an increased risk of dislocation, especially during the early postoperative period. Developing an appropriate immobilization and rehabilitation program suited to each patient will reduce the risk. Late dislocations are usually caused by a fall and may require open reduction. Prosthetic loosening, especially of the distal component, has been the most common late complication of total wrist arthroplasty and is related to the design of the implant. The Universal prosthesis has a unique distal component design that has demonstrated reliable long-term fixation. Dislocation has been the most common complication with the Universal prosthesis but appears to be related to excessive bone resection and failure to perform a complete closure of the capsule. Because the prosthesis is unconstrained, proper implant alignment and soft-tissue management are important

to its stability. In addition, patients with highly active synovitis and ligament laxity are not good candidates for this prosthesis. These operative indications and technical concerns have been applied equally to other joint arthroplasties for many years and should not be considered a limitation of wrist arthroplasty but rather an application of orthopedic principles.

Although wrist replacement has historically had a higher complication rate than arthrodesis, wrist arthrodesis is not without complications. A complication rate of 14% to 29% has been reported, with up to 65% of patients requiring plate removal (40,42). Zachary and Stern reported 45 soft-tissue and 29 bone and joint complications in 73 cases (43).

An overall survival of 91% in the initial series of Universal wrist arthroplasty with up to 10-year follow-up shows that a total wrist replacement with a sound design can be predictable and durable (31,41). However, as advocated for all other joints commonly treated by arthroplasty, precise handling of both the bone and soft-tissues will be necessary to achieve satisfactory results. Surgeons interested in performing this procedure should have a sound knowledge of wrist anatomy and understand the technical features specific to wrist arthroplasty.

SALVAGE OF A FAILED TOTAL WRIST ARTHROPLASTY

Revision arthroplasty, arthrodesis, and resection arthroplasty are options for salvaging a failed total wrist arthroplasty due to imbalance, loosening, or instability. The decision to perform a revision depends on the integrity of the bone and soft-tissues. Patients with poor bone stock or inadequate capsular tissue are not indicated for revision arthroplasty. Conversion to a newer prosthetic design that has better implant fixation should be considered. Iliac crest bone graft may be needed to fill defects and re-establish the basic architecture of the carpus. When using the Universal total wrist prosthesis, the graft can be transfixed to the remaining carpus using the carpal component fixation screws. An established infection should be treated by implant removal and either primary or delayed conversion to an arthrodesis. Resectional arthroplasty for prosthetic loosening or sepsis is an option but it causes significant loss of power and the overall outcome is unpredictable (2,44).

Salvaging a failed total wrist arthroplasty by arthrodesis has generally been successful. Lorei et al. reported on 9 failed arthroplasties, including 8 Trispherical and 1 Volz, with mechanical problems being the most common reason for failure (4). Five wrists underwent conversion to an arthrodesis, all of which achieved a painless, solid fusion after one operation at an average of 4.8 months. Beer and Turner reviewed 12 patients who underwent arthrodesis for failed arthroplasty, 8 of which were silicone implants (45). A tricortical iliac crest bone graft and intramedullary Steinmann pins were used. Seven wrists fused. Four developed a pseudoarthrosis at the graft-metacarpal junction and one at the graft-radius junction. There were 17 complications in 9 patients; however, all patients had markedly decreased pain and satisfactory function. Based on this experience, they recommended the use of more rigid internal fixation techniques (Figs. 13.17 and 13.18). In a review of wrist implant failures, Cooney et al. described four failures due to infection, chronic imbalance, or loosening treated by external fixation and bone grafting (44). There were no nonunions despite sepsis or wide excision of the carpus. Although a large block of autogenous iliac crest graft is typically used to fill the defect, femoral head allograft has been used successfully and reduces the operative morbidity (46).

Revision arthroplasty is an option for aseptic loosening if there is adequate bone stock or if bone grafting is feasible. The capsule is usually thickened and must be widely released to allow wrist flexion and extraction of the components. If there has been substantial subsidence, lengthening of the wrist flexors and extensor tendons may be required for exposure and revision. To remove a well-fixed, cemented component from the radius, the dorsal cortex can be finely split and delicately pried open to gain access to the cement mantle and proximal stem so the entire construct can be disimpacted as a unit. However, if possible, it is preferable to preserve cortical continuity when a revision arthroplasty is being considered.

In a series of 13 failed total wrist replacements of various designs treated by revision total wrist arthroplasty using the

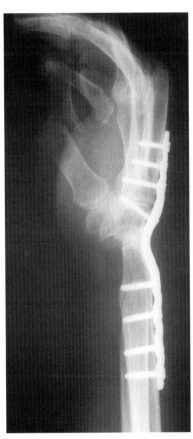

FIGURE 13.18. Total wrist arthrodesis performed for a failed Swanson implant.

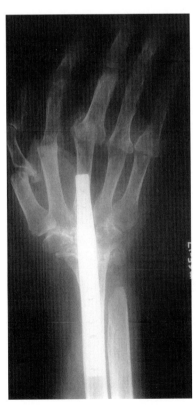

FIGURE 13.17. Total wrist arthrodesis performed for a failed Swanson implant.

Biaxial prostheses, 8 wrists had a functional arthroplasty, 2 wrists had undergone further revision for loosening, 1 wrist was fused, and 2 implants were loose but still in place at an average follow-up of 5.6 years (5). Cobb and Beckenbaugh reviewed the results of 10 revision arthroplasties using a custom Biaxial prosthesis with a multipronged distal component. At an average 3.8-year follow-up, 2 patients had undergone wrist arthrodesis, 1 for distal component loosening and the other for periprosthetic fracture, while the other 8 were functioning satisfactorily (26).

The decision to proceed with revision arthroplasty is difficult and must be weighed against the risk of further surgery for repeat failure. Although conversion to an arthrodesis is usually technically successful and preferred by surgeons, patients will often prefer revision arthroplasty despite the higher risks, especially if they have an arthrodesis of the opposite wrist.

ACKNOWLEDGMENTS

I would like to thank Tracy L. Chapman B.S. for her help in preparation of this manuscript and our continuing study of total wrist arthroplasty.

REFERENCES

1. Brase DW, Millender LH. Failure of silicone rubber wrist arthroplasty in rheumatoid arthritis. *J Hand Surg* 1986;11A:175–183.
2. Ferlic DC, Jolly SN, Clayton ML. Salvage for failed implant arthroplasty of the wrist. *J Hand Surg* 1992;17A:917–923.
3. Jolly SL, Ferlic DC, Clayton ML, et al. Swanson silicone arthroplasty of the wrist in rheumatoid arthritis: a long-term follow-up. *J Hand Surg* 1992;17A:142–149.
4. Lorei MP, Figgie MP, Ranawat CS, et al. Failed total wrist arthroplasty. *Clin Orthop* 1997;342:84–93.
5. Rettig ME, Beckenbaugh RD. Revision total wrist arthroplasty. *J Hand Surg* 1993;18A:798–804.
6. Comstock CP, Louis DS, Eckenrode JF. Silicone wrist implant: long-term follow-up study. *J Hand Surg* 1988;13A:201–205.
7. Swanson AB. Flexible implant arthroplasty for arthritic disabilities of the radiocarpal joint. A silicone rubber intramedullary stemmed flexible hinge implant for the wrist joint. *Orthop Clin North Am* 1973;4:383–394.
8. Fatti JF, Palmer AK, Mosher JF. The long-term results of Swanson silicone rubber interpositional wrist arthroplasty. *J Hand Surg* 1986;11A:166–175.
9. Stanley JK, Tolat AR. Long-term results of Swanson Siliastic arthroplasty in the rheumatoid wrist. *J Hand Surg* 1993;18B:381–388.
10. Peimer CA, Medige J, Eckert BS, et al. Reactive synovitis after silicone arthroplasty. *J Hand Surg* 1986;11A:24–38.
11. Smith RJ, Atkinson RE, Jupiter JB. Silicone synovitis of the wrist. *J Hand Surg* 1985;10A:47–60.
12. Rosello MI, Costa M, Pizzorno V. Experience of total wrist arthroplasty with siliastic implants plus grommets. *Clin Orthop* 1997;342:64–70.
13. Meuli HC. Arthroplasty of the wrist. *Clin Orthop* 1980;149:118–125.
14. Meuli HC. Meuli total wrist arthroplasty. *Clin Orthop* 1984;187:107–111.
15. Meuli HC, Fernandez DL. Uncemented total wrist arthroplasty. *J Hand Surg* 1995;20A:115–122.
16. Meuli HC. Total wrist arthroplasty. *Clin Orthop* 1997;342:77–83.
17. Volz RG. The development of a total wrist arthroplasty. *Clin Orthop* 1976;116:112–120.
18. Volz RG. Total wrist arthroplasty, clinical review. *Clin Orthop* 1984;187:112–120.
19. Lamberta FJ, Ferlic DC, Clayton MC. Volz total wrist arthroplasty in rheumatoid arthritis: A preliminary report. *J Hand Surg* 1980;5:245.
20. Dennis DA, Ferlic DC, Clayton ML. Volz total wrist arthroplasty in rheumatoid arthritis: A long-term review. *J Hand Surg* 1986;11A:483–489.
21. Menon J. Total wrist replacement using the modified Volz prosthesis. *J Bone Joint Surg* 1987;69A:998–1006.
22. Gellman H, Hontas R, Brumfield RH, et al. Total wrist arthroplasty in rheumatoid arthritis. *Clin Orthop* 1997;342:71–76.
23. Figgie HE III, Ranawat CS, Inglis AE, et al. Preliminary results of total wrist arthroplasty in rheumatoid arthritis using the trispherical total wrist arthroplasty. *J Arthroplasty* 1988;3:9–15.
24. Figgie MP, Ranawat CS, Inglis AD, et al. Trispherical total wrist arthroplasty in rheumatoid arthritis. *J Hand Surg* 1990;15A:217–222.
25. Cobb TK, Beckenbaugh RD. Biaxial total-wrist arthroplasty. *J Hand Surg* 1996;21A:1011–1021.
26. Cobb TK, Beckenbaugh RD. Biaxial long-stemmed multipronged distal components for revision/bone deficit total-wrist arthroplasty. *J Hand Surg* 1996;21A:764–770.
27. Hamas RS. A quantitative approach to total wrist arthroplasty: Development of a "precentered" total wrist prosthesis. *Orthopedics* 1979;2:245–255.
28. Beckenbaugh RD. Arthroplasty of the wrist. In: Morrey BF, ed. *Joint replacement arthroplasty.* New York: Churchill Livingstone, 1991:195–215.
29. Beckenbaugh RD. Total wrist arthroplasty. In: Cooney WP, Linscheid RL, Dobyns JH eds. *The wrist: Diagnosis and operative treatment,* vol. 2. St. Louis: Mosby, 1998:924–944.
30. Radmer, et al. Wrist arthroplasty with a new generation of prostheses in patients with rheumatoid arthritis. *J Hand Surg* 1999;24A:935–943.
31. Menon J. Universal total wrist implant: Experience with a carpal component fixed with three screws. *J Arthroplasty* 1998;13:515–523.
32. Goodman MJ, Millender LH, Nalebuff EA, et al. Arthroplasty of rheumatoid wrist with silicone rubber: an early evaluation. *J Hand Surg* 1980;5:114–121.
33. Vicar AJ, Burton RI. Surgical management of rheumatoid wrist fusion or arthroplasty. *J Hand Surg* 1986;11A:790–797.
34. Kobus RJ, Turner RH. Wrist arthrodesis for treatment of rheumatoid arthritis. *J Hand Surg* 1990;4:541–546.
35. Hastings H. Total wrist arthrodesis for post traumatic conditions. *Indiana Hand Cent Newsletter* 1994;1:14.
36. Millender L, Jalebuff E. Arthrodesis of rheumatoid wrist. *J Bone Joint Surg* 1973A;55:1026–1034.
37. Carroll R, Dick H. Arthrodesis of the wrist in rheumatoid arthritis. *J Bone Joint Surg* 1971A;53:1365–1369.
38. Mannerfelt L, Malmsten M. Arthrodesis of the wrist in rheumatoid arthritis: a technique without external fixation. *Scand J Plast Reconstr Surg* 1971;5(2):124–130.
39. Van Gemert JG. Arthrodesis of the wrist: a clinical, radiographic and ergonomic study of 66 cases. *Acta Orthop Scand Suppl* 1984;210:1–146.
40. Field J, Herbert TJ, Prosser R. Total wrist fusion. *J Hand Surg* 1996;21;4B:429–433.
41. Menon J. Total wrist arthroplasty for rheumatoid arthritis. In: Saffer P, Amadio PC, Foucher, eds. *Current practice in hand surgery.* London: Martin Dunitz, 1997:209–214.
42. Clendenin MB, Green DP. Arthrodesis of the wrist: complications and their management. *J Hand Surg* 1981;6:253–257.
43. Zachary BV, Stern PJ. Complications following AO/ASIF wrist arthrodesis. *J Hand Surg* 1995;20A:339–344.
44. Cooney WP, Beckenbaugh RD, Linscheid RL. Total wrist arthroplasty: problems with implant failures. *Clin Orthop* 1984;187:121–128.
45. Beer TA, Turner RH. Wrist arthrodesis for failed wrist implant arthroplasty. *J Hand Surg* 1997;22A:685–693.
46. Carlson JR, Simmons BP. Total wrist arthroplasty. *J Am Acad Orthop Surg* 1998;6:308–315.

DISTAL RADIOULNAR JOINT

KEITH A. GLOWACKI AND WILLIAM H. BOWERS

HISTORICAL PERSPECTIVE

Over the last two decades, and especially in the last 10 years, extremely important information has surfaced about many of the areas of the distal radioulnar joint (DRUJ). These areas, at one time referred to as the "low back" pain of the upper extremity, have now become the focus of numerous clinical and basic science studies (1–115).

A complete chapter on the distal radioulnar joint would have to include acute injuries of ligamentous and bony structures with the associated surgical repairs of those problems. Delayed diagnosis and subsequent reconstruction for chronic instability and chronic abnormalities resulting from factors would also be included. Finally, posttraumatic, degenerative, and inflammatory (rheumatoid) arthritis deformities would include reconstructive, resection arthroplasty, replacement arthroplasty, and salvage procedures. The focus of this chapter will be the arthritic disorders and treatment of late results after acute injuries. Salvage procedures such as hemiresection, Darrach, Sauve-Kapandji, and joint replacement will be discussed at length.

Painful derangements of the DRUJ and TFCC are more commonly recognized and treated. Diagnosis remains difficult and is often delayed. A systemic approach to diagnosis is most important. We propose an algorithm for management of disorders of the DRUJ including an authors' preferred section (Table 14.1).

The supervising physician must possess a thorough knowledge of the anatomy and function of this area. A careful and thorough history will direct a similar physical examination. Diagnosis continues with various imaging modalities. These include plain radiographs, CT scans, MRI, arthrograms, and motion series. Included in the evaluation are differential injections and diagnostic arthroscopy. Standard x-ray projections of the wrist plus various positions and grip loading views can help delineate ligamentous structures and give clues to the possibility of disruption. Arthrography as well as arthroscopy have long been used to evaluate chronic ligament tears, as well as changes in the joint cartilage. Selective anesthetic blocks may also give insight into the patient's cause for pain and functional loss. Technetium bone scans may be used as a screening tool to focus further studies. Computed

tomography of the radioulnar joint is now utilized extensively for evaluating articular alignment, arthrosis, and DRUJ dorsal or volar instabilities. Standard scans may include axial, sagittal, and coronal views in three different positions (supination, neutral, and pronation). MRI is being used more frequently due to the advent of extremity coils and new advances in the software. The addition of enhancing substances with MRI studies makes them much more informative. There is no doubt that arthroscopy as a diagnostic tool will continue to become more popular and more effective in both treatment and diagnosis for further planning of reconstructive and arthritic surgeries.

Arthritis of the DRUJ may be the cause of severe disability and pain. There exists a choice of procedures for treatment in this area but there is no one procedure that treats each patient in the best fashion. Once a very thorough history and physical examination have been performed and the diagnostic tests have been evaluated, it is the surgeon's clinical judgment that leads to the appropriate surgery.

Table 14.1 is a summary of the authors' recommendations for management of the arthritic disorders of the distal radioulnar joint. Each of these conditions will be discussed in this chapter from the viewpoint of joint dysfunction as a whole.

ANATOMY

The anatomy of the DRUJ and associated ligaments is complex, and a thorough understanding is necessary to manage the pathologic conditions that we will discuss further. It is well-known that the stability is achieved by articular contact and ligamentous stabilizers. The DRUJ articulation is trochoid, as is that of the proximal radioulnar joint. The shallow sigmoid articular notch has dimensions that are on the average 1.5 cm or so volar and 1 cm proximal to distal (Fig. 14.1). The notch has three distinct margins: dorsal, distal, and palmar. The dorsal margin is acutely angular in cross-section and palmar less so. The carpal (distal) margin is the junction between the notch and distally facing lunate facet. The two are separated by the attachment of the triangular fibrocartilage to the radius. The articulation of the ulnar head with the sigmoid notch is not congruous inasmuch as the radius of the sigmoid notch. Viewed from within the radioulnar joint, the styloid attachment appears folded. Between the folds, vessels enter the TFCC. This intra-articular fold and its vascular hilum have been termed the ligamentum subcruentum (Fig. 14.2C). The folded appearance is actually the confluence of the TFC and a V-shaped ligament, which extends from the styloid hilar area to twin insertions on the volar surface of the lunate and triquetral bones (Figs. 14.2A–C).

The peripheral margins of the triangular cartilage consist of thick lamellar collagen adapted to bear tensile loading (31). These are often referred to as the dorsal and palmar radioulnar ligamentous margins. The thin central portion, occasionally referred to as the articular disc, is chondroid fibrocartilage, a type of tissue seen in structures that bear compressive loads (20,21). The load-bearing function of the TFC is a subject of much discussion and controversy (13,16, 32,33). Compressive force across the carpal-ulnar articulation is partially transmitted through the center of the TFC to the ulnar dome. The same force tends to separate the radius and ulna (particularly in a neutral or negative variant wrist). The TFC resists this tendency, thus converting some of the compressive loading to tensile loading within the lamellar collagen of the periphery of the TFC (31). The TFC is assisted in meeting this functional demand by the muscular action of the pronator quadratus and interosseus membrane. The rest of the load is accepted by the ulnar dome. The distribution of the load is greatly influenced by the length of the ulna relative to the radius (ulnar variance), and this variance changes with grip and forearm position. Palmar and Werner have shown experimentally that in the neutral variant, 80% of the static axial load is borne by the radius, whereas 20% is borne by the ulna. If relative ulnar length is increased 2.5 mm, the load borne by the ulnar increases to 40% (16). The significance of the negative variant is unknown, but some of the force is probably converted to tension. The picture becomes more complicated when grip forces are applied as the forearm is rotated. Rotational movement of the radius-TFC complex over the ulnar dome allows a variety of load scenarios, as well

as constantly changing marginal ligament tension (Fig. 14.3). For instance, in pronation, load transmission through the lunate to the ulnar columns is via an infinitely negative ulnar variant. The load may be transmitted via tensile loading of the volar marginal ligament. In midrotation and supination, the load may be transmitted directly to the ulnar dome of the compressive loading. This variable loading may account for the location and nature of the tears seen in the TFC by Chidgey and others (20,21).

The marginal ligaments of the TFC are important, not only in load transference from the carpus to the ulna but also in the stability of the radioulnar joint. The stability of this joint as understood by Ekenstam, Hagert, and the senior author is depicted in Figure 14.3 (2,3,19,32,34–39). The joint is stable in the extremes of rotation, or the compressive forces between the radius and ulna are resisted by the reciprocal tensile forces developed within the opposite TFC marginal ligament.

A recent experimental study of pressure relationships within the joint with rotation seems to corroborate this theory (40). In this study, the pressure concentrates dorsally in pronation and palmarly and supination. The palmar margin of the TFC is taut in pronation, with tension developing as the dorsal margin of the radius and the ulnar articular surface are compressed. Should the palmar margin become torn, dorsal subluxation of the distal ulna would occur in pronation. Similarly, the dorsal margin of the TFC becomes taut in supination, while the palmar margin of the sigmoid notch and the ulnar articular surface are compressed. Should the dorsal margin become torn, palmar subluxation might occur. The integrity of the osseous shape of the convexity of the ulna articular surface and margins of the sigmoid notch obviously play corresponding roles (40).

An alternative view of the relative importance of the portions of the TFCC in stabilizing the DRUJ were expressed by Linscheid (41,42) and supported by Schuind and Van der Heijden (43). Linscheid noted that the dorsal margin ligament of the TFC was tight in pronation (41,42). At this posi-

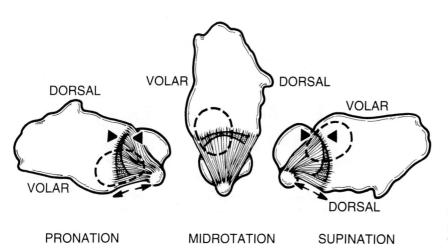

FIGURE 14.3. In pronation the volar portion of the TFC is under tension (*small arrows*) with compression on the dorsal surface (*large arrows*). Disruption of the volar TFC would, therefore, allow dorsal displacement of the ulna in pronation. In supination the opposite occurs. The dotted line represents the load transmission of the lunate to the TFCC in that position.

tion the ulnar head was compressed against the dorsal surface of the sigmoid notch. As supination occurs, the ulnar head seats firmly against the palmar surface of the sigmoid notch with a rolling, sliding motion. At this point, the palmar marginal ligament is taut. This theory was eloquently discussed by Van der Heijden, who corroborated the findings of Schuind (31). Both noted that the palmar marginal ligament of the TFC was significantly longer than its dorsal counterpart (mean of 3.2 mm longer; range, 1.9–7.9 mm) and insert together in the ulnar fovea. This theory suggests that in pronation, if the dorsal ligament is incompetent, dorsal displacement of the ulnar head would occur. This is partially supported by a study by Kihara et al. (44) in 1995, who demonstrated that subluxation did occur under each of these conditions. However, true dislocation did not occur until both dorsal and palmar marginal ligaments, as well as the pronator quadratus and interosseus membrane, became unstable. In Van der Heijden's study, the ulnocarpal ligaments were removed before testing, which perhaps influences some of the observations that forces generated on the carpus by the flexors in power grip caused displacement (43). This is seen in rheumatoid arthritis when progressive destruction of this ligament occurs. The styloid attachment of the complex provides a mechanism for stable, flexible attachment of the radiocarpal unit to the ulna, thereby permitting stable forearm rotations.

These two structures (TFC and ulnocarpal ligaments) are morphologically distinct and have individual roles even though the complex functions as a unit. The individual role of the combined ulnocarpal ligaments is to provide a stable connection between the ulna and volar-ulnar carpus (43,45). This ligament resists dorsal displacement of the distal ulna relative to the carpus in the radiocarpal unit. Destruction of this ligament as is commonly seen by attenuation in rheumatoid arthritis will allow volar displacement of the carpus in relation to the distal ulna, a condition even more obvious in pronation (the supinated carpal unit of rheumatoid arthritis).

Stability of the radioulnar and carpal unit is additionally influenced by the configuration of the sigmoid notch, the "slope" of the ulnar dome, the interosseus membrane, the extensor retinaculum, and the dynamic forces of the ECU and pronator quadratus, as well as by the dorsal carpal ligament complex (46). The latter can be visualized as a "star" centered over and blending with the dorsal peripheral margin of the TFCC. The proximal and distal legs are the ECU sheath extending from the ECU groove to the dorsal base of the fifth metacarpal. The radial legs are the proximal and distal radiotriquetral ligaments and the dorsal radiocarpal ligament. The ulnar leg is a wide ligament band proceeding from the center of the star around the ulnar aspect of the triquetrum distal to the styloid and attaching to the pisotriquetral joint capsule (Fig. 14.4).

The DRUJ capsule is uniformly thin and cannot be construed to offer stability in the usual sense. Dorsally, the capsule is minimally reinforced by the obliquely passing radiotrique-

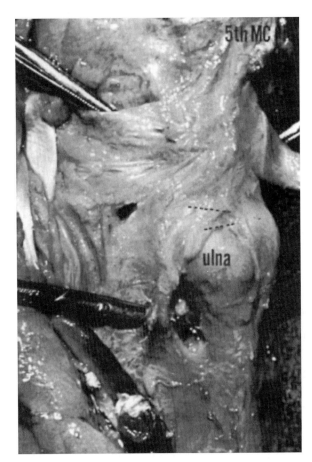

FIGURE 14.4. The dorsoulnar wrist ligament complex. The TFC is shown in dotted lines.

tral capsular ligament. It offers no coverage to the ulnar head. Spinner and Kaplan have called attention to the importance of the ECU musculotendinous unit in stabilizing the joint (10). The emphasis is warranted but should be shared by both the rather strong sheath system through which it runs and the strong volar ligament complex. Johnson and Shrewsbury (47) have demonstrated that the dual structure of the pronator quadratus stabilizes the radioulnar joint actively by maintaining coaptation of the ulnar head in the notch in pronation and passively by viscoelastic forces in supination.

INDICATIONS/CONTRAINDICATIONS

Posttraumatic and degenerative osteoarthritis of the distal radioulnar joint, although etiologically different, present similar problems with conservative and surgical treatment. The differential diagnosis for pain at the DRUJ includes arthritic deformities, instability, ulnocarpal impaction, subluxations, dislocations, DRUJ instability, and inflammatory conditions, i.e., rheumatoid arthritis. We will focus on the arthritic deformities involving the distal radioulnar joint.

Arthritis of the distal radioulnar joint is a common cause of disability and severe pain. In an area where pathoanatomic processes are only gradually becoming well-defined clinical entities, one must methodically gather data until a decision becomes very clear. Only then can treatment be rendered. Each patient needs to be assessed as to whether surgery will improve quality of life and which procedure will perform that goal the best.

The selection of a treatment option is often based on the occupational demands of the patient, and therefore, a careful work history is essential before any sequence of diagnostic maneuvers. It is critical to obtain a thorough understanding of the wrist motion, repetitions, and load to which the results of the surgical procedure will be subjected. After this is achieved, history taking should include age, dominance, symptom characteristics, and provocative questions designed to firmly fix in the examiner's mind the mechanism of injury or symptom production. The DRUJ is one of several structures on the ulnar side the wrist in which pathology can occur. Each of these areas needs to be examined to first decide whether the DRUJ is the source of patient disability. Specific palpation is most important because of the intimate location of these joints and their supporting structures. Palpation should be methodical and is often assisted by pressure with the eraser end of a pencil. Each joint is then individually stressed and manipulated to detect crepitation, pain, or snapping. The patient should then be asked to duplicate the motion that causes the symptoms, and this should be confirmed by the examiner's direct maneuvers. For example if the pronated, dorsiflexed wrist is rotated into supination and the patient experiences pain, this suggests possible stylocarpal impingement.

The predominating symptom of degenerative arthritis of the DRUJ is pain. The location is most commonly over the dorsal ulnar aspect of the wrist. Pain at the extremes of pronation and supination is often found. There is also commonly limited motion nearing these extremes. Only when the physician passively attempts to obtain full pronation or supination will the pain and crepitus then be felt. A history of symptom development is of a slow gradual increase in nature. Each area of the DRUJ including the ECU tendon, the distal ulna, the ulnar styloid, the DRUJ, the lunotriquetral ligament, the pisotriquetral joint, the triquetrohamate, radioulnar, and ulnocarpal ligaments must all be checked in turn. Frequently each of these joints may be individually injected with a local anesthetic in order to verify relief of the patient symptoms. Pre- and post-injection grip strength improvement of over 50% is frequently a good sign that the area in question represents the patient's pathology. Fluoroscopy with either a portable or stationary imaging device can allow a needle to be placed directly in the area of question. This allows for more reproducible diagnosis of various disorders.

Screening X-rays are obtained. It is important for a standardized technique to be performed in obtaining X-rays. This is increasingly important because the radioulnar joint and carpal pathologies are defined in terms of measurements (variance, carpal height, scapholunate angle and intercarpal distance), and these measurements are then used for surgical decision making. A standard zero rotation PA and lateral X-ray in neutral deviation is obtained (Fig. 14.5). Various motion series including ulnar deviation and radial deviation are usually supplemented for wrist series (Fig. 14.6). Provocative tests including certain positions, such as a clenched fist and full pronation and supination views, are added to supply more information regarding an instability pattern or arthritic process. A PA view of the wrist in degenerative arthritis shows narrowing of the joint space, sclerosis of the articular surfaces, and cyst and spur formation. Radioisotope scans may be very helpful in evaluating severe pain syndromes (48). Focal uptake makes subsequent films or arthrography more valuable as attention can be directed to the specific areas. Computed tomography with or without digital reconstruction has proved its clinical usefulness in evaluating subluxation and dislocation of the DRUJ (1,48–53). Its advantages are that it does not require precise positioning and can be done through a plaster cast, although films of the normal side are recommended. Digital reconstruction (54) is a technique that takes CT data and constructs a picture in any desired plane, not just a cross-section. The construction is limited only by the interpolation required for the area between scanned cuts. Recently developed CT programs allow the reconstruction of data so that a three-dimensional facsimile is obtained. Manipulation

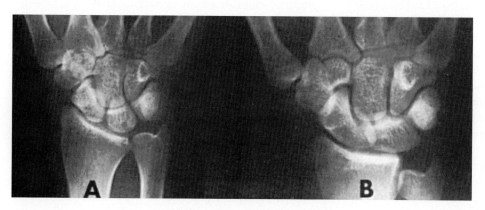

FIGURE 14.5. X-rays demonstrating positive (**A**) and negative (**B**) ulnar variance.

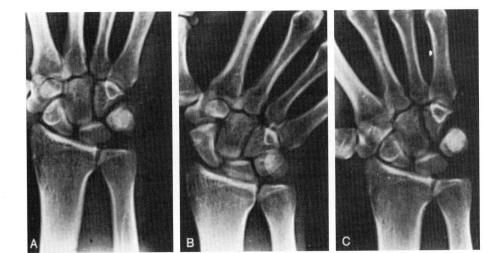

FIGURE 14.6. A standard zero rotation PA x-ray of the wrist (**A**), ulnar deviation (**B**), and radial deviation (**C**).

of these images can then be performed to either simulate surgical procedures or to view the joint from all aspects. Although not widely available, the technique has tremendous promise. Other diagnostic techniques include arthrography, arthroscopy, and magnetic resonance imaging. Arthrography is used commonly to determine wrist ligament pathology but also in degenerative cases. Frequently arthritic conditions of the DRUJ can be accompanied by associated ligamentous tears including the scapholunate, lunotriquetral, and TFCC areas. There is some debate as to whether or not triple versus single injection arthrography is as effective as wrist arthroscopy in diagnosis. Both are used rather commonly. It would be recommended that the physician be present upon the injection of contrast material. In this way a more dynamic view may be obtained of the path and course of the dye during fluoroscopy. This technique adds more detail and information to the diagnostic data, but positive findings do not prove causal relationships in all cases. Reinus et al. have noted a poor correlation of positive arthrographic findings with the initial pain symptoms or with plain film findings such as positive ulnar variance (57). Recent studies question the relevance of positive arthrograms because of a high incidence of symmetric lesions on both the symptomatic and asymptomatic sides and a poor correlation of physical examination and arthrographic findings (34,55–57).

Magnetic resonance imaging is now frequently combined with enhancing gadolinium for diagnosis of soft-tissue pathology as well as bony pathology. This technique is coming into its own. Newer, smaller extremity coils are becoming used specifically to evaluate the wrist. As the software to analyze these images also improves, this technique will be much more frequently used. This technique will be able to provide noninvasive, not radiating, real-time images of small joints and their ligaments. This most likely will replace arthrography as the gold standard.

Arthroscopy is more commonly being used over the last 5 to 10 years as not only a diagnostic but a therapeutic technique. There is no substitute for a direct visualization of a torn or degenerative area. The therapeutic extent to which arthritic disorders may be treated is still somewhat limited. This field will continue to expand and progress over the years. The DRUJ is a less predictably entered joint. On occasion, DRUJ loose bodies or chondromalacia can be seen and treated by those skilled in access (58). This field is far from static, and its maturity is eagerly anticipated.

PREOPERATIVE PLANNING

Surgical alternatives for the conditions of posttraumatic and degenerative osteoarthritis are: (a) excision of the distal end of the ulna by using the classic techniques popularized by Darrach; (b) one of the many modifications of this technique; (c) hemiresection arthroplasty and matched resection; (d) resection and replacement, arthrodesis, and/or creation of the proximal ulnar pseudoarthrosis to restore rotation (Sauve-Kapandji); or (e) other salvage procedures. A review of the indications, techniques, complications, and outcomes will be discussed.

In 1912 William Darrach (59) presented at the New York Surgical Society a patient with an unreduced palmar dislocation of the distal ulna treated by resection of its lower inch. He credited Dr. Kirby Dwight with the idea, although the procedure was first mentioned by DeSault (60) and later by Moore (61), Von Lesser (62), Lauenstein (63), Van Lannep (64), and Angus (65). The procedure now carries his name and has withstood the test of time and critical review over the years (66–72). This ablative-type procedure is the prototypical type of which several variations and subsequent new procedures will be discussed.

The patient type indicated for the original Darrach procedure is (a) the rheumatoid patient who has intractable pain at the distal radioulnar joint; (b) the rheumatoid or non-rheumatoid patient with an uncorrectable deformity due to subluxation on the distal radioulnar joint with or without extensor tendon ruptures (Caput Ulnae syndrome); and (c) the nonrheumatoid patient who has painful arthritis of the DRUJ characterized by marginal osteophytes, articular incongruity, and debris. Several areas somewhat controversial for this technique are those that involve loss of pronation, supination, ulnocarpal impingement, and failed previous DRUJ stabilization procedures.

In rheumatoid arthritis the ulnar compartment contains proliferative synovitis in the DRUJ, which stretches the ulnocarpal ligament complex. This results in changes referred to as Caput Ulnae syndrome. This syndrome is the result of destruction of the ligamentous complex. Dorsal dislocation of the distal ulna occurs with supination of the carpus on the hand and volar subluxation of the ECU. The ulnar side ligaments become stretched and subsequently allow this deformity to occur. This syndrome is seen in many rheumatoid patients who undergo hand surgery. This results in weakness and pain and is aggravated by forearm rotation. The tendon subluxation sets up a scenario for possible rupture of extensor tendons.

AUTHORS' PREFERRED METHOD: DORSAL APPROACH TO DISTAL RADIOULNAR JOINT

The following descriptive dorsal approach to the DRUJ is utilized for most of the procedures described further in this chapter.

The keys to exposure are the ECU and EDM tendons (Fig. 14.7). As the ECU enters the retinacular compartment it lies on top of the ulnar styloid in any position of forearm rotation. The EDM changes from muscle to tendon as it enters the retinacular compartment. The first centimeter of

this tendon lies on the radial attachment of the TFCC. The ulnar head can be made to pass between these two tendons if the arm is pronated. For exposure of the major portion of the ulnar articular surface, this procedure is begun in full pronation. The incision is begun laterally three finger breadths proximal the styloid along the ulnar shaft and curves gently around the distal side of the head to end dorsally at the midcarpus. For further extension distally it can be curved back ulnarly (Fig. 14.8A). The incision lies just dorsal to the dorsal sensory branch of the ulnar nerve, which must be found and protected from vigorous retraction or pressure during the procedure. As the skin flaps are developed, dorsal veins are retracted rather than cut if possible, and dissection is carried to the obliquely lying extensor retinacular fibers. Beneath the proximal border of the retinaculum the capsule of the ulnar head passes between the extensor digiti minimi and ECU tendons. A V-shape portion of ulnar shaft disappears proximally between the deep lying EIP muscle belly (Fig. 14.8B).

The proximal and ulnar half of the extensor retinaculum is reflected radially to uncover the ECU and EDM tendons. The base of this flap is the septum between the EDM and EDC compartment. Care is taken to not enter the EDC compartment. The EDM is retracted to reveal the dorsal margin of the sigmoid notch of the radius and TFCC (Fig. 14.8C–D). The capsule is sharply detached from the radius, with a 1 mm cuff for later repair. The capsule is then reflected toward the ulna to expose the ulnar head. A small lamina spreader may be used to view the sigmoid notch. To better expose the underside of the TFCC, the forearm should be brought into neutral rotation and a nerve hook or small right angle retractor used to expose this area. Loupe magnification is helpful

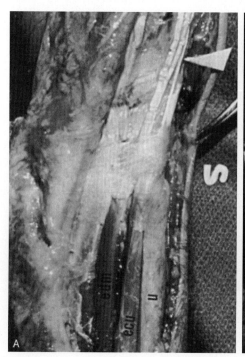 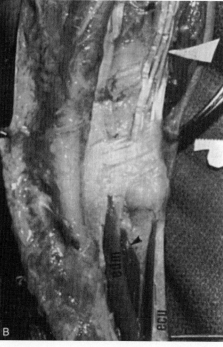

FIGURE 14.7. A. Exposure of the dorsum of the distal radioulnar joint in full supination. Note the extensor carpi ulnaris (ECU) and extensor digiti minimi (EDM) are adjacent. (U, ulnar shaft). **B.** The same specimen now fully pronated. The ulnar head passes between the ECU and EDM. Note the arrow pointing to the extensor indices proprius muscle belly.

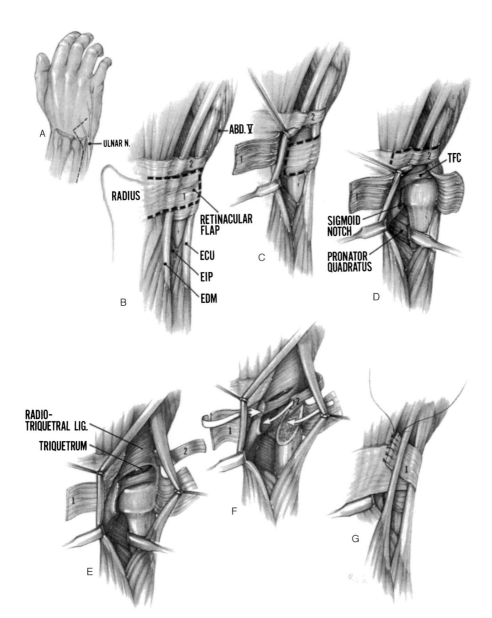

FIGURE 14.8. **A.** Operative approach of the distal radioulnar joint showing the incision and location of the ulnar sensory nerve. **B.** The dorsal retinacular structures and outline of the first retinacular flap. **C.** The proximal retinacular flap (1) and capsular incision (*dotted line*). **D.** The capsular flap reflected with exposure of the sigmoid notch. **E.** The retinacular flap (2) is developed and reflected to expose the radiotriquetral ligaments and TFC. Care is taken to reflect the ECU in its sheath as a unit to avoid potential dorsal destabilization. **F.** The ulnar head has been resected and the capsular flap covers the cancellous region exposed. The dorsal capsule is sutured to the volar capsule as interposition material. Retinacular flap (2) is used to cover the radioulnar articulation by suturing it to the previous capsular attachment on the radius. **G.** The first retinacular flap (1) is used to stabilize the ECU tendon. This step is unnecessary if the ECU was left undisturbed.

for observing changes in the TFCC. To further expose the TFCC, as this is frequently performed in these ablative procedures, both the EDM and ECU can be released from the retinacular compartment. This can be accomplished by reflecting the distal half of the extensor retinaculum opposite that of the first flap. The retinaculum is divided along the EDM septum, and the base of this flap is the attachment of the ECU compartment nearest the ulna. The ECU, where its groove is most pronounced, lies 1 to 2 mm ulnar to the attachment of the TFCC. The ECU should only be released fully if it is pathologically involved. The unviolated sixth compartment should be subperiosteally dissected from the ulnar shaft for exposure without disturbing its stabilizing function.

When the extensor digiti minimi and ECU are reflected to either side, one observes the transverse line fibers of the dorsal radiotriquetral ligament (Fig. 14.8E). This ligament may

be incised along its course for a good look at the lunate and triquetral surfaces of the TFCC. A triangular base flap may be elevated. For excellent exposure of the styloid, the forearm is carried to full supination with the groove of the ECU used to mark its dorsal base. The reflected capsule may be used as an interpositional arthroplasty flap if arthritis dictates partial distal ulnar resection. The ECU should be returned to its styloid groove, and the first retinacular flap can be used to stabilize dislocation of the tendon if necessary (Fig. 14.8F–G). Alternative retinacular flaps have been described by others (10,73).

The intact DRUJ surfaces and ulnocarpal joint structures cannot be fully explored by a single approach because of the intimacy of contact between the radius and ulna and the TFCC. This approach allows visualization of the dorsal 60% of the ulnar head and carpal base of the TFCC, the lunotriquetral ligament, the triquetrum, the prestyloid recess, and most of the DRUJ synovial cavity. If carefully dissected and replaced, none of this exposure should alter joint mechanics or stability. It is the procedure of resection that ultimately uncouples the rotational unit of the distal radioulnar joint. As discussed in the complication section, this leads to many of the instability problems and impingement frequently seen.

TECHNIQUE: DARRACH PROCEDURE

The ulna is approached by an incision that is extended proximally from the ulnar styloid process. The subcutaneous approach to the bone is done by separating the ECU and FCU tendons, with care taken to avoid the dorsal cutaneous branch of the ulnar nerve. The periosteum is incised and reflected from the distal 3 cm of the ulna. An osteotomy is made 2.5 cm or less proximal to the styloid or at the level of the proximal extent of the sigmoid notch. The author prefers to do the osteotomy by pre-drilling the cortex and then completing the cut with the saw, sharp osteotomes, or a bone cutter. Alternatively, a power saw can be used. The distal fragment is then dissected free, and the ulnar styloid process is osteotomized at its base and left in situ. The periosteal sleeve is closed to provide a firm attachment for the styloid process and ulnar collateral ligament, which will prevent abduction laxity. The wound is closed in layers, as instructed by Darrach. A splint is applied and active motion is encouraged in 24 hours. Dingman (69) and more recently DiBenedetto (74), Nolan and Eaton (70), and Tulipan et al. (72) have reviewed the procedure with regard to the technical points of extraperiosteal or subperiosteal resection, the obliquity of the cut, whether or not to remove the styloid, and the amount of bone to be resected. Dingman's study suggested that none of these factors other than the amount of bone resection was a critical determinant of a good outcome. He suggested that only the ulna adjacent to the sigmoid notch of the radius be removed. His preference was that the styloid process be left in situ and resection be subperiosteal, because those patients in whom regeneration had occurred appeared to have had better results. The shorter period of immobilization after surgery, the sooner the patient returned to work. The authors agree with these findings, particularly on the amount of ulnar resection and, in fact, the development of the hemiresection arthroplasty arose out of the attempts to preserve as much of the ulnar shaft component as possible (see hemiresection arthroplasty section).

COMPLICATIONS

The Darrach procedure is not without difficulties (32,71,75, 76). Increased ulnocarpal translocation, although theoretically possible, is not shown in patients unless they have had the radiocarpal ligaments disrupted by trauma or rheumatoid arthritis. This would be a contraindication to a Darrach procedure unless a stabilizing procedure was combined such as a radiolunate fusion. There are some reports of decreased grip strength although the authors have noticed increased grip strength in patients in whom the procedure has been appropriately used.

The Darrach procedure does destroy the bony support for the TFCC. In addition to creating ulnocarpal instability, it creates "unstable" rotation of the radiocarpal unit around the ulnar axis. With muscular action, the ulnar stump abuts the radius and irritates the overlying tissues. This may be seen as painful snapping and cause rupture of tendons, or both. There are no excellent salvage procedures for the painful instability of a too short Darrach resection. Some options are found in certain modifications used to improve the Darrach procedure. Forearm bracing has found some limited success in long-term usage. For these reasons, use of the Darrach procedure today should be very selective. Given the newer techniques available for posttraumatic arthrosis, most reserve the Darrach procedure for only the lowest demand patients, such as rheumatoid arthritics. In some of those situations the procedure should be combined with a radioulnar fusion or other radiocarpal stabilization procedures (71).

TECHNICAL MODIFICATIONS

To mitigate the instability created by the Darrach excision, a variety of modifications have been proposed. Swanson has replaced the distal ulna with a silicone cap, which provides a focus about which ligament reconstruction may take place (77,78). Its greatest proven application is in the rheumatoid DRUJ. Disruption and dislocation of the implant are problems as well as silicone synovitis (79,80). Blatt and Ashworth (81) have sutured a flap of the volar capsule to the dorsal ulnar stump to hold it down. Leslie et al. (82), O'Donovan and Ruby (83), and Webber and Maser (84) suggested tethering the distal stump with a distally based strip of the ECU. The intact portion of the ECU is then stabilized in a permanent dorsal position as Spinner and Kaplan have suggested (10). Kessler and Hecht (85) suggested dynamic stabilization of the ulnar stump by looping a strip of tendon around the distal ulnar stump and the ECU and tying the two together. Many other authors have used variations of ECU, FCU, or both threaded through ligaments and/or the canal to stabilize the ulnar stump (86–88). We have used some of these procedures with success in failed Darrach procedures. A further adjunct in the management of an unstable distal ulnar stump may be the pronator advancement flap of Johnson (89). A variation on the direction of pronator interposition has been used with success by Ruby et al. (90). Kleinman and Greenberg (91) have used both ECU tenodesis and pronator interposition with pins to salvage failed Darrach procedures. Bieber, Bell, and Minami all recommend that procedures not be done in younger, nonrheumatoid patients (67,92,93).

Reoperation on such patients rarely is successful. Hartz and Beckenbaugh reported good results performing the Darrach procedure with 82% of patients having good or excellent results and improvement of grip strength (94). Some recent reports have not been uniformly positive. Field et al. (95) found only half of 36 patients had a satisfactory result. Most continued with pain and weakness. The presence of osteoarthritis was most associated with a poor outcome. Because of these problems with the ablative procedure, further procedures were designed to help deal with the unfortunate uncoupling of the radius and ulna distal axis.

PARTIAL RESECTION ARTHROPLASTIES

The problems associated with the Darrach operation were improved upon by Bowers (96) in 1985, and Watson et al. (97) in 1986. Both proposed a limited resection of the articulating surfaces of the distal ulna. The ulnar styloid axis and soft-tissue attachment to TFC were left intact. These were operations designed to handle the resultant shaft instability found after many Darrach procedures. Partial resection arthroplasties require more surgical skill and attention to detail. Adequate resection is important to prevent postoperative impingement between the remaining ulnar shaft and radius. Despite meticulous techniques radioulnar convergence still occurs. This is the result of forearm rotation and gripping secondary to muscular contraction.

HEMIRESECTION INTERPOSITION TECHNIQUE

This procedure is an outgrowth of what Dingman (69) described as the best Darrach procedures, i.e., those in which minimal resection was followed by regeneration of the ulnar shaft within the retained periosteal sleeve. The articular ulnar head is resected only leaving the shaft/styloid relationship intact. An interposition of tendon, muscle, or capsule is placed in the vacant DRUJ synovial cavity to limit contact of the radial and ulnar shafts, which tend to approach each other after the procedure as mentioned (Fig. 14.9). The procedure supposes an intact or reconstructable TFCC. It should not be used in situations in which ulnar variance is positive unless the ulna is shortened as part of the procedure. This avoids a common problem of stylocarpal impingement. A majority of cases in patients with rheumatoid arthritis with TFCC will be unreconstructable. Here a modified Darrach procedure coupled with radiolunate arthrodesis is a good choice. Another alternative is the Sauve-Kapandji procedure, which is discussed later. An additional contraindication is preoperative evidence of ulnocarpal translation.

AUTHORS' PREFERRED TECHNIQUE

The initial exposure is as illustrated in Figure 14.8 and as described earlier. There is no need to enter the radiocarpal joint or expose the carpal surface of the TFC unless pathology is suspected therein. The retinacular flaps are developed for exposure and to conserve tissue for dorsal stabilization of the ECU (proximal flap) or augmentation of the deficient TFCC (second or distal flap.) If not needed for these purposes, the flaps may be reattached, used for deep cover of the arthroplasty site, or excised. The ECU should not be removed from its retinacular compartment if it is stable. Subperiosteal reflection of the compartment is possible and allows excellent exposure of the distal ulnar area. When returned to its position, the ECU will assume its stabilizing function. Stabilization of the ECU is done only if it is displaced palmarly or is unstable in the compartment. In these instances the ECU is freed to its insertion in the fifth metacarpal. The proximal flap is then used to create a sling. This technique is similar to that recommended by Spinner

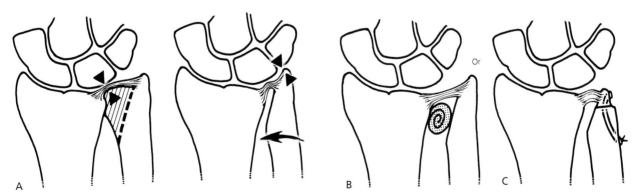

FIGURE 14.9. **A.** The hemiresection technique used in ulnocarpal impaction syndrome. The arrows represent stylocarpal impingement, a condition caused by approximation of the radius and ulna when the articular dome is removed. **B.** Interposition or **C.** shortening are necessary to fix this impingement. This should be considered in every hemiresection case and fluoroscopic image used to determine intraoperatively if necessary.

and Kaplan (10). It varies in that after the flap is passed around the ECU, the distal end is sewn to the fourth compartment wall distal to its takeoff. This ensures a sling rather than a noose (see Fig. 14.8G).

After development of the retinacular flaps, the DRUJ capsule is detached distally, radially, and proximally. This exposes the articular surface. A synovectomy is done, and the ulnar articular surface and subchondral bone are removed with small osteotomes and rongeurs. Inadequate bone removal is the most likely technical error at this point (98). Large osteophytes around the sigmoid notch and all of the bone of the ulnar head under the articular surfaces must be removed. The remaining shaft and styloid axis should be round in cross-section and resemble a tapering dowel. The volar portion of the head is particularly easy to miss in the depths of this incision. A complete synovectomy is then performed and the TFC carefully inspected. Lesions of the TFC will be readily apparent. If central perforations exist, they are now functionally inconsequential because of the resected ulnar head.

The decision about shortening, which was begun preoperatively with radiographic impressions about possible stylocarpal impingement, should be completed at this point. The radial and ulnar shafts should be compressed and rotated with the wrist ulnarly deviated. If there is any question about impingement, the ulna should be shortened. Shortening may be done through the metaphyseal base at the site of previous ulnar head or by more proximal osteotomy with plating. If the former site is chosen, fixation is accomplished with a compression interosseous wire loop (see Fig. 14.9C). The radioulnar space may be maintained by placing a carefully made ball of tendon about the size of the resected dome into the vacant DRUJ cavity (see Fig. 14.9B) and stabilizing into the dorsal/volar capsules with a few sutures. The material may be obtained from the palmaris longus, ECU, or FCU. This added interposition bulk adequately captures the radioulnar shaft approximation and therefore obviates stylocarpal impingement in borderline cases (zero variant, 1 mm).

Closure is accomplished as discussed in the approach to the joint. The ECU compartment is replaced in its original position or stabilized by using the sling. If no shortening is done, a postoperative short arm bulky dressing with dorsal and palmar plaster is applied. Finger motion is encouraged, and early antiedema and range of motion performed with occupational hand therapy. At two weeks, suture removal is accomplished, and a wrist splint allowing unrestricted rotation is applied for two more weeks.

If ulnar shortening is done in association with a hemiresection, the initial plaster reinforcement splint goes above the elbow and limits forearm rotation. This operative dressing is converted to a short arm cast with interosseous molding at two weeks. This allows slightly more rotation and is removed four weeks later (six weeks postoperatively). A wrist splint is then used for the transition to full use over the next several weeks. The osteotomy, if done at the site of the ulnar head

resection, will usually heal in six weeks. If the resection is done at the shaft level, the osteosynthesis should be protected with an Orthoplast forearm splint until full healing at approximately 12 weeks.

The operation has an inherent problem. If the articular surfaces are removed with sufficient bone to unload an abnormally loaded ulnocarpal articulation and avoid contact with arthritic or unstable radial and ulnar shafts in rotation, the biomechanical factor becomes obvious. The normal dome provides a stable seat for the radius to ride its rotational part. Absence of the seat allows the two shafts to come together, especially in power grip. The usual maximal migration of the radius and ulna toward one another is 0.75 cm in this operation. In a grip view, the distance measured from the radial styloid to the ulnar styloid may be 0.75 cm less than before surgery. If, on a preoperative x-ray view in neutral rotation, this amount of narrowing would allow the styloid to come within 2 mm of the ulnarly deviated carpus, one may anticipate impingement of the ulnar styloid on the carpus after the procedure. Some provision must be made, as mentioned, to performing an ulnar shortening in order to prevent the most common complication known as stylocarpal impingement.

The procedure cannot succeed if the TFCC is not a functional structure. This most often occurs, as mentioned, in rheumatoid arthritis or traumatic disruption. If the TFCC can be reconstructed and DRUJ arthritis exists, the hemiresection excels (93). The procedure will fail if stylocarpal impingement is not anticipated and prevented. Isolation of the ECU and sheath reconstruction by retinacular flaps are necessary only in rheumatoid patients with ECU instability. The procedure cannot restore stability in an unstable painful radioulnar joint. It simply substitutes a less painful instability. A correctly planned and performed arthroplasty using a hemiresection interposition technique may not alone restore rotation in long-standing contracture. Loss of flexibility in the ulnocarpal ligament complex as well as the interosseous membrane may preclude a good result even if the central arthritic obstruction is removed. This poor result can be anticipated in patients with a dystrophic forearm such as occasionally seen following trauma.

MATCHED DISTAL ULNAR RESECTION

In 1986 Watson described the matched ulnar resection as a treatment for the painful and compromised DRUJ (97). This is also a procedure introduced to address the complications inherent with the Darrach procedure. Similar to the previous hemiresection technique the preservation of the ulnar shaft styloid axis is maintained to decrease postoperative instability. The TFCC and ulnocarpal sling mechanisms are maintained as the DRUJ and distal ulnar dome are resected. According to Watson, scar tissue forms around the resected bone and stabilizing structures once this procedure is performed (97). The distal ulna is resected convexly at the DRUJ articular surface to "match" the corresponding radial metaphysis concavity. Three-quarters of the arc of the distal ulna is resected to avoid impingement in full pronation and supination. The increased interval between the shaft of the ulnar styloid and metaphysis of the distal radius prevents impingement. Indications for this procedure described by Watson include chronic subluxation, dislocation, or DRUJ incongruency (97). This includes patients with degenerative or posttraumatic arthritis, rheumatoid arthritis, and congenital anomalies. Patients with evidence of ulnocarpal impingement are also a contraindication to this procedure.

Watson uses a transverse incision made dorsally beginning approximately 2.5 cm proximal to the distal ulnar articular surface (97). Careful attention is employed to protect superficial nerves and veins. A portion of 5 to 6 cm of the distal ulna is resected, keeping a cuff of periosteum and ligamentous structures attached to the distal ulna. The ulna is resected in a long arc sloping to curve and match the opposing concave radius (Fig. 14.10). Fluoroscopic image is useful during this procedure but direct visualization of the interval under-supination and full pronation ensures adequate bone resection. The standard approach and closure is also performed after this procedure. It is possible to interpose or stabilize with structures such as pronator quadratus or capsule but it is not described by Watson.

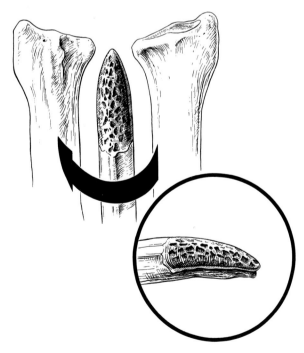

FIGURE 14.10. The resected DRUJ is fashioned to match the corresponding concave radial metaphysis as shown. (Reprinted with permission from Dr. Kirk Watson, Hartford, CT.)

Potential complications exist where the proximal portion of the sigmoid notch is more prominent than the distal portion. This proximal portion should be resected to avoid ulnar impingement (99). At times the dorsal and volar margins of the sigmoid notch are prominent and should also be resected to prevent impingement. Ulnocarpal impingement can be avoided if the resected ulna is no longer than the end of the adjacent radius.

SAUVE-KAPANDJI PROCEDURE

Distal radioulnar joint fusion with the creation of a proximal pseudoarthrosis to the fusion site is known as the Sauve-Kapandji procedure. In 1936 Sauve (100) and later Kapandji (101) proposed an operation describing this process. This procedure is described as a salvage-type procedure treating patients who have undergone unsuccessful distal ulnar surgery. The other salvage procedures are creation of a one bone forearm and a massive resection of the distal ulna. The Sauve-Kapandji procedure was advanced as an alternative management of DRUJ disorders previously treated by the Darrach distal ulna head resection.

Patients who are considered for this surgery have already undergone multiple procedures about the distal ulna. They will remain symptomatic with a painful DRUJ, instability, degenerative arthritis, or rheumatoid arthritis. They may have severe functional loss of pronation and supination. This procedure provides for restoration of malrotation by excisional arthroplasty of the ulna just proximal to the fusion site.

The most frequent complication arising from the use of this technique and many of the others is still instability of the distal ulnar stump. There are numerous stabilization techniques described. Comparison of all these techniques has been difficult and somewhat unreliable. According to Goncalves (102), the Sauve-Kapandji procedure offers the advantages of avoiding potential progressive ulnar translation of the carpus as found in rheumatoids, ulnar deviation and subsequent instability with pain and weakness of grip. By preserving the ulnar base against the distal radius as it continues from the sigmoid notch, these potential complications are avoided.

Indications are similar to those for the Darrach procedure and especially when dealing with a younger, more vigorous population. Indications include (a) osteoarthritis or severe chondromalacia of the DRUJ, (b) posttraumatic ulnocarpal impingement associated with distal radioulnar joint arthrosis, (c) younger rheumatoid arthritic patients with ulnar translocation in addition to DRUJ disease, (d) rheumatoid arthritis patients who may need a stable radioulnar surface for support of an arthroplasty or implant, and (e) nonrheumatoid patients with distal radioulnar joint subluxation or dislocation when other options such as ulnar shortening or reconstruction are not feasible. Recently, many others have expressed satisfaction with this procedure (101–107).

OPERATIVE TECHNIQUE

The technique for the Sauve-Kapandji procedure was well described by Taleisnik (108). A longitudinal incision is preferred and placed in the space between the ECU and FCU tendons 2 to 3 cm proximal to the prominence of the head to just distal to the styloid. The extensor carpi ulnaris retinaculum and subsheath are left undisturbed. The neck of the ulna is exposed and the periosteum removed in the area of the planned ulnar resection and pseudarthrosis. The ulna head is grasped with a large towel clip for better control. This will serve to manipulate in the case where an ulnar shortening secondary to positive variance is indicated. An osteotomy is performed transversely no more than 2 mm proximal to the articular margin of the distal ulna (Fig. 14.11). One to 1.5 cm of ulna is then excised. If there is a need to perform an ulnar shortening into the notch, the ulnar head needs to be recessed proximally until it faces the sigmoid cavity of the radius. Neutral rotation is usually selected. The ulna is then hinged away from the radius, exposing the opposing radioulnar articular surfaces. The areas are decorticated down to cancellous bone. The head is then placed against the radius and pinned with either K-wires (.0625 or .045 inch types), or with screws. Bone graft can be packed into this portion when fixation is complete. Usually bone graft can be taken from the excised portion of the ulna. Next the pronator quadratus is brought into the pseudarthrosis gap and sutured to the sheath of the ECU, as described by Sauve and Kapandji (100, 101). If the ulnar stump still appears unstable, particularly in pronation, a capsular flap can be brought over the dorsal end of the ulna in a manner similar to that described by Blatt and Ashworth (81) or an FCU or ECU tenodesis (86–88) procedure may be considered (Fig. 14.12). The pronator quadratus

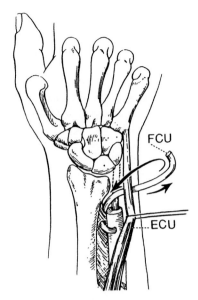

FIGURE 14.12. Stabilization of the ulnar stump using the FCU. (Reprinted with permission from Tsai TM, Stillwell JH. Repair of chronic subluxation of the distal radioulnar joint using flexor carpi ulnaris tendon. *J Hand Surg* 1984;9B:289–293.)

is usually sutured through drill holes made in the dorsal margin of the ulna. A 3.0 nonabsorbable suture passed through 0.035 K-wire holes is performed. This fusion should be protected approximately six weeks with a short arm splint though motion is allowed a few days after surgery, and progression of motion continues depending on the level of pain. Usually three to four weeks postoperatively one of the two K-wires may be removed if this fixation was used. A second wire is removed after the fusion appears solid in six to eight weeks.

Rothwell et al. (109) advocate a simplified technique for this procedure. A modification does not involve excision of the periosteum over the pseudarthrosis site, the pronator quadratus is not advanced into the defect, and superficial portions of the sheath overlying the ECU are sutured to the periosteum as their means of stabilization. With early reported good results this technique is less complicated and shows promising results. Further follow-up is needed. In this study arthrodesis was found in 78% of their patients despite no decortication (109).

Many others have reported favorable results regarding the classic Sauve-Kapandji procedure. Taleisnik has reported a surgical technique and results in 24 patients with greater than 1 year follow-up (108). Elimination of pain, restoration of forearm rotation, and few complications led him to express satisfaction with the procedure. The theoretically predictable complications of unstable proximal ulnar stump were observed in only 3 of the 24 patients. Minami et al. (110) reported favorable results in patients undergoing this technique for osteoarthritis of the DRUJ. Despite some of their patients showing evidence radiographically of an unstable ulnar shaft and convergence, this did not correlate with poor

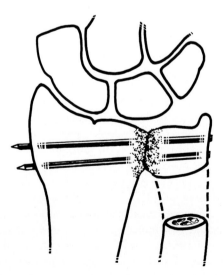

FIGURE 14.11. The Sauve-Kapandji procedure as described by Taleisnik. (Reprinted with permission from Taleisnik J. The Sauve-Kapandji procedure. *Clin Orthop* 1992;275:110–123.)

postoperative functional results and pain. Taleisnik reported that less favorable results were found in some patients with posttraumatic distal ulnar instability (108). He reported the need for reoperation in a minority of patients for stabilization of the proximal ulnar stump. Attention to the indications when selecting appropriate patients and a careful surgical technique will give the most consistent results.

Radioulnar Arthrodesis

Radioulnar arthrodesis and the creation of a one bone forearm is used as a means of treating failed surgery about the distal ulna. This is a major salvage procedure used as a last resort for stabilization of a forearm. If a stable forearm is paramount and rotation can be sacrificed, the technique of Carroll and Imbriglia (111,112) is trustworthy. A dorsal curvilinear incision is made over the DRUJ. The exposure continues as described previously (see Fig. 14.8). The periosteum is stripped from the ulna just proximal to the articular surface. The dorsal radioulnar ligaments are stripped sharply and if the distal ulna is still remaining, the articular cartilage is removed with osteotomes. If the distal ulna has been removed or a part of the distal ulna is missing, the remaining portion of the distal ulna is decorticated. The radius is then prepared with a drill and small osteotomes. A notch is made in the ulnar aspect of the distal radius where the distal ulna can be slotted. The corticated notch in the radius depends on the length of the ulna. It is manually compressed into the notch with the forearm held in 10° to 15° of pronation. Bone graft has been recommended at this point (Fig. 14.13). When the surgeon is satisfied with the position, K-wires are driven from

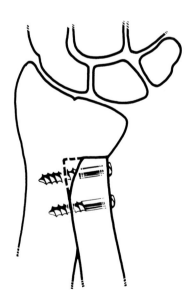

FIGURE 14.13. Distal radioulnar arthrodesis as described by Carroll and Imbriglia. (Reprinted with permission from Carroll RE, Imbriglia JE. Distal radioulnar arthrodesis. *Orthop Trans* 1979; 3:269.)

the ulna into the radius and two lag screws, 3-0 cannulated or 4 mm compression type, are driven from the outer aspect of the ulna through the cortices of the radius. The compression aspect of the technique is very important because the ulna tends to distract laterally. Simple K-wire fixation is not recommended, nor does single screw fixation seem able to provide enough strength. Occasionally a plate and screws may be used as well. The forearm is fixed in either neutral position or slight pronation and is immobilized in surgery until bony union is present. A long arm cast is applied and immobilization is continued for approximately eight weeks.

Peterson et al. (113) reported the Mayo Clinic experience with the operation. Their union rate was 68%, with 69% of patients achieving good or excellent results. The 32% nonunion rate did not correlate with a poor clinical result.

One-bone forearm creation is, at this point, used as the last possible salvage procedure. With new research and techniques regarding distal ulna arthroplasty we may find this procedure reserved for only severe complications following distal ulna resections and surgery.

EXTENSIVE DISTAL ULNA RESECTION

Cooney et al. indicated generally favorable results with an extensive resection of the distal ulna (114). The experience and results have come mainly from tumors involving the distal ulna. They reported some problems with instability and convergence of the radius and the ulna such as those found undergoing a Darrach procedure (114). The subcutaneous approach is carried out to the ulna and the resection is performed.

Results indicate functional relief of pain after the extensile resection of the distal ulna may be good or excellent in most patients. This study found a high percent of normal grip strength was preserved and 80% to 90% of range of motion remained in all planes. There was no correlation to grip strength, range of motion, and the amount of ulna resected. These results are encouraging; however, this extensive resection is again an extreme form of salvage procedure (114). Further studies and results with outcomes are needed.

ULNAR HEAD PROSTHETIC ARTHROPLASTY

Another form of salvage and possibly eventually an initial treatment for distal radioulnar joint arthrosis is a combined ulnar head prosthesis with soft-tissue procedure. The previous partial resections and procedures described inevitably all will compromise this function of an intact normal distal radioulnar joint. The instability manifested after a procedure to deal with instability, arthrosis, and various other disorders may be addressed by replacement of an ulnar head prosthesis recreating the forces in the sigmoid notch, the length of the ulnar shaft and repairing the soft-tissues accordingly to create

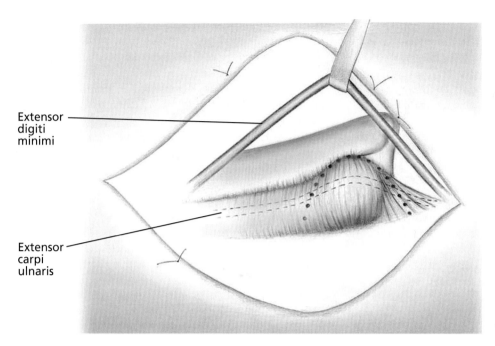

Extensor
digiti
minimi

Extensor
carpi
ulnaris

FIGURE 14.14. The capsular reti-nacular flap is marked out as shown with the dotted line.

a strong envelope. This procedure is performed by only a handful of surgeons around the world at this time. There is no other reliable procedure to deal with post-resection insta-bility in the chronically incapacitated patient in whom multi-ple surgical procedures have been attempted. There is a need for a reliable procedure to address this common problem associated after excisional arthroplasty. This can be thought of as a salvage at this point but may develop into a more reli-able and primary procedure with longer follow-up and favor-able outcomes (115).

This is a porous-coated titanium stem that supplies an interference fit with the medullary canal of the ulna. The stem has a range of different collar sizes, but it is recom-mended to adjust length to a 2 mm ulnar minus variant. In cases with excessive shortening of the ulna, a custom prosthe-sis is recommended. A ceramic (zirconium oxide) head was chosen as the articulating surface. The procedure is per-formed through a dorsal approach with an ulnar-based cap-suloretinacular flap. The flap begins at the bed of the EDM tendon, where the capsule attaches to the rim of the sigmoid

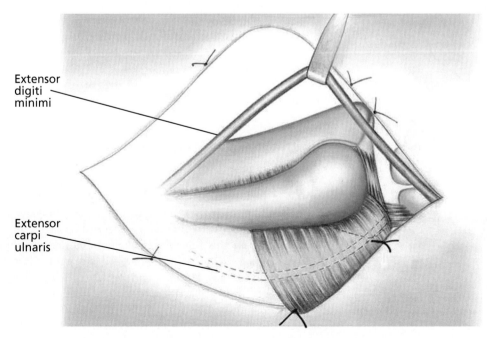

Extensor
digiti
minimi

Extensor
carpi
ulnaris

FIGURE 14.15. Retracting the flap allows exposure of both the DRUJ and ulno-carpal joints. The sixth com-partment should not be opened as it forms the base of the flap (ex-tensor carpi ulnaris).

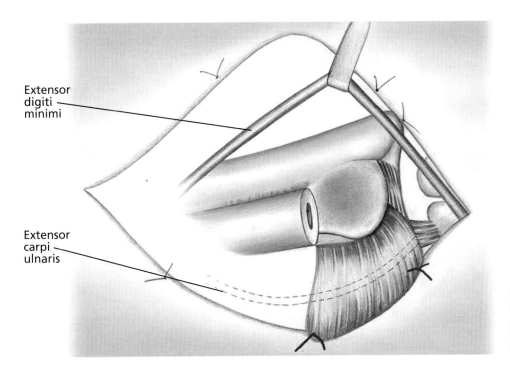

Extensor
digiti
minimi

Extensor
carpi
ulnaris

FIGURE 14.16. Following resection of the ulnar head, the TFC is carefully inspected. Soft-tissue flaps may be used to reinforce or repair a torn fibrocartilage.

fossa (Fig. 14.14). This is elevated as a full thickness layer including capsule and extensor carpi ulnaris with retinaculum. This is carefully freed from the dorsal surface of the TFCC and its bony attachments to the ulna. An important portion of this procedure is a careful inspection of the TFCC and either repair or reconstruction as necessary using local soft-tissue, flaps, or reconstruction (Fig. 14.15). The ulnar cut is performed using fluoroscopic image to verify the appropriate position of a trial component into the remaining sigmoid notch. At times the sigmoid notch needs to be reamed to fit the appropriate sized head. It is recommended to place the largest head possible for both stability but also allow soft-tissue closure without tension (Fig. 14.16). After reaming the ulnar shaft a trial prosthesis is used to check which sides of head and stem restores optimal length and stability (Fig. 14.17). Adjustments can be made with a reaming

device or bur to the sigmoid notch if necessary to create a seat for the ulnar head. The flap is then sutured back onto the triangular fibrocartilage with nonabsorbable sutures and advanced over the prosthesis. This is reattached to the dorsal rim of the sigmoid fossa either through drill holes or with anchoring devices under sufficient tension to restore stability to the ulna and to the carpus (Fig. 14.18). Postoperatively the patient is placed into an above-elbow splint and a removable splint fabricated for use of approximately six weeks after surgery. The splint is allowed to be removed for active joint mobilizing exercises under the supervision of therapists (Fig. 14.19).

The results of a multicenter study following 23 patients for an average of 27 months follow-up showed improvement of pronation averaging 140, supination 260, and grip strength 26%. Stability and pain reduction were achieved in all patients but one, where due to an infection the prosthesis

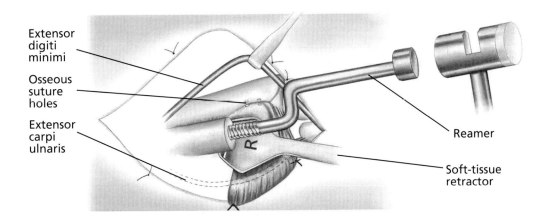

Extensor
digiti
minimi

Osseous
suture
holes

Extensor
carpi
ulnaris

Reamer

Soft-tissue
retractor

FIGURE 14.17. With the soft-tissue retractor in place, the ulnar shaft is then reamed for a tight fit. The slotted hammer is used to extract the reamer.

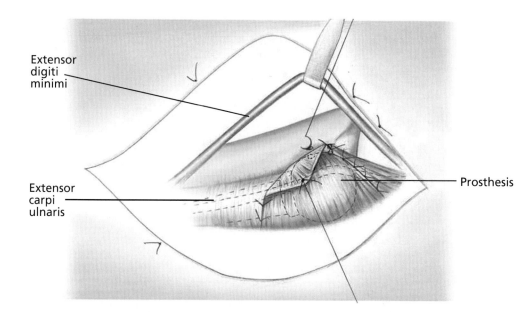

Extensor digiti minimi

Extensor carpi ulnaris

Prosthesis

FIGURE 14.18. After placing the prosthesis, the capsular flaps are closed to stabilize with non-absorbable mattress sutures. The flap is advanced until it is tight enough to provide complete stability while still allowing for full ROM. Pronation by the assistant can facilitate reduction and closure. Sutures passed through the sigmoid notch dorsal aspect of a size zero nonabsorbable suture material is recommended.

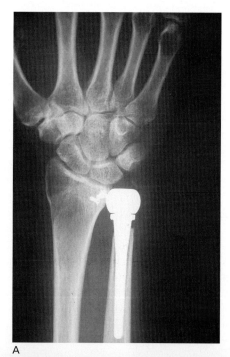

A

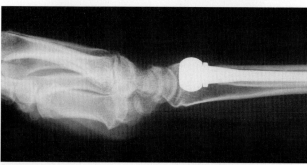

B

FIGURE 14.19. Postoperative X-rays showing the prosthesis in good position of a posterior/anterior (**A**) and lateral (**B**) view.

had to be removed. The overall satisfaction and pain reduction with these clinical results show that replacement of the ulnar head is an option for restoring stability and function in patients who have previously undergone partial or total excision of the ulnar head. Further follow-up is recommended in long term, but early encouraging results are found by these authors (115).

REFERENCES

1. Cone RO, Szabo R, Resnick D. Computed tomography of the normal radioulnar joints. *Invest Radiol* 1983;18:541–545.
2. Ekenstam F. *The distal radioulnar joint—an anatomical, experimental, and clinical study* [dissertation]. Uppsala: Faculty of Medicine, 1984;505:1–55.
3. Ekenstam F. The anatomy of the distal radioulnar joint. *Clin Orthop* 1992;275:14–18.
4. Pirela-Cruz MA, Goll SR, Klug M, Windler D. Stress computed tomography analysis of the distal radioulnar joint: a diagnostic tool for determining translocational motion. *J Hand Surg* 1991;16A:75–82.
5. Lewis OJ, Hamshere RJ, Bucknill TM. The anatomy of the wrist joint. *J Anat* 1970;106:539–552.
6. Kauer JMG. The articular disc of the hand. *Acta Anat* 1975;93:590–605.
7. Kauer JMG. Functional anatomy of the wrist. *Clin Orthop* 1980;149:9–20.
8. Kauer JMG. The distal radioulnar joint: anatomical and functional considerations. *Clin Orthop* 1992;275:37–45.
9. Kaplan EB. *Functional and surgical anatomy of the hand*, 2nd ed. Philadelphia: JB Lippincott, 1965:114–140.
10. Spinner M, Kaplan EB. Extensor carpi ulnaris. Its relationship to stability of the distal radio-ulnar joint. *Clin Orthop* 1970;68:124–129.
11. Palmer AK. Symposium on distal ulnar injuries. *Contemp Orthop* 1983;7:81.
12. Palmer AK. Triangular fibrocartilage complex lesions: a classification. *J Hand Surg* 1989;14A:594–606.

13. Palmer AK, Glisson RR, Werner FW. Relationship between ulnar variance and triangular cartilage complex thickness. *J Hand Surg* 1984;9A:681–683.

14. Palmer AK, Levinsohn EM, Kuzma GR. Arthrography of the wrist. *J Hand Surg* 1983;8:15–23.

15. Palmer AK, Werner FW. The triangular fibrocartilage complex of the wrist: Anatomy and function. *J Hand Surg* 1981;6:153–161.

16. Palmer AK, Werner FW. Biomechanics of the distal radioulnar joint. *Clin Orthop* 1984;187:26–34.

17. Palmer AK, Werner FW. Glisson RR, Murphy DJ. Partial excision of the triangular fibrocartilage complex. *J Hand Surg* 1988;13A:391–394.

18. Taleisnik J. The ligaments of the wrist. *J Hand Surg* 1976;1:110–118.

19. Ekenstam F, Palmar AK, Glisson RR. The load on the radius and ulna in different positions of the wrist and forearm. *Acta Orthop Scand* 1984;55:363–365.

20. Chidgey LK. Histologic anatomy of the triangular fibrocartilage. *Hand Clin* 1991;7:249–262.

21. Chidgey LK, Dell PC, Bittar E, Spanier S. Tear patterns and collagen arrangement in the triangular fibrocartilage. *J Hand Surg* 1987;16A:1084–1100.

22. Mikic ZD. Age changes in the triangular fibrocartilage of the wrist joint. *J Anat* 1978;126:367–384.

23. Mikic ZD. Arthrography of the wrist joint: An experimental study. *J Bone Joint Surg* 1984;66A:371–378.

24. Mikic ZD. Detailed anatomy of the articular disc of the distal radioulnar joint. *Clin Orthop* 1989;245:123–132.

25. Mikic ZD. The blood supply of the human distal radioulnar joint and the microvasculature of its articular disc. *Clin Orthop* 1992;275:29–36.

26. Mikic ZD. Treatment of acute injury of the triangular fibrocartilage complex associated with distal radioulnar joint instability. *J Hand Surg* 1995;20A:319–323.

27. Mikic ZD, Some L, Somer T. Histologic structure of the articular disc of the human distal radioulnar joint. *Clin Orthop* 1992;275:29–36.

28. Biyani A, Mehara A, Bhan S. Morphological variation of the ulnar styloid process. *J Hand Surg* 1990;153:352–354.

29. Bowers, WH, Zelouf D. Treatment of chronic disorders of the distal radioulnar joint. In: Lichtman DM, ed. *The wrist and its disorders*, 2nd ed. Philadelphia: WB Saunders, 1997.

30. Bowers WH. The distal radioulnar joint. In: Green DP, ed. *Operative hand surgery*, 4th ed. New York: Churchill Livingstone, 1999:986–1032.

31. Schuind F, An K-N, Bergland L, et al. The distal radioulnar ligaments: A biomedical study. *J Hand Surg* 1991;16A:1106–1114.

32. Ekstam F, Engvist O, Wadin K. Results from resection of the distal end of the ulna after fractures of the lower end of the radius. *Scand J Plast Reconstr Surg* 1982;16:177–181.

33. Werner, FW, Palmer AK, Fortino MD, Short WB. Force transmission through the distal ulna: Effect of ulnar variance, lunate fossa angulation, and radial and palmar tilt of the distal radius. *J Hand Surg* 1992;17A:423–428.

34. Hagert C-G. Functional aspects on the distal radioulnar joint (abstract). *J Hand Surg* 1992;4:585.

35. Hagert C-G. The distal radioulnar joint. *Hand Clin* 1987;3:41–50.

36. Hagert C-G. The distal radioulnar joint in relation to the whole forearm. *Clin Orthop* 1992;275:56–64.

37. Hagert C-G. Distal radius fracture and the distal radioulnar joint—anatomic considerations. *Hand Chir Mikrochir Plast Chir* 1994;26:22–26.

38. Bowers WH. Surgical procedures for the distal radioulnar joint. In: Lichtman DM, ed. *The wrist and its disorders*. Philadelphia: WB Saunders, 1988:232–243.

39. Bowers WH. Instability of the distal radioulnar articulation. *Hand Clin* 1991;7:311–327.

40. Ishii S, Werner FW, Short WH, Palmer AK. Pressure distribution in the distal radioulnar joint. Paper presented at: 51st annual meeting of the American Society for Surgery of the Hand; October 1996; Nashville, TN.

41. Linscheid RL. Symposium on the distal radioulnar joint. *Contemp Orthop* 1983;7:81.

42. Linscheid RL. Biomechanics of the distal radioulnar joint. *Clin Orthop* Feb. 1992;275:46–55.

43. Van der Heijden EPA, Hillen B. A two dimensional kinematic analysis of the distal radioulnar joint. *J Hand Surg* 1966;21B:824–829.

44. Kihara H, Short WB, Werner FW, et al. The stabilizing mechanisms of the distal radioulnar joint during pronation and supination. *J Hand Surg* 1995;20A:930–936.

45. Weisner L, Rumelhart C, Pham E, Comtet JJ. Experimentally induced ulnocarpal instability. *J Hand Surg* 1996;21B:24–29.

46. Tolat AR, Stanley JR, Trail IA. A cadaver study of the anatomy and stability of the distal radioulnar joint in the coronal and transverse planes. *J Hand Surg* 1996;21BB:587–594.

47. Johnson RK, Shrewsbury MM. The pronator quadratus in motions and instabilazation of the radius and ulna at the distal radioulnar joint. *J Hand Surg* 1976;1:205–209.

48. Bastillas J, Vasilas A, Pizzi WF. Bone scanning in the detection of occult fractures. *J Trauma* 1981;21:564–569.

49. Burk DL Jr, Karasick D, Wechsler RJ. Imaging of the distal radioulnar joint. *Hand Clin* 1991;7:263–275.

50. King GJ, McMurtry RY, Rubenstein JD, Gertzbein SD. Kinematics of the distal radioulnar joint. *J Hand Surg* 1986;11A:798–804.

51. Mino DE, Palmer AK, Levinsohn EM. The role of radiography and computerized tomography in the diagnosis of subluxation and dislocation of the distal radioulnar joint. *J Hand Surg* 1983;8:23–31.

52. Space TC, Louis DS, Francis I, Braunstein EM. CT findings in distal radioulnar dislocation. Case report. *J Comput Assist Tomogr* 1986;10:689–690.

53. Weigl K, Spira E. The triangular fibrocartilage of the wrist joint. *Reconstr Surg Traumatol* 1969;11:139–153.

54. Roberts D, Ram C, Udupa J, et al. Computerized 3-D image reconstruction from computerized tomographic scans. Abstract 136. Paper presented at: Second Congress of the International Federation of Societies for Surgery of the Hand; 1983; Boston.

55. Hardy DC, Totty WC, Carnes KM, et al. Arthrographic surface anatomy of the carpal triangular fibrocartilage complex. *J Hand Surg* 1988;13A:823–829.

56. Cantor RM, Stern PJ, Wyrick JD, Michaels SE. The relevance of ligament tears or perforation in the diagnosis of wrist pain: An arthrographic study. *J Hand Surg* 1994;19A:945–953.

57. Reinus WR, Hardy DC, Totty WG, Gilula LA. Arthrographic evaluation of the carpal triangular fibrocartilage complex. *J Hand Surg* 1987;12A:495–503.

58. Leibovic SJ, Bowers WH. Arthroscopy of the distal radioulnar joint. *Orthop Clin North Am* 1995;26:755–757.

59. Darrach W. Forward dislocation at the inferior radioulnar joint, with fracture of the lower third of the shaft of the radius. *Ann Surg* 1912;56:801.

60. Desault M. Extrait d'un memoire de M. Desault sur la luxation de l'extremite inferieure du radius. *J Chir* 1791;1:78.

61. Moore EM. Three cases illustrating luxation of the ulna in connection with Colles fracture. *Med Rec NY* 1880;17:305–308.

62. Lesser L Von. Zur Behandlung fehlerhaft geheilter Bruch den karpelen radiusepiphyse. *Centralbl Chir* 1887;15:265–270.

63. Lauenstein C. Zur Behandlung de nach karkpaler Vonderarm-Fraktur zuruckbleibenden Starung und Supinations-Bewegung. *Centralbl Chir* 1887;23:433.

64. Van Lannep GA. Dislocation forward of the head of the ulna at the wrist joint. Fracture of the styloid process of the ulna. *Mahneman Monthly* 1897;32:350–354.

65. Angus. Dislocation of the head of the ulna caused by a "backfire" in starting a motor car. *North Humberland Durham Med J* 1908–1909;18:23.

66. Albert SM, Wohl MA, Rechtman AM. Treatment of the disrupted radioulnar joint. *J Bone Joint Surg* 1963;45A:1373–1381.

67. Bieber EJ, Linscheid RL, Dobyns JH, Beckenbaugh RD. Failed distal ulna resections. *J Hand Surg* 1988;13A:193–200.

68. Boyd HB, Stone MM. Resection of the distal end of the ulna. *J Bone Joint Surg* 1944;26:313–321.

69. Dingman PVC. Resection of the distal end of the ulna (Darrach operation). An end result study of twenty-four cases. *J Bone Joint Surg* 1952;34A:893–900.

70. Nolan WB, Eaton RG. A Darrach procedure for distal ulnar pathology derangements. *Clin Orthop* 1992;275:85–89.

71. Rowland SA. Stabilization of the ulnar side of the rheumatoid wrist following radiocarpal arthroplasty and resection of the distal ulna. *Orthop Trans* 1982;6:474.

72. Tulipan DJ, Eaton RG, Eberhart RE. The Darrach procedure defended. Technique redefined and long-term follow-up. *J Hand Surg* 1991;16A:438–444.

73. Linscheid RL, Dobyns JH. Rheumatoid arthritis of the wrist. *Orthop Clin North Am* 1971;2:662.

74. DiBenedetto MR, Lubbers LM, Coleman CR. Long term results of the minimal resection Darrach procedure. *J Hand Surg* 1991;16A:445–450.

75. Minami A, Ogino T, Minami M. Treatment of distal radioulnar disorders. *J Hand Surg* 1987;12A:189–196.

76. Nanchahal J, Sykes, PJ, Williams RL. Excision of the distal ulna in rheumatoid arthritis. Is the price too high? *J Hand Surg* 1996;21B:189–196.

77. Swanson AB. Implant arthroplasty for disabilities of the distal radioulnar joint. Use of a silicone rubber capping implant following resection of the ulnar head. *Orthop Clin North Am* 1973;4:373–382.

78. Swanson AB. *Flexible implant arthroplasty in the hand and extremities.* St. Louis: CV Mosby, 1973:275.

79. Gould JS, Nicholson B. Prosthetic replacement of the distal ulna. Abstract 47. Paper presented at: Second Congress of the International Federation of Societies for Surgery of the Hand; 1983; Boston.

80. McMurtry RY, Paley D, Marks P, Axelrod T. A critical analysis of Swanson ulnar head replacement arthroplasty: Rheumatoid versus nonrheumatoid. *J Hand Surg* 1990;15A:224–231.

81. Blatt G, Ashworth CR. Volar capsule transfer for stabilization following resection of the distal end of the ulna. *Orthop Trans* 1979;3:13–14.

82. Leslie BM, Carlson G, Ruby LK. Results of extensor carpi ulnaris tenodesis in the rheumatoid wrist undergoing a distal ulnar excision. *J Hand Surg* 1990;15A:547–551.

83. O'Donovan TM, Ruby LK. The distal radioulnar joint in rheumatoid arthritis. *Hand Clin* 1989;5:249–256.

84. Webber JB, Maser SA. Stabilization of the distal ulna. *Hand Clin* 1991;7:345–353.

85. Kessler I, Hecht O: Present application of the Darrach procedure. *Clin Orthop* 1970;72:254–260.

86. Golcher JL, Hayes MO. Stabilization of the remaining ulna using one-half of the extensor carpi ulnaris tendon after resection of the distal ulna. *Orthop Trans* 1979;3:330–331.

87. Breen TF, Jupiter J. Tenodesis of the chronically unstable distal ulna. *Hand Clin* 1991;7:35–363.

88. Tsai TM, Stillwell JH. Repair of chronic subluxation of the distal radioulnar joint using flexor carpi ulnaris tendon. *J Hand Surg* 1984;9B:289–293.

89. Johnson RK. Stabilization of the distal ulna by transfer of the pronator quadratus origin. *Clin Orthop* 1992;275:130–132.

90. Ruby LK, Ferenz CC, Dell PC. The pronator quadratus interposition transfer: An adjunct to distal radioulnar joint resection arthroplasty. *J Hand Surg* 1996;21A:60–65.

91. Kleinman WB, Greenberg JA. Salvage of the failed Darrach procedure. *J Hand Surg* 1995;20A:951–958.

92. Bell MJ, Hill RJ, McMurtry RY. Ulnar impingement syndrome. *J Bone Joint Surg* 1985;67B:126–129.

93. Minami A, Kaneda K, Itoga H. Hemiresection-interposition arthroplasty of the distal radioulnar joint associated with repair of triangular fibrocartilage complex lesions. *J Hand Surg* 1991;16A:1120–1125.

94. Hartz, CR, Beckenbaugh RD. Long-term results of resection of the distal ulna for posttraumatic conditions. *J Trauma* 1979;19:219–226.

95. Field J, Majkowski RJ, Leslie IJ. Poor results of Darrach's procedure after wrist injuries. *J Bone Joint Surg* 1993;75B:53–75.

96. Bowers WH. Distal radioulnar joint arthroplasty: The hemiresection-interposition technique. *J Hand Surg* 1985;10A:169–178.

97. Watson HK, Ryu J, Burgess R. Matched distal ulnar resection. *J Hand Surg* 1986;11A:812–817.

98. Wicks B, Fletcher D, Palmer AK. Failed Bowers procedure (HIT technique). Paper presented at: 45th annual meeting of the American Society for Hand Surgery; September, 1990; Toronto.

99. Watson HK, Gabuzda GM. Match distal ulnar resection for posttraumatic disorders of the distal radioulnar joint. *J Hand Surg* 1992;17A:724–730.

100. Sauve K. Nouvelle technique traitement chirurical des luxations recidivantes isolees de l'extremite inferieur du cubitus. *J Shir (Paris)* 1936;47:589–594.

101. Kapandji IA. The Kapandji-Sauve operation: Its techniques and indications in nonrheumatoid disease. *Ann Chir Main* 1986;5:181–193.

102. Goncalves D. Correction of disorders of the distal radioulnar joint by artificial pseudoarthrosis of the ulna. *J Bone Joint Surg* 1974;56B:462–463.

103. Gordon L, Levinsohn DG, Moore SV, et al. The Sauve-Kapandji procedure for the treatment of posttraumatic distal radioulnar problems. *Hand Clin* 1991;7:397–403.

104. Johnson MK, Lawrence JF, Dionysian E. The Kapandji procedure for the treatment of the distal radioulnar joint in young patients. *Comtemp Orthop* 1995;31:291–298.

105. Millroy D, Coleman S, Ivers R. The Sauve-Kapandji operation. *J Hand Surg* 1992;17B:411–414.

106. Sanders RA, Frederik HA, Hontas RB. The Sauve-Kapandji procedure: A salvage operation for the distal radioulnar joint. *J Hand Surg* 1991;16A:1125–1129.

107. Vincent KA, Szabo RM, Agee JM. The Sauve-Kapandji procedure for the reconstruction of the rheumatoid distal radioulnar joint. *J Hand Surg* 1993;18A:978–983.

108. Taleisnik J. The Sauve-Kapandji procedure. *Clin Orthop* 1992;275:110–123.

109. Rothwell AG, O'Neill L, Cragg K. Sauve-Kapandji procedure for disorders of the distal radioulnar joint: A simplified technique *J Hand Surg* 1996;21A:771–777.

110. Minami A, Suzuki K, Suenaga N, Ishikawa J. The Sauve-Kapandji procedure for osteoarthritis of the distal radioulnar joint. *J Hand Surg* 1995;20A:602–608.

111. Carroll RE, Imbriglia JE. Distal radioulnar arthrodesis. *Orthop Trans* 1979;3:269.

112. Schneider LH, Imbriglia JE. Radioulnar joint fusion for distal radioulnar joint instability. *Hand Clin* 1991;7:391–395.

113. Peterson II CA, Maki S, Wood MB. Clinical results of the one-bone forearm. *J Hand Surg* 1995;20A:609–618.

114. Cooney WP, Damron TA, Sim FH, et al. En bloc resection of tumors of the distal end of the ulna. *J Bone Joint Surg* 1997;79A:406–412.

115. Van Schoonhoven J, Fernandez DL, Bowers WH, Herbert TJ. Salvage of failed resection arthroplasties of the distal radioulnar joint using a new ulnar head prosthesis. May 2000;25(3)436–438.

Index

Acutrak screw fixation in interphalangeal
 joint arthrodesis, 54–55, 55f
Adhesion molecules in rheumatoid arthritis,
 13, 16
Anesthesia
 in mucous cyst excision, 46, 46f
 in rheumatoid arthritis, 30
Anti-inflammatory drugs, nonsteroidal
 in osteoarthritis, 8, 20
  for carpometacarpal joints, 114
  for distal interphalangeal joints, 43–44
 in rheumatoid arthritis, 19
Arachidonic acid metabolites in rheumatoid
 arthritis, 19
Arthritis mutilans, 42, 42f, 94
 surgery in, 102
Arthrodesis. *See also specific anatomic sites*
 carpometacarpal joints, 114f, 114–115,
  115f
  in thumb, 107
 interphalangeal joints
  distal, 45, 47–56
  proximal, 66f, 66–67, 67f, 68f
 metacarpophalangeal joints, 34, 83–84
  in thumb, 100–102, 101f
 radioulnar, 191, 191f
 wrist
  limited, 121–137
  total, 155–163
Arthroplasty. *See also specific anatomic sites*
 carpometacarpal joints, 116f, 116–117,
  117f
  in thumb, 109, 109f
 distal radioulnar joints
  partial resection, 187–188
  ulnar head prosthesis, 191–194, 192f,
   193f, 194f
 interphalangeal joints
  distal, 45, 56f, 56–57
  proximal, 68–71, 69f, 70f
 metacarpophalangeal joints, 33–34, 34f,
  82–83, 84–89
  in thumb, 102, 104
 wrist
  limited, 140–153
  total, 166–175
Arthroscopic surgery
 proximal row carpectomy, 150–151
 radial styloidectomy, 142–143, 143f

B-cells in rheumatoid arthritis, 14, 17
Basilar joint arthritis. *See* Carpometacarpal
 joints
Bone structures in osteoarthritis, 6, 41
Bouchard's nodes, 4, 41, 42f
Boutonnière deformity, 34, 34f, 35f
 in thumb, 92–93, 93t
 surgery in, 97–102, 98f–101f

Capitolunate arthrodesis, 126, 127
Carpal boss, 112
 differential diagnosis of, 113
 surgery in, 117
Carpal tunnel syndrome, and wrist
 arthrodesis, 157, 163
Carpectomy, proximal row, 144–151, 146f,
 147f
 arthroscopic, 150–151
  indications, 150
  postoperative rehabilitation, 151
  results, 151
  technique, 150–151
 capsular interposition with, 148–149,
  149f, 150f
  indications, 148
  postoperative rehabilitation, 148–149
  results, 149
  technique, 148
 complications of, 151
 indications for, 144–145
 postoperative rehabilitation in, 147
 radial styloidectomy with, 141, 142
 results of, 147, 148t
 salvage procedures, 151
 technique of, 145–147, 146f, 147f
Carpometacarpal joints, 111–118
 arthrodesis, 114f, 114–115, 115f
 arthroplasty
  partial resection in, 117
  silicone interposition in, 116–117,
   117f
  tendon interposition in, 116, 116f
 carpal boss in, 112, 113
  surgery in, 117
 complications of surgery, 117–118
 nonoperative therapy, 114
 postoperative rehabilitation, 118
 preoperative planning, 112–114
 radial rays, 111, 112f

thumb, 106–110. *See also* Thumb joints
 ulnar rays, 111, 112f
Cartilage
 characteristics of, 5, 5f
 in osteoarthritis, 5–6
Cerebral palsy, total wrist arthrodesis in, 156
Chondroitin sulfate in osteoarthritis, 8
Classification
 of osteoarthritis, 3–4, 4t
 of rheumatoid arthritis, 29–30
Collagen in articular cartilage, 5, 15
Collagenase in rheumatoid arthritis, 19, 19t
Corticosteroid injections
 in carpometacarpal arthritis, 114
 in distal interphalangeal joint arthritis, 44,
  44f
 in rheumatoid arthritis, 30
COX-2 inhibitors in distal interphalangeal
 joint arthritis, 44
Cyclophosphamide in rheumatoid arthritis,
 20, 20t
Cysts
 mucous, in distal interphalangeal joint, 44,
  44f, 57
  excision of, 46, 46f–47f, 57, 59
 subarticular, in osteoarthritis, 6
Cytokines in rheumatoid arthritis, 17–18, 18t
 and anti-cytokine therapy, 22

Darrach procedure in distal radioulnar joint
 arthritis, 186
Dendritic cells in rheumatoid arthritis, 13
Distal interphalangeal joint arthritis, 41–62
 arthrodesis in, 45, 47–56
  absorbable screws or implants, 56
  Acutrak screw insertion, 54–55, 55f
  bony preparation, 49–50, 49f–50f
  closure, 56
  complications, 50t, 60–61
  external fixation, 56
  fixation, 50–51, 51f
  Herbert screw insertion, 53–54, 54f
  interosseous wiring, 52, 52f
  joint exposure, 47–49, 48f
  postoperatve rehabilitation, 59–60
  results, 57f, 57–59, 58f
  standard screw insertion, 52–53,
   52f–53f
  tension band fixation, 55

Distal interphalangeal joint arthritis,
  continued
  arthroplasty in, 45, 56f, 56–57
    bony preparation and implant insertion,
      56–57
    complications, 61–62
    postoperative rehabilitation, 60
    results, 58
  debridement in, 46
  historical aspects of, 41–42
  mucous cyst in, 44, 44f
    excision of, 46, 46f–47f, 57, 59
  nonoperative treatment of, 43–44, 44f
  preoperative planning in, 45–46, 46f
  surgery in, 44–62
    salvage procedures, 62, 62f
Distal radioulnar joint arthritis, 177–194. *See
  also* Radioulnar joint arthritis, distal
Drug therapy
  in distal interphalangeal joint arthritis,
    43–44
  in osteoarthritis, 8, 20
  in rheumatoid arthritis, 20t, 20–22, 21t
    perioperative considerations with, 30–31

Endothelial cells in rheumatoid arthritis,
  15–16
Epidemiology
  in osteoarthritis, 4, 4t
  in rheumatoid arthritis, 10
Erosive osteoarthritis, 41
Etanercept in rheumatoid arthritis, 21t, 22

Fibrillation affecting cartilage, 6

Gamekeeper's deformity of thumb, 94
Genetic factors in rheumatoid arthritis,
  11–13
Glucosamine sulfate in osteoarthritis, 8
Gold therapy in rheumatoid arthritis, 20, 20t,
  21
Gout, 42
Granulocyte-macrophage colony-stimulating
  factor in rheumatoid arthritis, 18, 18t

Heat therapy for distal interphalangeal joints,
  43
Heberden's nodes, 4, 41, 42f
Herbert screw fixation in interphalangeal
  joint arthrodesis, 53–54, 54f
  in thumb, 97, 97f
HLA-DR alleles in rheumatoid arthritis,
  11–13, 12t
Hyaluronan injections in osteoarthritis, 8
Hyaluronic acid in synovial fluid, in
  osteoarthritis, 6

Immunogenetic factors in rheumatoid
  arthritis, 11–13, 12f
Infectious agents in rheumatoid arthritis,
  10–11, 11t, 14–15
Interferon-[g] in rheumatoid arthritis, 17, 18t
Interleukins
  IL-1 in rheumatoid arthritis, 17, 18t
    inhibition of, 22
  IL-6 in rheumatoid arthritis, 18, 18t

Interphalangeal joints
  distal. *See also* Distal interphalangeal joint
    arthritis
    arthritic conditions, 41–44
    surgery in arthritis, 44–63
  proximal. *See also* Proximal interphalangeal
    joint arthritis
    rheumatoid, 34f, 34–35, 65–66
    surgery in arthritis, 66–73
  thumb
    rheumatoid, 92–95
    surgery in arthritis, 95–97

Kienböck's disease, 123f, 144, 144f, 145f
  arthrodesis in, 121
  proximal row carpectomy in, 144

Laboratory findings
  in osteoarthritis, 8
  in rheumatoid arthritis, 30
Leflunomide in rheumatoid arthritis, 21, 21t
Leukotrienes in rheumatoid arthritis, 19
Loose body formation in osteoarthritis, 6
Lunocapitate arthrodesis, 126, 127
Lunotriquetral arthrodesis, 126, 127, 135,
  135f
  technique, 132, 132f

Macrophages in rheumatoid arthritis, 17
Metacarpophalangeal joints, rheumatoid, 33f,
  33–34, 34f, 75–89
  anatomy in, 75
  arthrodesis in, 83–84
  arthroplasty in, 82–83
    joint replacement, 84–89, 85f–89f
    perichondrial graft, 83
    resection interposition, 82–83
  disease progression in, 75–78
  nonoperative treatment of, 78
  preoperative planning in, 78–79
  surgery in, 79–89
  synovectomy in, 79–82, 80f
    crossed intrinsic transfer, 81
    extensor mechanism realignment, 81
    outcomes, 82
    postoperative care, 81–82
  thumb surgery in, 97–104
  ulnar drift in, 75–76, 76f
Metalloproteinases in rheumatoid arthritis,
  19, 19t
Methotrexate in rheumatoid arthritis, 20,
  20t, 21
Methylprednisolone in rheumatoid arthritis,
  20, 20t
Molecular basis of osteoarthritis, 5–6
Monoclonal antibody therapy in rheumatoid
  arthritis, 21, 21t, 22
Mucous cysts in distal interphalangeal joint,
  44, 44f, 57
  excision of, 46, 46f–47f, 57, 59

Nerve decompression in rheumatoid arthritis,
  32
Nodules, rheumatoid, 33
Nonoperative management
  in carpometacarpal arthritis, 287

in distal interphalangeal arthritis, 43–44,
  44f
in osteoarthritis, 8
in rheumatoid arthritis, 19–22, 20f, 20t,
  21t, 30
  in metacarpophalangeal joints, 78

Osteoarthritis
  bone structures in, 6, 41
  carpometacarpal joints in, 111–118
  cartilage in, 5f, 5–6
  classification of, 3–4, 4t
  clinical features of, 7f, 7–8, 8f
  distal interphalangeal joints in, 41–62
  distal radioulnar joints in, 181–183
  epidemiology of, 4, 4t
  molecular basis of, 5–6
  nonoperative management of, 8
  pathophysiology of, 3–9
  proximal interphalangeal joints in, 65–66
  synovial fluid in, 6
  in thumb, 92
    at carpometacarpal joint, 106–118
  in wrist, 121
Osteophytes, 5–6

Pannus, rheumatoid, 14
Pathophysiology
  of osteoarthritis, 3–9
  of rheumatoid arthritis, 10–22
Perioperative evaluation in rheumatoid
  arthritis, 30–31
Physical examination
  in osteoarthritis, 7
    carpometacarpal joints, 113
    distal interphalangeal joints, 42
  in wrist arthritis, 156–157
Pisotriquetral arthroplasty, 151–153, 152f
  complications of, 153
  indications for, 151
  results of, 152–153
  salvage procedures, 153
  technique of, 151–152
Platelet-derived growth factor in rheumatoid
  arthritis, 18
Posttraumatic arthritis, 6, 42
  distal radioulnar joint, 181–182
  proximal interphalangeal joint, 65–66
  proximal row carpectomy in, 144
  total wrist arthrodesis in, 155–156
Prostaglandins in rheumatoid arthritis, 19
Proximal interphalangeal joint arthritis
  arthrodesis in, 66f, 66–67, 67f, 68f
    bone grafting, 67, 73
    postoperative rehabilitation, 72
    results, 71
  arthroplasty in, 68–71, 69f, 70f
    complications, 72–73
    joint replacement, 68–69, 69f
    postoperative rehabilitation, 72, 72f
    results, 71f, 71–72
    surface replacement, 69f, 69–71, 70f
  historical aspects of, 65
  preoperative planning in, 66
  salvage procedures in, 73
Psoriatic arthritis, 42, 42f

Radial deviation in osteoarthritis of thumb, 7f
Radial styloidectomy, 141–144
Radiocarpal arthrodesis, 126–127, 127f, 128, 135f
  results, 135–136
  technique, 132f, 132–134, 133f–134f
Radiography
  carpal boss view of wrist, 113, 113f
  in distal interphalangeal joint arthritis, 42–43, 43f
  in distal radioulnar joint arthritis, 182, 182f, 183f
  in osteoarthritis, 7, 7f, 8f
  in rheumatoid arthritis, 29, 33f, 34f
    in wrist, 168f
  in thumb basilar joint arthritis, 106, 107f
Radionuclide scans in osteoarthritis, 8, 43, 113
Radioulnar joint arthritis, distal, 177–194
  anatomy in, 177–181, 179f, 180f, 181f
  Darrach procedure in, 186
    complications, 186
    modifications, 186–187
  distal ulnar resection in
    extensive, 191
    matched, 188–189, 189f
  dorsal approach in, 184f, 184–186, 185f
  hemiresection interposition technique in, 187, 187f
  historical aspects of, 177
  indications for surgery in, 181–183, 182, 183f
  management recommendations in, 178t
  partial resection arthroplasties in, 187–188
    dorsal approach, 187–188
  preoperative planning in, 183–184
  radioulnar arthrodesis in, 191, 191f
  rheumatoid, 33
  Sauve-Kapandji procedure in, 189–191, 190f
  and total wrist fusion, 157, 163
  ulnar head prosthesis in, 191–194, 192f, 193f, 194f
Remicade in rheumatoid arthritis, 22
Rheumatoid arthritis
  classification and staging of, 14, 14t, 29–30
  in distal radioulnar joint, 183–184
  epidemiology of, 10
  etiology of, 10–11, 11t
  goals of surgery in, 27
  HLA-DR alleles in, 11–13, 12t
  infectious agents in, 10–11, 11t, 14–15
  in metacarpophalangeal joint, 75–89, 76f, 77f
  nonoperative treatment of, 19–22, 20f, 20t, 21t, 30
  pathogenesis of, 14–19, 15f
  pathology in, 13–14
  principles of surgery in, 27–29
  in proximal interphalangeal joint, 65–66
  psoriatic arthritis with, 42f
  surgery in
    general considerations in, 27–36
    relative merits of procedures in, 29, 29t
    in thumb joints

interphalangeal, 95–97
metacarpophalangeal, 97–104
in wrist
  preoperative radiographs, 168f
  total arthrodesis in, 156, 157–158, 158f
  total arthroplasty in, 169
Rheumatoid factors, 15

Salvage procedures
  in interphalangeal joint arthritis
    distal, 62, 62f
    proximal, 73
  in pisotriquestral arthroplasty, 153
  in proximal row carpectomy, 151
  in radial styloidectomy, 144
  Sauve-Kapandji procedure in distal radioulnar arthritis, 189–191, 190f
  in thumb metacarpophalangeal arthritis, 104
  for wrist
    in limited arthrodesis, 136–137
    in total arthroplasty, 174–175, 175f
Sauve-Kapandji procedure in distal radioulnar arthritis, 189–191, 190f
Scaphocapitate arthrodesis, 124, 127, 135, 135f
  technique, 130, 130f
Scaphoid nonunion advanced collapse, 124–125, 141, 144
Scapholunate joint
  advanced collapse, 124f, 124–125, 125f, 140, 141f, 144, 155
  arthrodesis, 126
  dissociation, 122f, 123–124
Scaphotrapezium-trapezoid arthritis, 122–123, 123f
  thumb carpometacarpal arthritis with, 108–109, 109f
Scaphotrapezium-trapezoid arthrodesis, 122–124, 123f, 127, 134, 135f
  technique, 129–130
Splints
  in carpometacarpal arthritis, 114
  in distal interphalangeal arthritis, 43
  postoperative
    in metacarpophalangeal joint replacement arthroplasty, 88–89, 89f
    in proximal interphalangeal joint arthritis, 72, 72f, 73
    in proximal row carpectomy, 147, 148–149, 151
    in synovectomy of metacarpophalangeal joint, 81–82
    in total wrist arthroplasty, 173, 174
  in rheumatoid arthritis, 30
Staging of rheumatoid arthritis, 14, 14t
Stromelysin in rheumatoid arthritis, 19, 19t
Styloidectomy, radial, 141–144
  arthroscopic, 142–143, 143f
    indications, 142
    postoperative rehabilitation, 143
    results, 143
    technique, 143
  complications of, 144
  indications for, 141–142
  ligamentous injury with, 141, 142f
  postoperative rehabilitation in, 143

proximal row carpectomy with, 141, 142
  results of, 142
  salvage procedures, 144
  technique, 142
Swan-neck deformity, 34, 35f, 76f, 77, 77f
  in thumb, 93–94, 94t
  surgery in, 102
Swanson silicone wrist implant, 166, 167f
Synovectomy
  in metacarpophalangeal joint arthritis, 79–82, 80f
    in thumb, 97
  in rheumatoid arthritis, 31–32
    in wrist, 33
  in thumb joints, 95, 97
Synovial fluid in osteoarthritis, 6
Synovial membrane
  in osteoarthritis, 6
  in rheumatoid arthritis, 13–14
Synovitis in rheumatoid arthritis, 13, 15

T-cells in rheumatoid arthritis, 13, 16f, 16–17
  and anti-T-cell therapy, 21–22
Tendons in fingers, normal anatomy of, 35f
Tenosynovectomy in rheumatoid arthritis, 31, 32f, 32–33
Thumb joints
  boutonnière deformity, 92–93, 93t
    surgery in, 97–102, 98f–101f
  carpometacarpal arthritis, 106–110
    arthrodesis in, 107
    arthroplasties in, 109, 109f
    clinical features of, 106, 107f
    ligament reconstruction in, 108
    radiographic staging of, 106, 107f
    scaphotrapezium-trapezoid arthritis with, 108–109, 109f
    trapezial excision with tendon interposition in, 108f, 108–109
  interphalangeal arthritis, 95–97
    arthrodesis in, 95–97, 97f
    synovectomy in, 95
  metacarpophalangeal arthritis, 97–104
    arthrodesis in, 100–102, 101f
    arthroplasty in, 102, 104
    extensor reconstruction in, 97–100, 98f–101f
    postoperative rehabilitation in, 103–104
    results of surgery in, 103
    salvage procedures in, 104
    synovectomy in, 97
  swan-neck deformity, 93–94, 94t
    surgery in, 102
Tidemark zone, characteristics of, 5, 5f
Time sequences for surgery, 28, 78–70
Tournicot, finger, 46, 46f
Trauma
  carpometacarpal joints, 111
  and osteoarthritis development, 6, 42. *See also* Posttraumatic arthritis
  wrist, 121
Tuberculosis, total wrist arthrodesis in, 155
Tumor necrosis factor-α in rheumatoid arthritis, 17, 18t
  inhibition of, 22

Ulnar drift in metacarpophalangeal joint arthritis, 75–76, 76f
Ulnocarpal impaction syndrome, hemiresection interposition technique in, 187, 187f
Universal Total Wrist prosthesis, 168, 168f, 169f

Virus infections, rheumatoid arthritis in, 11, 11t
Volz wrist prosthesis, 166–167, 167f

Wrist
  distal radioulnar joint disorders, 177–194
  limited arthrodesis, 121–137
    capitolunate, 126, 127
    complications, 136, 136f
    four-bone, 124, 125, 127, 130–131, 131f, 135, 135f
    intercarpal, 126
    lunotriquetral, 126, 127–128, 132, 132f, 135, 135f
    midcarpal, 122–126
    postoperative rehabilitation, 136
    preoperative planning, 127–128
    radiocarpal, 126–127, 127f, 128, 132f, 132–134, 133f–134f, 135f, 135–136
    results, 134–136
    salvage procedures, 136–137
    scaphocapitate, 124, 127, 130, 130f
    scapholunate, 126
  scaphotrapezium-trapezoid, 122–124, 123f, 127, 129–130, 134, 135f
    techniques, 128–134
    universal dorsal approaches, 128f, 128–129, 129f
  limited arthroplasty, 140–153
    historical aspects, 140–141
    pisotriquetral, 151–153, 152f
    proximal row carpectomy, 144–151
    radial styloidectomy, 141–144, 142f
  midcarpal instability, 125
  rheumatoid arthritis, 33, 33f
    and metacarpophalangeal joint alignment, 33f, 33–34, 34f
  scaphoid nonunion advanced collapse, 124–125
  scapholunate advanced collapse, 124f, 124–125, 125f
  scapholunate dissociation, 122f, 123–124
  surgical decision making, 156f
  total arthrodesis, 155–163
    capitate-radius technique, 158–159, 159f
    and carpal tunnel syndrome, 157, 163
    Carrol and Dick technique, 158, 158f, 159f
    complications, 163
    compression plate fixation, 160
    contraindications, 156
    and distal radioulnar joint symptoms, 157, 163
  dorsal approach, 160f, 160–162, 161f, 162f
    Haddad-Riordan radial approach, 159, 160f
    historical aspects, 155
    indications, 155–156
    joints to be fused, 157
    pin fixation in rheumatoid patients, 157–158, 158f
    position of fusion, 157
    postoperative rehabilitation, 163
    preoperative planning, 156–157
    results, 162–163
  total arthroplasty, 166–175
    complications, 174
    historical aspects, 166–168
    indications and contraindications, 169
    operative technique, 170f, 170–173, 171f, 172f
    postoperative rehabilitation, 173–174
    preoperative planning, 169
    results, 172
    salvage procedures, 174–175, 175f
    Swanson silicone implant, 166, 167f
    Universal Total Wrist prosthesis, 168, 168f, 169f
    Volz prosthesis, 166–167, 167f
  ulnar translocation of carpus, 126

Zig-zag deformity in rheumatoid arthritis, 28, 28f, 76f, 78